Biomedical Technology and Human Rights

BIOMEDICAL TECHNOLOGY
AND HUMAN RIGHTS

Eugene B. Brody

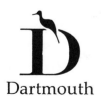

Dartmouth

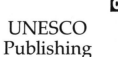

UNESCO
Publishing

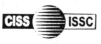

ISSC

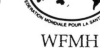

WFMH

Published jointly by the United Nations
Educational, Scientific and Cultural Organization
75700 Paris
France

and
Dartmouth Publishing Company Limited
Gower House
Croft Road
Aldershot
Hants GU11 3HR
England

Dartmouth Publishing Company
Old Post Road
Brookfield
Vermont 05036
USA

in association with
The International Social Science Council (ISSC)
1 rue Miollis
75015 Paris, and

The World Federation for Mental Health (WFMH)
1201 Prince Street
Alexandria
Virginia 22314–2971
USA

A CIP catalogue record for this book is available from the British Library

Library of Congress Cataloging-in-Publication Data
Brody, Eugene B.
    Biomedical technology and human rights / Eugene B. Brody.
        p.   cm.
    Includes bibliographical references and index.
    ISBN 1–85521–373–7 (Dartmouth): $46.95 – ISBN 92–3–102806–5
(UNESCO)
    1. Medical ethics. 2. Bioethics. 3. Medical innovations–Moral
and ethical aspects. I. Unesco. II. Title.
R724.5757   1993
174'.25–dc20

© UNESCO 1993
UNESCO ISBN: 92–3–102806–5
Darmouth ISBN: 1 85521 373 7

Printed in Great Britain at the University Press, Cambridge

Contents

Preface

UNESCO's interest in the complex issues now known under the term 'bioethics' is not recent. In the early 1970s, this subject area made its appearance as an important focal point for reflection on the social and cultural changes brought about by scientific and technological progress. A symposium on the 'Problems and positive results of scientific research in molecular genetics' organized at that time by UNESCO examined the potential scope for genetic manipulation applied to the solution of problems of vital concern to humanity. It drew attention to the acceleration of genetic erosion and suggested the creation of an international network of 'seed banks' to ensure the preservation of genetic resources, notably of plants.

A further symposium was organized in 1975; it was attended by eminent biologists and philosophers and led to the appearance, in 1978, of a work entitled *Biology and Ethics* by Bruno Ribes, published by the organization in French, English and Spanish.

In 1984, UNESCO undertook an analysis of 'human rights *vis-à-vis* recent scientific and technical progress'. This activity aimed at further examining the possibilities of an increased protection of human rights taking into account new dangers which had arisen or which could occur. An international symposium was to study, *inter alia*, questions related to brain research, biological and neurophysiological experimentations on human beings and genetic manipulations.

UNESCO entrusted the International Social Science Council (ISSC) with the task of organizing, in March 1985, this first international symposium (Barcelona I). This meeting, held in co-operation with the International Council of Scientific Unions (ICSU) and the International Council of Philosophy and Human Sciences (CIPSH), adopted 'Conclusions and recommendations' for further research.

On this basis, UNESCO asked the ISSC to prepare a study surveying the branches of the clinical and biomedical sciences that may have an impact on human rights. In addition, UNESCO requested the World Federation for Mental Health (WFMH) to set up a multidisciplinary, international working party to study the impact of new human reproductive technologies on the rights of women. These two studies were examined during a second international symposium (Barcelona II) in November–December 1987.

The recommendations of this second symposium highlighted a number of important points. First, the vulnerability of underprivileged groups in face of recent advances in science and technology. To take two examples, members of underprivileged groups rarely have access to *in vitro* fertilization techniques, one major reason being a lack of information. Conversely, the practice known as 'surrogate motherhood' is liable to worsen further the situation of women belonging to the underprivileged groups.

The symposium then turned its attention to a problem which is causing increasing concern to the public, namely the impact of compulsory or voluntary medical screening on human rights. With reference to screening, it called particular attention to:

- the possibility that it may lead to a temptation to adopt certain forms of eugenics;
- the potential for destruction of the private life of individuals or of the life of a couple which may, for example, stem from genetic screening to overcome infertility;
- the dramatic repercussions of compulsory screening in the case of certain jobs – for example on the right to work – and once again on the temptation to resort to eugenics as a means of adapting individuals to the needs of the labour market;
- the acceleration of the evolution of an illness or other physical or mental handicap through a process known to medical and psychological research as a self-fulfilling prophecy.

Lastly, the symposium stressed the need for a detailed study of the problems created by organ transplantation and the commercialization of human organs and tissues.

The following four areas were highlighted as appropriate subjects for future research:

- the impact of compulsory or voluntary screening on human rights;
- the implications for human rights of transactions involving body parts and human foetuses;
- the impact of surrogate motherhood on the rights of women and on the rights of the child; and
- the potential impact of the expanding bio-engineering industry on human rights.

The time has come to define some international guiding principles with a view to orienting the evolution of science and medicine, particularly in the field of human genetics.

With this in mind, in 1992 UNESCO started preparatory work for the elaboration of an international instrument for the protection of the human genome. This task will be accomplished by an International Consultative Committee on Bioethics created by UNESCO in early 1993, but which will bear fruit in 1994.

In the meantime, in order to make available the results and findings of the above meetings, in particular Barcelona I and II, as well as subsequent research commissioned by the Organization, UNESCO and the ISSC entrusted to Dr Eugene B. Brody, Secretary-General of the WFMH, the preparation of the present book. UNESCO wishes to thank the author for having accepted this task and believes that this publication will increase the knowledge of problems in this area and the awareness of the general public and decision-makers of the issues at stake.

UNESCO
February 1993

Author's Foreword

The impetus for this volume originated in the International Symposium on Biomedical Technology and Human Rights held in Barcelona in March 1985, organized by the International Social Science Council (ISSC) in response to a request from UNESCO's Division of Human Rights and Peace. The summary of the 1985 Symposium constitutes Appendix 1.

As a consequence of the Symposium, UNESCO and ISSC commissioned the World Federation for Mental Health (WFMH) to convene a Working Group to consider the impact of the new reproductive technologies on the rights and roles of women. Meetings in Paris in July 1986, and in Rhode Island, USA, in March 1987 resulted in a report, *Reproductive Technologies and the Rights and Roles of Women*, submitted in June 1987. A third discussion group convened by WFMH for ISSC and UNESCO in Barcelona from 30 November to 2 December 1987 reviewed the June 1987 report, as well as a document prepared for ISSC by the author of this volume entitled *Domains of Biomedical Research and Technology Bearing on Human Rights*. Finally, a document, *Human Rights Aspects of Transactions in Body Parts and Human Foetuses*, prepared by the author on commission for UNESCO, delivered in December 1989 and issued in April 1990, became a working paper for a UNESCO European meeting on bioethics. These papers constitute a background for this volume.

I express my gratitude to Dr Stephen Mills, Deputy Secretary General of ISSC, and Dr Georges Kutukdjian, Progamme Specialist for UNESO's Division of Human Rights and Peace, who have acted as my most supportive liaisons with their organizations. It is also a pleasure to acknowledge the context for this work provided by the philosophy and goals of WFMH, a body I have served as President from 1981 to 1983 and Secretary-General since that time. The World Federation for Mental Health is the world's only international, non-governmental coalition of individual and organized professionals of all disciplines, citizen volunteers, former patients, and self-help groups accredited as a consultant in mental health to all the UN's major agencies. At the time of writing it is active through its committees in relation to many of the world's health-related problems, especially those which cross international boundaries, maintains a presence at all UN headquarters, and is represented in

104 countries. Its approach to health issues across political, social and cultural boundaries is consistent with its founding declaration at the Third International Congress on Mental Health in London on 21 August 1948. That declaration, entitled 'Mental Health and World Citizenship', proclaimed 'The idea of the "world citizen" . . . an informed, reflective, responsible allegiance to mankind as a whole . . . built on free consent and on the respect for individual and cultural differences'. This was conceived in terms of a 'common humanity'.

Only four months later, on 10 December 1948, the still fledgling United Nations proclaimed its Universal Declaration of Human Rights which is reprinted as Appendix 2 of this volume. That Declaration, in many ways, espoused the same goals as WFMH through the powerful concept of 'the human family'. This concept touches the universal desire to be part of an overarching community while still retaining the individual and cultural diversity and individual autonomy which are part of being fully human. More specifically, the Declaration's particular articles enumerate rights to education, the benefits of science, mental and physical health, and freedom from involuntary medical/scientific experimentation. Its chief author, René Cassin (1887–1976), was especially concerned with the possible effects of biological and behavioural research on human rights. In 1969 he urged consideration of how scientific advances 'might be channelled into beneficial applications, and whether limits should be imposed on some directions of investigation' (Rosenzweig, 1985, revised 1989). But his concern with protecting the rights of human beings was combined with a sense that such protection should not impose unjustified restrictions on research.

In the years which have passed since 1948 most developed countries have developed ethical codes or regulations to guide investigators working with human subjects, and these have provided a focus of international consultation for members of the world scientific, clinical and ethical communities. In 1989 WFMH adopted a Declaration of Human Rights and Mental Health, intended as a guide to other NGOs, governments and the intergovernmental system in their continuing efforts to follow the goals of the 1948 UN Declaration. This WFMH Declaration appears as Appendix 3 of this volume.

International initiatives and collaboration in health and science are made easier by the worldwide nature of the non-governmental biomedical and other scientific communities. Despite restrictions imposed by some sovereign states upon their clinicians and scientists on grounds of 'national security', the similar interests and values of members of this international network tend to override their diverse political, social and cultural identities. Similarly, despite discouraging instances in which attempts have been made to subvert them for political ends, the agencies of the United Nations which have the best records regarding international collaboration and achievement are those dealing with health and science. It is through international collaboration in health and science that the UN and the family of NGOs have the best chance, in Kantian terms, of creating a moral human community dedicated to the protection of human rights. The preservation of these rights is inherent in the World Health Organization's (WHO) definition of health as a state of physical, psychological and social well-being.

In 1978 the World Health Assembly of WHO, meeting in Alma Ata, Kazakhstan and attended by a few NGOs including WFMH, proclaimed 'Health for All by the Year 2000'. Realizing that goal as the twenty-first century arrives will require deliberate attention to the rights to health and well-being embodied in the UN's 1948 Declaration of Human Rights and those elaborations which have followed it. It will require particular attention to the consequences of advancing biomedical science and technology, including the questions which they raise.

The present volume is addressed, on the eve of a new century, to the global clinical and scientific, as well as the intergovernmental, communities. It is hoped that its publication will help bring the reality of human rights closer to the ideals espoused by men and women of good will everywhere.

Eugene B. Brody, MD
January 1993

1 Health in the Context of International Human Rights

The Concept of Human Rights

'Human' Rights as a Code of Interpersonal Behaviour

'Human rights' as an often reiterated slogan usually refers to the content of one of several legal or quasi-legal codes of behaviour. All indicate what is permissible and expected, or not permissible, in the treatment of one human being by another. All codes are specific in their prohibition of massive identity violations, such as torture, but shade into ambiguity regarding the discretionary granting of power or privilege by one person to another. An example is informed consent for non-experimental medical treatment; the patient is given the privilege of knowledge about a usually esoteric area, and the power to refuse the treatment overriding the recommendation of the professional.

In the area of expectations, for economic, social or health support, or the range of more technical medical therapies, another source of ambiguity becomes apparent. This is the blurring of rights with privileges and obligations. At this point the sense of formally articulated codes of behaviour merges into the complex of informal beliefs and attitudes about what is acceptable in the relationships between individuals and between groups. These have varied with historical periods and, particularly in the twentieth century, with culture (including religion and ethnicity), national identity, and socio-economic status. They typically differ in regard to relationships between members of the same family, friendship network and community, and those with others defined as strangers.

Global Values for the Human Family

The formal, twentieth-century value context of international medical practice and research is that of the United Nations Universal Declaration of Human Rights. Proclaimed on 10 December 1948, its Preamble describes 'all members of the human family' as possessing

1

an 'inherent . . . dignity' and 'equal and inalienable rights'. Prominent among these rights is 'a standard of living adequate for the
health and well-being of [the person] himself and of his family'. This
standard unequivocally encompasses a right to health, as it includes
'medical care and necessary social services' (Article 25.1). Nearly
twenty years later it was specifically reaffirmed in the Covenant on
Economic, Social and Cultural Rights: 'The States Parties to the
present Covenant recognize the right of everyone to the enjoyment of
the highest obtainable standard of physical and mental health' (UN
1966a, Article 12.1).

Mental health had already been the subject of a declaration from a
non-governmental source. On 21 August 1948, four months prior to
the UN Declaration, a call to 'Mental Health and World Citizenship'
headed a declaration by the Third International Congress on Mental
Health. The World Federation for Mental Health, a global non-
governmental organization born at that Congress, stated that 'The
ultimate goal of mental health is to help [people] live with their
fellows in one world.' The idea of the 'world citizen' was meant to
convey the notion of a 'common humanity', 'an informed, reflective,
responsible allegiance to mankind as a whole . . . a world community
built on free consent and on the respect for individual and cultural
differences' (World Federation for Mental Health, 1948).

International acceptance of a universal concept of human rights
implies acceptance of an allegiance to humankind as a whole, of a
human family. This represents a step away from the particularity of
the UN's rigid observance of the national sovereignty of Member
States, inviolate within their own borders. None the less, in the late
twentieth century, despite the beginning efforts of UN 'peace-
keeping' forces, nation–states and ethnic groups continue to insist on
their own pre-eminent status; despite disclaimers they override the
concept of a human family with rights allotted simply because of
shared human status. While all human beings have a sense of self,
and profound attachments to their particular extended family and
community, these are not automatically extended to unfamiliar
humans, to strangers. On the contrary, it is usual for one group to try
to deprive other groups of their rights.

Self-concepts and Definitions of the Human: the Universal and the Particular

Assertions about the 'rights' of human beings derive from some view
about the nature of being human. This involves questions for which
scientifically valid answers are not forthcoming. What does it mean to
be a human being? What is the meaning of sentient, reflective life? Do
organisms which are self-aware and reflective have a legitimate claim
to rights or privileges beyond those granted to presumably non-

reflective organisms such as infra-human primates, animals or plants?

All answers to questions of meaning and rights may be understood as social constructions, artefacts of culture – a society's socially inherited blueprint for living (Kluckhohn, 1944) with its core of values. Within particular contexts people give themselves the kind of culturally compatible answers which are essential to maintaining the structure of their lives. Thus, preliterate and preindustrial peoples often designated themselves as 'the' or the 'chosen' people. Their own centrality in the universe, prior to their contact with Europeans, was taken for granted.

The rights formulations of industrialized societies also reflect a community's shared assumptions about the nature of its human members and the surrounding world and universe of which they are a part. They reveal their self-concepts, need for self-esteem, and need for a sense of purpose and meaning in life. In the industrialized or modern world, however, unlike the preliterate world, concepts of self and humanity are informed by science with its reductionist pressure away from the subjective towards the objective. Objectivizing one's self is taken in the contemporary world as a necessary prerequisite to self-mastery and goal-attainment. High-technology medicine emphasizes its practitioners' sense of their own power, and pushes them towards an objectivized perception of their patients as decontextualized biological systems, and away from engagement with them as persons. Again, this is in the service of their mastery over disease and disability. As elements of the contemporary identity – that of the 'post-modern' age (Engelhardt, 1991) – late twentieth-century self-concepts reflect the tension between what Taylor (1989) described as the 'neutral stance toward the world . . . adopted from the demands of "science" ' (p. 8), and that stemming from a sense of self: 'we should treat our deepest moral instincts, our ineradicable sense that human life is to be respected, as our mode of access to the world in which ontological claims are discernible' (p. 8). Whether this stance has an ultimate theistic or secular basis it acknowledges 'some ground in human nature or the human predicament which makes human beings fit objects of respect' (Taylor, 1989, p. 10), a respect which implies the attribution of 'rights' as well as privileges, and presumably of obligations.

A being entitled to the respect essential to self-esteem is assumed to have an intrinsic worth or 'dignity' and to be self-determining within finite limits. There can be no freedom of will or body outside the strictures imposed by humankind's biological nature, and all peoples encounter limits imposed by particular cultural (including moral) frameworks, in some instances translated into law. These pervade every aspect of ministering to suffering persons. Convictions about particular moral issues are deeply invested with emotion. In the United States, perhaps the most intense emotional responses have been aroused in relation to reproductive health (as, for example, abortion, contraception and artificial reproduction), the medical extension of life in comatose or mentally impaired persons, and euthanasia. Engelhardt (1991) directly confronts the problem of particular versus universal moralities in determining the permissible in health care. He regards secular humanism as 'central to our contemporary moral and cultural challenge: justifying a moral framework that can be shared by moral strangers in an age of both moral fragmentation and apathy' (p. xi). Secular humanism is seen as a philosophical solution to 'the diverse character of traditional, especially religious, moral accounts, and their conflicting implications for health care. . . . There is a natural hope that we may share enough together simply as humans in order to justify a common bioethics' (Engelhardt, 1991, p. xi). Without a common moral framework available to be shared by 'moral strangers', Engelhardt suggests that health care policies, inevitably alien to some sectors of the population, will be imposed on all according to the moral vision of the reigning political authority.

An International Right of Equal Opportunity: Natural, Absolute and Inherent?

In contrast to the traditional societies of the less industrialized and often non-literate world, or of the non-Judeo–Christian societies, the rights concept of the industrialized Christian West (exemplified mainly by Western Europe, the United Kingdom, North America, Australia and New Zealand) has long been the subject of formal analysis. While it still has an aura of ambiguity under circumstances other than those of gross violation it carries a presumption of ontological validity. Human beings in the industrial democracies – growing up with the expectation of self-improvement, in a social structure encouraging the ideal of upward mobility – are socialized to feel that they possess certain 'natural' or 'inherent' freedoms and entitlements simply by virtue of being human. 'The fundamental normative load carried by natural rights – that persons ought to be guaranteed a core of personal security and autonomy – is almost irresistible' (Meyers, 1985, p. 1). This understanding is translated in some measure into the welfare provisions of many states concerned with the just, that is fair or equitable, treatment of their citizens.

The idea of an innate dignity as a central justification for granting individual rights bridges the legal and natural–moral conceptions of human status (Forsythe, 1989). The connection of rights with a justice essential to dignity, basic to the kind of contemporary thinking which led to the health and welfare provisions of the UN's 1948 Universal Declaration, was contained in Justinian's *Institutiones*: 'Justice is the constant and perpetual will of giving to each his own right (*ius suum*)'. Golding (1984, pp. 124–5; 1981) notes that the identification of *ius* with *dignitas*, worth, or *meritum*, dessert or worth, derives from Cicero whose definition of justice is cited by Placentinus: 'Justice is that condition of the mind which, with the common utility being preserved, gives to each his own *dignitas*' (*De Inventione*, II, 53, 160).

The idea of worth is also inherent in Kant's view of human beings as rational, self-aware, self-legislating moral agents and members of a moral community; it implies that their acts are voluntary and purposive, and, therefore, *worth* attaining: 'An ineluctable element of worth . . . is involved in the very concept and context of human purposive action' (Gewirth, 1984, p. 23).

However, the actuality of human dignity in varying contexts is influenced by the fact that societies, worldwide, are not characterized by an equitable and publicly visible distribution of entitlements, goods, liberties or self-esteem (Rawls, 1971). The existing inequality of access to life's goods, including health, can, paradoxically, be seen as compatible with another Western value, that of a right of equal access to opportunity. This permits consequences essential for survival, the realization of latent capacities, and the attainment and maintenance of human status or personhood (Brody, 1976, p. 553). But equitable 'opportunity', with its implication of self-reliance and personal achievement as the route to the good life, is not identical with the principle of equal access to the world's variably limited resources. In this sense the scientifically influenced Western value system may contain potential contradictions; while not necessarily incompatible with the ideal, it does not imply the sweeping promises for care and support contained in the United Nations Universal Declaration of Human Rights. It suggests, rather, that an autonomous, striving individual – with sufficient competence – should be able to take advantage of an open opportunity structure to achieve the good things of life, including health care. A right to become as fully developed an individual as possible (part of that of equal opportunity) implies both the opportunity to relate to others and the concept of a dignity innate to human individuals.

The Cultural Context of Rights and Obligations

The Individual and the Collective

In contrast to the predominantly Judeo–Christian West with its complex societies, stress on individual autonomy and personal responsibility, persons from non-Western cultures, as well as the less industrialized, traditional agrarian areas of much of the world, may have quite different views of human rights, privileges, and obligations. For them collective values attributing importance to familial responsibility, reciprocity and lineage are often more important. This has been true largely for traditional societies in the less developed world, for those of the East such as Japan, and for theocracies, mainly Islamic, in which industrialization co-exists with the persistence of peasant and traditional life. It has been repeatedly observed, for example, both among preindustrial peoples and in technically advanced Japan, that, in contrast to the Western view of autonomy–independence–self-determination as a right, high value is attached to moral and emotional interdependence and conformity to perceived family and community needs and norms. This suggests less attribution of individual responsibility on the basis of acquired behavioural standards and greater power to control individual behaviour invested in societal structures. Triandis (1990), for example, regards the relative emphasis on individualism and collectivism as the most important dimension of cultural differences in social behaviour. In the collectivist societies he notes that doing 'right' typically requires conforming to the wishes of established authority figures, while in the former creative, innovative, self-reliant independent action is considered desirable. Increasing cultural complexity, with economies based on functional specialization, bringing different lifestyles, conflicting norms and world-views, may encourage cultural movement towards individualism (Triandis, 1990, p. 44). Under these circumstances personal decisions must be made on the basis of individual, usually subjective, factors rather than the historically transmitted norms of a particular collectivity. In these settings, for example, autonomy and independence for adolescents do not have the high value accorded them in the United States.

In the West, however, the collective point of view continues to emerge in varying form. Thus, in relation to health care, the philosophy of communitarianism emphasizes the importance of community-based goals which may require the subordination of individual desire to the broader conception of what is best for the group. Emanuel's liberal communitarianism (1991) offers a vision of how small communities might arrive at a shared concept of what is best for all members of the group and organize community health plans to deliver medical care in accordance with that concept. It is not suggested that the shared vision of any particular small community can have universal applicability. However, such communities in widely different cultures could, given the resources and freedom from authoritarian rule, organize locally acceptable health plans which conform in some, though not in all, respects with the Universal Declaration of Human Rights.

Unconscious Mental Processes in Cultural Context

A culturally relativistic view of rights, as discussed above, is not totally, or necessarily, antithetical to that of an absolute, inherent or natural human endowment. A community's agreed-upon concept of rights is always a social construction. The expression of a particular claim as a right inevitably, if in language alone, reflects the social and cultural context, the values of the particular society, in which it is put forth. The interpretation by any individual of the community concept also, inevitably, reflects personal biography within that context. Devereux (1956) proposed that the 'relative degree of importance which a culture assigns to various defense mechanisms' and its basic demand patterns 'permits certain impulses, fantasies and the like to become and to remain conscious, while requiring others to be repressed' (p. 6).

Such a formulation permits a culturally specific understanding of unconscious determinants of concepts of right and wrong, the essence of being human, and whatever are considered rights owed to one by virtue of human status. It also adds to the idea of rights as conscious claims that of the claim itself, as an expression of unconscious mental processes influenced by cultural context.

The idea of the 'psychic unity of mankind' bears on this thesis. Espoused by Geza Roheim (1950), a psychoanalytically trained ethnologist, it assumes that cross-cultural equivalences in myth and folklore, the common use of universal symbols, and common mechanisms – across cultures – of individual defence reflect common human problems. Roheim's field studies were aimed at discovering evidence of unconscious universals in all human groups. While his conclusions were not unequivocally accepted, most contemporary psychoanalysts recognize that the greater the socio-cultural similarity between them and their patients, the more able they are to empathize with the patient's experience. Many feel that empathy is always possible through the discovery of some common developmental experience. Kracke (1979), on the basis of work with Amazonian Indians, demonstrated to his satisfaction that human similarity, even between individuals from dramatically different cultural backgrounds, could be established by discovering the concepts or language in which subjective observations could be discussed. It should be noted that he discovered the concepts and language of subjectivity within a relationship. He lived with the tribe for a prolonged period, shared their ordeals and the grief of death, and became an important purveyor of medicines for them. Such discovery may not be possible in a brief, delimited interview. Even with shared arousal, the presumed human capacity for empathy, based on shared structural and developmental features, does not always seem able to traverse the gulf to another person from a different culture and from a different socio-economic stratum.

Cultural Universals

Intermediate between the natural rights position and that of cultural relativism is that of cultural universals (Renteln, 1990). These are convergences between the moral systems of all human cultures. The presupposition is that all cultures have ideals which contain moral principles, and that these cultural ideals are not fixed or immutable. Instead they evolve, and in the course of evolution (especially in the contemporary era of advanced transportation and communication technologies) the likelihood is that there will be increasing convergence between them. This reflects a process of cultural diffusion.

Health Rights and Knowledge Transfer across Cultural Boundaries

The communicative and empathic challenge to human rights is greatest when patient and clinician, or technology controller and a population to be screened or surveyed, are from different ethnic, cultural, or socio-economic backgrounds. Then it is the professional's responsibility to try to understand that differing background, including its healers and other support systems. If necessary, bicultural clinicians and investigators should be recruited to consult or work actively on the problem at hand. This is now the accepted approach in most US centres dealing with refugees and other migrants. In some instances the bicultural helper need not be professionally trained, but a trusted member of the patient's own community. Within the same culture someone who, him or herself, has been sick or has undergone the procedure in question, may be the best counsellor. The effort is always to empower the patient to share the hard decisions about using the forbidding and expensive technology at the clinician's command.

Patient or community empowerment is especially difficult and important when the technology in question has been transferred from an industrialized to a less developed setting. Under these circumstances an appreciation of community and cultural as well as individual rights is essential. Without a thoroughgoing analysis prior to the transfer, the community is at risk of unintended non-beneficial effects of having the new technology within it. Aside from general issues of interhuman and intercultural communication it is a truism that the definition of disease or illness, how the body (and the mind) function, and how they should be dealt with (if at all) vary widely from one people to another. Variations in function are not uniformly perceived as diseases requiring medical 'treatment'. Persons perceive themselves and their inner structures in ways which influence not only their self-reports, but their experience of illness. The transfer of technology may lead to familiar discomforts or disabilities being redefined as illness or disease requiring investigation and treatment.

The process of introducing new biomedical technology and its trained operators from a complex individualistic culture into a less complex collectivist community cannot leave the community unchanged. The symbolic and interactional context of life which contributes to any individual's sense of meaning and worth is altered. Further, those who introduce and manage the technology are figures of power, often perceived as outstripping that of local healers. This may place the rights, privileges and obligations of the entire community at risk. Under these circumstances an authentic process of informed consent for treatment with the new devices or procedures may be impossible. 'Informed consent' is difficult enough in the usual circumstances when the investigator–clinician, in contrast to the patient or subject, is healthy, educated, socially powerful and the master of esoteric knowledge. Even with an educated, sensitive patient the clinician's full disclosure can be perfunctory and assent almost reflexive under the pressure of fear and the desire to be well or whole. When the clinician must work out his/her own identity within a strange culture in relation to the patient as a cultural (or in Engelhardt's term, moral) stranger, and time is limited, it may be almost impossible. This is intensified when the doctor–patient relationship is one of a whole new range of relationships and experiences, and interpreters must be used to breach a language barrier. In every instance the personal history of the clinician (or technological decision-makers) constitutes a powerful and usually unidentified influence upon the interactions which generate the relevant data. This history includes not only idiosyncratic personal biography, but socialization into a profession and the meaning of the professional role in the clinician's or the investigator's society and culture of origin, as well as that in which he is now working. These factors will affect the clinician's response to such modal responses in the new culture as circumlocution, flattery or automatic acquiescence to authority.

It is evident that advocacy for health-preserving measures accepted in the Western industrial democracies may have differing significance in the developing world (Brody, 1981a). Incentives offered to very poor people in such countries, such as the distribution of transistor radios to young Indian males as an incentive for vasectomy, inevitably have an element of hidden coercion (Brody,

1976). Investigators from industrialized nations working in the poverty-stricken Third World have begun to face analogous issues. They wonder if differing value systems preclude their former assumption that the moral codes of research workers from an industrialized country are necessarily applicable to collaborative research carried out in different cultures or less industrialized nations (Angell, 1988). It has been questioned, for example, if informed consent, especially to procedures used by Western-trained scientist–clinicians, can be authentically applied to illiterate populations in countries without a democratic tradition (Barry, 1988). Ijesselmuiden and Faden (1992), in considering this problem, have reviewed

> the complex motivation behind decisions to conduct research in the developing world rather than in the West [including] such question-able factors as lower costs, lower risks of litigation, less stringent ethical review, the availability of populations prepared to cooperate with almost any study that appears curative in nature, anticipated underreporting of side effects because of low consumer awareness, the desire for personal advancement, and the desire to create new markets for pharmaceutical agents and other products (p. 833).

They conclude that, despite occasional problems in communication and the tendency of potential subjects of clinical trials to agree with anyone in authority, and to undertake any procedure with potential therapeutic value, there should be no substitute for first-person informed consent.

Social Organization and Human Rights

Individual Freedom and the Common Good

In the West the more common argument has concerned the value of individual freedoms versus behavioural restrictions deemed necessary to maintain the general welfare. Such individually imposed restrictions are publicly visible counterparts of the internal obligations of well-socialized citizens to behave in ways which further the well-being of the community.

The nineteenth-century English founder of utilitarian philosophy, Jeremy Bentham, was convinced that the concept of 'the rights of man' was irrevocably incompatible with the demands of the general good of society; he dismissed the former as 'anarchical fallacies'. Opposing is the view that the support of individual rights does not contradict the common good but, in fact, enlarges it. In the twentieth century, while 'violators of human rights will almost always take their actions to be promoting the general good', utilitarians, too, are beginning to recognize that a commonly and universally respected core of human rights protections will 'enhance human thriving and human happiness' (Gibbard, 1984, p. 93).

Still, the absoluteness of any individual right can be questioned on moral as well as legal grounds. In practice this appears to depend upon the nature or acts of the person about whom, or the circumstances under which, the question is raised. The 'stringency' of a murderer's right to life 'plummets toward zero' (Meyers, 1985, p. 3). Opposed, in this instance, are arguments against capital punishment in any society which supports every person's absolute right to life as well as recognizing the fallibility of human judgement and the possibility of mistaken death sentences. But there are no systematic arguments in favour of letting a murderer roam freely in the community without restraint. The major debate regarding alternatives to capital punishment has been between life-long incarceration which both protects the community and punishes the offender, and attempts at rehabilitation to be followed by restoration of freedom with varying degrees of monitoring. These contrasting solutions involve differing concepts of human rights (of both the offending individual and the community). They also have implications for biomedicine since they suggest different aetiologies of violent or anti-social behaviour.

Rights as Inalienable and Universal

Societies, as well as their cultures, have varied in their willingness to assign all human beings the status of persons with dignity and rights. Some have been excluded on the grounds that they did not have the souls essential to human status. A contemporary argument within the United States concerns the humanity of foetuses – should they have the same moral status and rights as independent, reflective adult humans, or do they represent 'a mere instance of human biological life morally on a par with other biological life of the same actual functional ability', which can be construed as part of a larger question 'about whether there is a deity who cares about fetuses or no God at all?' (Engelhardt, 1991, p. 15). Excluded from full human status with its associated rights at various times have been neonates prior to the age of nine days, mentally retarded individuals, cultural aliens, slaves, prisoners of war and devotees of non-majority religions. The Nazi category of 'life not worthy of life' included primarily persons defined as Jews, but also at times Gypsies, Poles, and psychotic, mentally defective or unproductive people.

Once an individual has been defined as human, rights have generally been granted on a non-categorical basis. Blackstone's *Commentaries on the Laws of England* (1765 *et seq.*) described 'the absolute rights of man' endowed 'as a free agent' with 'the natural liberty of mankind' (Golding, 1984, p. 123; 1981). The US Declaration of Independence proclaimed 'that all Men are created equal . . . endowed by their Creator with certain unalienable Rights'. But like universality and absoluteness, 'inalienability adopts the perspective of the right-holder rather than the right-respecter' (Meyers, 1985, p. 4). From this position health rights and other entitlements can never be lost, even in consequence of the right-holder's behaviour, and even if others can be justified in not granting them. As Hohfeld (1964) has noted, rights attributable to humans are primarily claims; they are expectations that other persons, groups or institutions will behave in ways ensuring that right-holders are not deprived of their freedoms and entitlements.

The Interpersonal Web of Health Rights and Obligations

The pragmatics of distributing scarce entitlements and permitting potentially damaging freedoms have led 'rights' to be described as 'solutions to problems of institutional design' (Gibbard, 1984, p. 94). This design, however, must take account of the fact that they exist in an interpersonal web. One person's or one group's rights are another's obligations: to supply the rightful entitlements or avoid infringing upon the rightful freedoms. Claims both for welfare rights or entitlements, and option rights or freedoms, assume an un-specified right of control over the behaviour of others. These include both the individuals and the institutions involved in the everyday activities of the community: 'All moral precepts, regardless of their greatly varying contents, are concerned with how persons ought to *act* toward one another' (Gewirth, 1984, p. 12). This view is com-patible with that of a right as a social construction, an artefact of culture with its core of values.

Within any particular socio-culture rights observance embodies the values of a particular historical moment. As noted in Chapter 2, even the US Bill of Rights is subject to interpretation by the Supreme Court, and advancing technology can change the meaning of such concepts as 'privacy'.

For physicians trained in Western medicine the primary accepted value has been the patient's right to beneficent treatment (couched in terms of medical responsibility for his or her best interest). This was recognized in the earliest Hippocratic, Chinese and Indian codes of medical ethics. It is central in the post-Second World War declar-ations of non-governmental groups, beginning with the Code of Nuremberg (1947), which arose from the medical exploitation of vulnerable, helpless prisoners by the Nazis.

Other codes of medical ethics have been the World Medical

Association's Declaration of Geneva (1948), the Indian Physicians' Code (1956), the Oath of the Soviet Physician (1971), the Principles of Ethics of the American Medical Association (1981), and the Council for International Organizations of Medical Sciences–UN Principles of Medical Ethics (1982). All are concerned with the rights and welfare of the individual patient; they are consistent with the Kantian tradition of respect for the single individual considered a member of a moral community. However, all medical codes embody an implicit paternalism which may be ultimately irreconcilable with the ideal of patient autonomy.

Welfare and Health Entitlements as Human Rights

The conviction that the right to health is 'a human right entitled to legal recognition' is a corollary to the proposition that governments have a duty to 'advance the enjoyment' of other freedoms and entitlements considered the right of each human being (Buergenthal, 1989, p. 3). As Roemer (1989) points out, however, 'obviously everyone cannot be assured perfect health'; since a right to health itself cannot be enforceable, 'it is more accurate to speak of the right to health care' (p. 17). State responsibility for individual and public health, that is, health as a legal 'right', was identified as early as the fourth century BC by Aristotle, who wrote of 'an absolute right to such a measure of good health as society, and society alone, is able to give' (Roemer, 1989, p. 17). State protection of access to care is implied in the introduction to a 1989 Draft European Declaration on the Rights of Patients as it refers to equity in health as a policy objective for Member States along with a commitment to ensure quality of care (WHO, 1989).

Militant Ethnocentrism and the Rights of Victims

Many perceptions of human rights focus on violations of the sense of self by political authorities or militant rebels. Their ordinarily taken-for-granted liberties and capacities have been forcibly taken away from them. Carried to extreme lengths, as in torture, these violations destroy whatever might be considered the essence of the persons against whom they are directed. To the degree that individuals have been targeted on categorical grounds, because they are members of a particular group, usually defined in political, racial, ethnic or religious terms, their social organization and culture are victims. Thus, the torture of leaders, with the other personal violations surrounding it (sudden seizure and imprisonment, harassment in all major life spheres), is a recognized method of destroying the integrity of targeted groups.

Most accounts of human rights violations, in contrast to failures to meet claims for support understood as a right, deal with the consequences of militant forms of ethnocentrism – seeing all who are not members of one's own group as inferior, dangerous and different to the point of not being fully human. Militant ethnocentrism has been central to the world-views of conquest-bent and colonizing groups throughout recorded history. Such conquerors have ranged from Genghis Khan, to North American settlers from Europe displacing the native Indians, to the British in India and Africa, to the totalitarian regimes of the twentieth century whose abuses are perpetrated against their own citizens. In every instance the dominant parties have reserved for themselves the 'right' of eminent domain. They have kept the good things of the earth, and destroyed the freedoms, lives, property, psychological and physical integrity, and personal and organizational prerogatives of opposing, colonized, defeated, enslaved or minority groups. Their victims are treated, if not actually regarded, as inferior or not fully human.

In a mild, and often unrecognized, fashion, ethnocentrism is a universal characteristic of members of all human groups. All divide their perceived world in some manner into 'we' and 'they', and members of one group, feeling themselves as 'we', have great difficulty empathizing with strangers who are perceived as 'they'. It is difficult to see the world through the other's eyes and 'they', often enough, are perceived as the enemy.

The Institutionalization of Human Rights in World Politics

An early step towards the contemporary institutionalization of human rights concerns was the 1894 Geneva Convention for victims of armed conflict. It affirmed the neutrality of medical personnel by allowing them to treat sick and wounded soldiers. This recognized the individual soldier as entitled 'to at least a minimum of respect for his essence as a person . . . even in war' (Forsythe, 1989, p.7). An identity as a human individual with implied rights to humane treatment was substituted for that of an impersonal combatant used by superior officers to pursue the goals of a militant state. The Convention was later revised through successive treaties aimed at the care of prisoners of war. The Swiss citizens who worked for it became the nucleus of what eventually grew into the International Committee of the Red Cross.

The League of Nations' attempts to protect human rights between 1919 and 1939 concerned mainly the well-being of minorities, workers and inhabitants of colonies, with some attention to refugees. In the same period a number of non-governmental organizations formed the Anti-Slavery League. With great effort, and still uncertain practical results in some parts of the world, the League influenced a large group of countries to adopt a 1926 Convention outlawing slavery, finally implemented in the 1950s (Forsythe, 1989).

This was a first breach of the principle of national sovereignty, a traditional basis of international relations. Still fiercely upheld by most Member States of the UN, this principle is, perhaps, the greatest obstacle to a universal standard of human rights. Both the UN General Assembly and world public opinion, however, appear to be moving away from a rigid view of national sovereignty. Reluctant nation–states are, very slowly, moving towards adopting international standards for the treatment of politically dissenting citizens, or refugees. Active regional human rights laws and bodies exist for Western Europe, the Americas, Africa and Europe as a whole. But, while Western Europe has a highly developed system, with all 21 Member States of the Council of Europe adhering to the European Convention on Human Rights which entered into legal force in 1953, the records of the other regions are less clear. The 1975 Helsinki Accord for Europe as a whole rarely mentions human rights, but emphasizes humanitarian principles. In most of the rest of the world the practical significance of rights instruments is determined largely by the degree to which their provisions have been incorporated into national law. 'The weak international control agencies, for the most part, exist to nudge states into national steps for promoting rights' (Forsythe, 1989, p. 46). But adherence to national restrictions is variable, and some laws seem to have been enacted largely for the benefit of world public opinion. Voluntary non-governmental organizations remain the most active and consistent world advocates for human rights.

The conflict between particular moral codes and the attempt to achieve a universal set of values began with the initial UN debates about the Universal Declaration of Human Rights. The Arab States strongly objected to the concepts of religious freedom and the right to move from one religious affiliation to another because they did not fit the strictures of the Koran. The Soviets were opposed to the Western emphasis on civil liberties, favouring instead material or welfare entitlements. These included such 'rights' as those to food, shelter, health care and employment.

At the intergovernmental level Article 55 of the United Nations Charter (UN, 1945) has become the basis for subsequent human rights instruments. It notes 'the principle of equal rights and self determination of peoples'. More specifically it committed the UN to promote 'higher standards of living . . . solutions of international economic, social, health and related problems, and international cultural and educational cooperation'.

This commitment was embodied in the 1948 Universal Declaration which was followed by treaties, called covenants, on civil and political (UN, 1966a), and economic, social and cultural (UN, 1966b) rights. By 1988, 86 states had pledged adherence to the civil and political and 90 to the economic–social–cultural covenant. The Political Covenant allows individuals to petition international organizations (NGOs) against their governments under certain conditions.

The 'tension between socio-economic and civil–political rights' (Forsythe, 1989, p. 14) embodied in the 1966 covenants was a concern for Western observers. Third World and Eastern-bloc leaders, in contrast to those of the industrial democracies concerned with individual freedoms, conceived human rights as welfare entitlements, in other words, to the social benefits of technological progress reflected mainly in the availability of basic necessities such as food and shelter. Their emphasis was on the obligations of the paternalistic state to provide its citizens with the wherewithal for survival. None the less, international law concerning individual freedoms with ramifications for health continued to develop. International Labour Organization treaties restricted forced and child labour; UN General Assembly treaties attempted to outlaw genocide and racial discrimination; a UNESCO treaty opposed discrimination in education. At least twenty-two basic human rights treaties, including one on refugees, were on the books by 1988 (UN, 1988). The Convention on the Rights of the Child, passed by the General Assembly on 20 November 1989, reflects the widespread twentieth-century disregard for children, as it places the age below which they should not be conscripted into armed forces at 15. Efforts to raise the limit to at least the age of 18 were defeated.

Human Rights in Relation to Health and Individual Medical Care

Societal Concerns

Public concern has accelerated with an awareness of unequal access to the benefits and unequal vulnerability to the possible harms of advancing technology. The access of individuals and groups to the benefits, and their vulnerability to the harms, are correlated with their relative power and status in society. Interest in this issue, therefore, is becoming part of a general concern with equal opportunity, equal worth and fair treatment.

Society and culture ultimately assert responsibility for life and death decisions made by their designated healers. This has intensified with the advent of technologies, such as artificial reproduction and genetic manipulation, which could modify the shared concept of what constitutes a human being. All biomedical technologies have the potential for changing the character of society itself. This is why, in the industrial democracies, increasing attention is being given to the value of an educated, informed community at large and public debate about the issues raised by new medical powers.

Individual Claims to Health Care: Justice, Autonomy, Self-esteem

Following Hohfeld (1964), all individual rights can be considered legitimate claims upon the community, understanding that communities do not have equal scientific, medical and health resources and that access to some may be restricted by particular moral systems. It is further understood that a presumed right to a service can impose an obligation on unwilling health care personnel. However, claims to demonstrably safe and effective health care are considered valid even if a lack of resources or cultural taboo makes their fulfilment impossible for anyone in the society, or only for members of particular social groups. So are claims to autonomy or freedom in respect to health care decisions valid, even in a context which submerges them. But the apparent validity of health care claims for expensive labour-intensive advanced biomedical technology raises another question: that is, how to distinguish a need, which might reasonably be considered part of publicly funded entitled health care, from desire for a special treatment which society is not obliged to supply.

Individual health, and the ability to care for one's self, especially with the proliferating products of biomedical research, requires a subjective sense of competence and autonomy, of self-esteem. This has been especially evident in studies of contraceptive use and non-use in developing societies in which women tend to be only partly literate and subordinated to men (Brody, 1981a). The physical availability of contraceptive or other health services to uninformed, traditional peoples is not sufficient to ensure their use. More complex technologies which require specially trained physicians to administer them are completely out of reach of most of the world's population and available only to the few with the means to pay for or the power to demand them. As Rawls (1971) noted, the interests of those most remote from decision-makers, the most disadvantaged or least powerful members of the society, tend to be submerged when policy, including health policy, is being formulated. In a fee-for-service economy affluent individuals can exercise their right to health care, and their claim on the physician provider is accompanied by a reward which ensures the rapid delivery of that care. The desirable contrast would be a social contract ensuring a favourable outcome, and an increased sense of personal worth, for society's least advantaged members. In most industrial countries, however, attempts to increase the health and welfare options, and self-esteem, of the least advantaged members of society have inspired resistance from taxpayers unwilling to assume the necessary additional costs.

Ethics Decision-making Bodies

A major societal response to the challenge of advancing biomedical technology has been the still-emerging discipline of bioethics. That discipline, professionalized and institutionalized, has become the property not only of philosophers, including ethicists and religious scholars, but of lawyers and judges and, by extension, legislators and other policy-makers. These are all holders of societal power. In sharp contrast the persons whose survival and integrity may depend upon (or be impaired by) the new technologies are relatively powerless. This may contribute to a certain scepticism about the committees or commissions and their members. As Engelhardt (personal communication) has noted, they are sometimes arenas for the chronic struggle between secular and religious forces for control of the public morality. Ingelfinger (1973), for example, doubted the logic of institutions providing more than the broadest medical ethical guidelines, feeling that 'the onus of decision-making ultimately falls on the doctor' (p. 914). He was also concerned with the potential com-prof medical research and rising public distrust of physicians as consequences of the meticulous and possibly trivial delineation of ethical issues put at risk by medical objectives. Questions still arise about the possibly unnecessary inhibition of research, and the irrelevance of abstract rules when human needs must immediately be met in the cauldron of hospital practice. Lo (1987) has examined committee composition and process, wondering if hospital ethics committees always, in fact, proceed in an ethical manner. Some seem, for example, to function mainly as social–emotional supports for clinicians, or to reduce the possibility of legal liability for malpractice. Only a few allow patients to bring their own cases to the committee, allow patients and families to attend meetings, or even welcome representation by nursing staff (who are often more intimately familiar with patients as persons than the attending physicians). Other issues concern the committee appeal and review process, pressure for consensus, the adequacy of primary data, and innovative and imaginative ways of reaching agreement. However, while Lo (1987) suggests that the question of whether ethics committees are useful is an empirical one, this may not recognize the consciousness-raising and educational value of the review process regardless of the outcome in a particular case.

Bioethics commission pronouncements inevitably reflect the

cultural predilections of the societies of which they are part. In the Western industrialized democracies which have given rise to them, these include the ethic of respect for individuals with emphasis on the 'right-making' principles of autonomy, beneficence, and justice. However, they pay little attention to the immediate socio-cultural matrix of medical care in which the cases referred to them arise. It is possible, while recognizing the self-protective efforts of society and culture, to consider a more elastic construal of human rights which is patient, culture and society oriented in relation to biomedical technology, and which also takes account of personal attachments and relationships. Contemporary laws which attempt to deal with the new human problems posed by the capacities of biomedical technologies vary between local, provincial and national entities and are in a state of flux and development.

Clinical Practice Concerns

Successive reconceptualizations of human rights tend to follow technological development and clinical practice rather than the reverse. There can be no realistic conception of the hazards posed to human dignity by a particular diagnostic or therapeutic measure without understanding its nature, limitations and power. It can have the power to stigmatize as well as to heal and protect, and by identifying their particular biological characteristics can make individuals vulnerable to later discrimination. 'Ethical' condemnation of some current technologies may simply reflect ignorance of their usefulness, or failure to accurately predict their future benefits. The rights and wrongs of new possibilities offered by biomedical research are, to be sure, interpreted by tradition and religion as well as by bioethicists in the light of particular moral codes. But in the clinic and at the bedside, while constrained by cultural and legal concerns, the interaction of the human needs of patient, family and doctor tends to generate a relational and empathic conception of human rights. With increasing information and the rise of consumerism in the industrial democracies, patients and their families have become more involved in the biomedical decisions which affect them. They tend to make their judgements more on the basis of existing relationships with loved ones in need of help than of autonomy–beneficence–justice in the abstract. This may even involve, as noted in Chapter 4, the use of other human beings as means rather than ends in themselves. Others can be sources of body parts to ensure the survival of persons who already have affectional bonds with the older and more powerful arrangers of the life-sustaining situation.

The clinician, faced with decisions about using newly available technological powers, now has unsolicited consultation from non-clinical professionals. But it is the clinician who, in the final analysis, is engaged with patient and family in the struggle to protect life, physical and psychological integrity and human rights. In this setting it is the clinician's task to try to see the world through the patient's eyes. It is also his responsibility to be aware of his own excitement and his wish to utilize the new technology, and to be omnipotent and omniscient, in so far as it may not benefit the patient. Achieving such self-awareness may require consultation in the decision-making process.

Informed Consent and Free Access to Medical Information

The concept of 'informed consent' of subjects raised in the 1948 UN Universal Declaration of Human Rights was emphasized as an indispensable requirement for human clinical research by the Nuremberg Code (1947) and the Declaration of Helsinki (1964). It became routinized in the Western industrial democracies in the mid-1970s (Faden and Beauchamp, 1986); it is now a basic requirement for patients receiving accepted though possibly hazardous treatments, as well as those who are given experimental therapies or are acknowledged subjects of clinical research. It has different operational meanings for the clinician who must obtain it from a patient before engaging in a procedure, a lawyer who may view it as the basis of a liability, or the patient who grants it. As a legal doctrine it varies with jurisdiction. As an ethical doctrine it is based on the premise that 'the patient is an autonomous person who is entitled to make treatment decisions based on relevant, factual information and perhaps advice provided by a doctor or other care-provider' (Lidz et al., 1984, p. 4). The patient must be entitled to refuse as well as consent, and is expected to act as a 'free agent'.

'Informed consent', in the view of many clinicians accustomed to work under pressure to make rapid decisions with inadequate information, is an ideal which, given the psychological needs of sick persons for direction and care, their vulnerability to even unintended persuasion, and the physician's own need for action, can never be totally achieved. It is requested and experienced differently in an authoritarian (if it is, indeed, used) than an egalitarian setting, and for a literate, urban, middle-class patient familiar with the consumer's rights movement than for a semi-literate farmer or labourer. The health practitioner is separated from the latter by socio-economic status and power as well as by esoteric knowledge. It is particularly difficult to evaluate the consent of prisoner volunteers to participate in research as subjects: 'Coercion . . . flows from the deeply intrusive, literally totalitarian character of prisons.' Prisoners, additionally, are poor, bored, and so preoccupied with eventual release that they will usually do anything which might hasten the date (Cohen, 1979).

Sometimes efforts at informed consent fail because of lack of scientific knowledge. Treatments often have undesirable effects which are unknown at the time of prescribing. Some drugs which appear to have no side-effects will produce them when a third factor becomes active. The difficulties are compounded when patient and physician share an uncritical enthusiasm for a medication which is effective and for which no side-effects have been identified, even though available data suggest that they might emerge. An example was DES, diethylstilboestrol, widely used for many years to prevent miscarriages during pregnancy, and used, in limited fashion, as therapy for psychotic depressions with post-menopausal onset. It was not until a generation later that DES was blamed for cancer of the uterus and cervix in adult daughters of women who had used it (Fisher and Apfel, 1985), and more recently there are suggestions of similar cancers in their granddaughters. In 1989 US courts opened the way for DES manufacturers to be sued for damages resulting from the use of this product, although they, presumably, had had no reason at the time of manufacture to suspect its toxicity, and were not directly involved in prescribing it to patients.

As Lidz et al. (1984) note, informed consent as a set of legal rules continues to undergo slow metamorphosis. Although the concept emerged in the eighteenth century the first recognized legal case was begun in 1957. The nature of a physician's 'duty to disclose' and exceptions to it (emergency, incompetence, decision by proxy, 'therapeutic privilege') were mainly delineated in the 1960s and 1970s. This reflected in part the world human rights ferment combined with the health consumer movement growing in the 1960s. It led to widespread concern with the use of demented persons as subjects for trials with drugs of unknown efficacy and potentially hazardous effects, and in at least one instance with injected living cancer cells (Langer, 1966/1976). Objections were also being raised to the use of prisoner volunteers for drug trials, especially those requiring inoculation with typhoid and other organisms. Among the more widely discussed US instances were two involving discrimi-nated-against minorities. One, part of several studies carried out in the 1930s by the US Public Health Service, deprived poor, un-educated, rural Southern Black men of available therapy as part of a study of the clinical course and pathology of syphilis (Tuskegee Panel, 1973/1977). The retrospective conclusion that the study was ethically unjustified was not reached until 1973. The other investi-gation, beginning in 1956, used institutionalized retarded children as subjects in a study of viral hepatitis with consent presumably obtained from their parents (Gorovitz et al., 1976, pp. 123–42). These were among the instances prompting increased attention to a concept of informed consent in order to protect the rights of persons subjected to investigative therapies or other procedures.

Informed Consent and New or Experimental Therapies for Desperate Patients

The proliferation of new but unproven remedies has given rise to a relatively new type of human rights concern. It involves the conflict between, on the one hand, the need for valid clinical information requiring randomized clinical trials followed by a slow process of official approval and, on the other, the wishes of dying patients and their families, and their feeling that they have a 'right' to benefit from any new approach which can offer hope of survival. One proposed solution has been 'parallel tracking', allowing clinical trials to continue while unproved therapies are released to participating physicians for their use with particular patients in dire need and for whom there is no hope except this remote one to stave off death. Thus, the situations in which this issue arises are socially visible and emotionally difficult for all participants. In the past the main patient group interested in unproved treatments was that of cancer sufferers. More recently it has been AIDS patients. These last have become a political pressure group and have achieved some expanded access to unproved AIDS treatments, but the eventual consequences for clinical trials are unclear (Skerrett, 1990).

The definition of therapy as 'experimental' has also taken on new financial meaning as payment for treatments so defined is excluded by most insurance policies. As discussed in Chapter 8, this has given rise to disputes between patients feeling that their rights to care are being denied, physicians and insurance companies; physicians, understanding that reliable prediction of cure is impossible, are, none the less, aware that, given the multiple variables involved, a new therapy could, conceivably, produce disease remission. As a rule physicians are sensitive to the psychophysiological costs as well as the potential benefits of unproven treatments. They do not want to offer new therapies which pose risks significantly greater than the standard treatments covered by insurance payers. On the other hand, to the degree that the medical role, indeed the patient's welfare, requires maintaining hope, no therapy should be excluded from payment because of its experimental status. In this sense the patient may be said to have a right to whatever resource is available, regardless of cost.

Randomized trials have also been used in health services research, such as studies of early hospital discharge for various types of patients, of various settings for different types of procedures, or of systems of health care financing. In these instances it is difficult to obtain prior informed consent in order to maintain any particular individual's right to self-determination; presumed social benefits, such as basing care on outpatient rather than inpatient facilities, may serve political and policy agendas which do not benefit the patient, while the principle of justice is not upheld as particularly vulnerable populations, such as the indigent, tend to become the subjects of research. Health services research requires especially careful consideration of the rights of subjects and of population groups (Brett and Grodin, 1991).

In the industrial democracies public concern about informed consent, as discussed above and in Chapter 2, and the evolution of social institutions to protect patients' rights, have not removed the tension between the investigative and therapeutic roles of physicians. The argument between utilitarian and rights-based moral theories continues in respect of many of the technologies discussed in the following chapters, as well as of the widespread use of randomized clinical trials. While they can be defended in terms of the need for new and certain knowledge, randomized trials inevitably require some sacrifice of the interests of particular patients whose right to individual treatment is ignored in favour of the new knowledge to be gained. Debate continues with a recommendation for 'alternative methods for acquiring clinical knowledge' (Hellman and Hellman, 1991, p. 1589) versus the assertion that 'properly carried out, with informed consent, clinical equipoise, and a design adequate to answer the question posed, randomized clinical trials protect physicians and their patients from therapies that are ineffective or toxic' (Passamani, 1991, p. 1591).

Health Rights in United Nations Declarations

The United Nations Universal Declaration of Human Rights (1948) reflected the desire of most nations, primarily the Western ones, after a devastating world war and the atrocities of totalitarian regimes, to formulate a code of international values aimed at protecting the lives, identities and integrity of individual persons regardless of the particular country, culture or social organization in which they lived. Because of Nazi medical experimentation there was a special emphasis by the document's framers upon health care and medical research subjects. The efforts to satisfy everyone, however, from those in the industrial democracies concerned with political and civil liberties to those in the less developed world concerned with ensuring the necessities of life, resulted in a document which omitted almost no aspect of human welfare. It is so broad and all-inclusive as to invite its automatic dismissal as unachievable by national health agencies struggling with minimal resources. Further, it ignores the extent to which its universal dicta, especially those dealing with equality and women's self-determination, constitute a moral framework incompatible with the particular customs of much of the world. At the same time it has provided a basis for a series of derivative statements refining and elaborating particular elements. The process has continued to focus the attention of governments and non-governmental organizations upon human rights concerns; if continued it should, in due course, eventuate in a set of propositions which will have the force of international guidelines if not law.

Much of the Universal Declaration is concerned with health. At almost the same time that the Declaration was proclaimed the United Nations founded its specialized health agency, the World Health Organization, WHO. Over the years WHO's definition of health has become progressively refined until it now focuses on a state of 'well-being'. This implies rights both to health (implying preventive as well as health promotion measures) and health care, in the sense of access to reparative or curative facilities in case of disease, injury or disability.

The following inventory suggests the thinking of representatives of Member States to the UN. While the Declaration's freedoms and entitlements, and those of its derivative statements, are often stated in general terms, and have not been systematically enforced, they contribute to a growing body of international law and precedent. However, some freedoms restricted on vague public health grounds can be easily abused.

Freedom from inhuman treatment   A prohibition, 'No one shall be subjected to torture or to cruel, inhuman or degrading treatment or punishment' (UN, 1948, Article 5) was later elaborated to include a specific reference to medical research: 'In particular, no one shall be subjected without his free consent to medical or scientific experiment' (UN, 1966b, Article 7). This does not include informed consent to procedures which fit the customary criteria for medical treatment.

Health and welfare-related restrictions on freedom of speech, expression and information   While the right to freedom of expression articulated in the 1948 Declaration is reiterated in the Covenant on Civil and Political Rights (UN, 1966b), it is qualified in its Article 19.3(b) on public health among other grounds. The right 'to seek, receive and impart information and ideas of all kinds, regardless of frontiers' (Article 19.2) 'may be subject to certain restrictions . . . as are provided by law and are necessary' (Article 19.3) 'for respect of the rights or reputations of others' (Article 19.3(a)) or 'for the protection of national security or of public order, or of public health or morals' (Article 19.3(b)). Similar concern with 'the protection of public health or morals' is expressed in Article 22 concerning a right to freedom of association with others.

While these restrictions could be useful in preventing contagion of panic or infection, and in controlling such problems as substance abuse, their potential for misuse is clear. This is especially obvious in regard to the protection of 'reputations', 'security', 'order' and 'morals'. They could also be used to limit the freedom to generate, disseminate, and have access to medical information (Brody, 1975a, 1975b).

As in the case of persons detained on grounds of mental disorder, both individual rights and the general good would be served by clearly separating therapeutic from police-power restrictions. The European Convention on Human Rights (Council of Europe, 1978) is more specific in this respect. Its Article 5.1 states: 'Everyone has the right to liberty and security of person. No one shall be deprived of his liberty except to prevent the spreading of infectious diseases, of persons of unsound mind, alcoholics or drug addicts or vagrants.' In order to avoid the danger of abusing these restrictions significant specification must be combined with flexibility in interpretation. Another loophole for abusive governments, or for states concerned with migrant newcomers, is the freedom to define such concepts as 'unsound mind' or 'vagrants' to suit their own purposes.

Freedom of personality development and the promotion of certain attitudes   The 1948 Declaration's Article 26.2 begins: 'Education shall be directed to the full development of the human personality'; it stresses the importance of education to promote general tolerance and respect. Article 29.1 states: 'Everyone has duties to the community in which alone the free and full development of his personality is possible.'

These statements are open to interpretation, especially in the light of advancing informational and educational technologies. On the one hand they may be taken as protection for the right to optimal development of one's personality and unique identity. On the other hand, while noting the importance of interpersonal respect and, presumably, tolerance for certain forms of unconventional behaviour, they open the door for subtly coercive educational programmes ('brainwashing') directed towards the production of people with particular attitudes prescribed by the community of origin.

Freedom from gender discrimination   Gender discrimination is clearly antithetical to a person's free and informed access to biomedical technologies. Article 1 of the 1948 Declaration refers to 'all human beings' as 'born free and equal in dignity and rights'. Article 2 includes sex among the distinctions which shall not be made in regard to entitlements to rights and freedoms. Article 16 refers to 'men and women of full age' as having 'the right to marry and to found a family' and 'entitled to equal rights as to marriage, during marriage and at its dissolution'. The Covenant on Civil and Political Rights (UN, 1966b) reiterates freedom from sex distinctions and (Article 3) emphasizes 'the equal rights of men and women to the enjoyment of all civil and political rights'. It goes beyond these (Article 23) to ensure that in case of dissolution of marriage 'provision shall be made for the necessary protection of any children'. Other United Nations instruments bear on freedom from gender discrimination with particular reference to women's health. In this respect it may be noted that the UN review, *The World's Women 1970–1990*, published in 1991, documents the persisting inferior position of women in the world. It presents data ranging from the higher illiteracy rates for young women than men, with the widest gaps in Africa and southern and western Asia, to the almost exclusive abortion of female (in contrast to male) foetuses in Bombay by parents who had identified the foetal gender through amniocentesis.

Entitlements to the benefits of science and basic health care   The 'right freely . . . to share in scientific advancement and in its benefits' (UN, 1948, Article 27), was later rephrased as 'the right of everyone . . . to enjoy the benefits of scientific progress and its applications' (UN, 1966a, Article 15.1). These are particular aspects of the more broadly stated rights included in the 1948 Declaration: 'a standard of living adequate for the health and well-being of himself and of his family, including . . . medical care and necessary social services' (Article 25.1); and 'special care and assistance' in conditions of 'motherhood and childhood' (Article 25.2). The Covenant on Civil and Political Rights (UN, 1966b) specifies rights to 'safe and healthy working conditions' (Article 7(b)) and 'rest, leisure and reasonable limitation of working hours' (Article 7(d)), both of which have a clear bearing on health. All the health-related rights come together again in the Covenant on Economic, Social and Cultural Rights (UN, 1966a) Article 12.1: 'The States Parties to the present Covenant recognize the right of everyone to the enjoyment of the highest obtainable standard of physical and mental health.'

Children's health entitlements and security rights   The general basis of later instruments in this area was the Declaration of the Rights of the Child (UN, 1959). To its provisions have been added (UN, 1966b) that children have rights comparable to adults; that 'every child shall be registered immediately after birth and shall have a name' (Article 24, paragraph 2); and that 'every child has the right to acquire a nationality' (Article 24, paragraph 3). The last two are relevant to the new technologies of artificial reproduction. The Covenant on Economic, Social and Cultural Rights (1966a) reiterates some of these entitlements and adds others which bear on health, such as a child's right to protection 'from economic and social exploitation' and 'employment in work harmful to their morals or health or dangerous to life or likely to hamper their normal development' (Article 10, paragraph 3). These covenants can be labelled as expressions of internationally institutionalized hypocrisy in so far as they conceal the existence of several million children described as occupying the virtual status of slaves. These include child indentured labourers within the untouchable caste in India, and those reportedly without rights in several other countries. While they are not slaves the street children of Latin America and Asia, conservatively estimated at fifty million, are regular victims of exploitation.

Article 12.1, recognizing the right 'to the enjoyment of the highest obtainable standard of physical and mental health' (paragraph 1), lists essentials 'to achieve the full realization of this right' (paragraph 2). They include 'the provision for the reduction of the stillbirth rate and of infant mortality and for the healthy development of the child [2(a)]; the improvement of all aspects of environmental and industrial hygiene [2(b)]; the prevention, treatment and control of epidemic, endemic, occupational and other diseases [2(c)]; the creation of conditions which would assure to all, medical services and medical attention in the event of sickness' (2(d)). These were further affirmed and elaborated in the 20 November 1989 Convention on the Rights of the Child (UN, 1989).

Women's health rights in relation to personal fertility control   The 1948 UN Declaration affirmed a right to plan a family (Article 16). In 1967 the General Assembly's Declaration on the Elimination of Discrimination against Women stated that in order to ensure women's right to work they should be provided with paid maternity leave and necessary services including child care facilities (Article 10.2), but that measures taken to protect them in certain occupations 'for reasons inherent in their physical nature shall not be regarded as discriminatory'.

More than twenty years later (Schmidt, 1989) a US federal appeals court ruling that an employer may bar all fertile women from jobs posing a potential risk to an unborn child raised alarm as the policy was viewed as sex discrimination denying women access to high-paying, if hazardous, jobs. However, on 20 March 1991 the US Supreme Court ruled that employment practices aimed at foetal protection illegally discriminated against women by requiring them, and not males, to choose between having children and (for some women of child-bearing age) undergoing sterilization, in order to keep their jobs (*International Union* v. *Johnson Controls Inc.*, 1991).

In 1969 'the right of couples to determine the number and spacing of their children freely' was reaffirmed by the UN along with the 'right of . . . access to the relevant information, means and methods for implementation of such decisions' (Economic and Social Council, 1969). WHO, trying to reconcile possible contradictions inherent in the concepts of reproductive freedom and restraint, stated that family planning is a 'way of thinking and living that is adopted voluntarily . . . by individuals and couples' (WHO, 1973). It did not discuss a right to reproduce to the extent made possible by nature. A UN symposium (1974) came closest to this issue when it referred to 'the necessity of defining the scope of the right [to procreate] as well as the right not to procreate'. The International Convention on the Elimination of Discrimination Against Women (UN, 1979), put into force in September 1981, also recommended access to family planning services, including voluntary sterilization and abortion. Additionally, it required States Parties to remove barriers restricting unmarried men or women from obtaining such services, and to eliminate rules requiring spousal authorization for them. The spirit of the 1979 Convention was re-emphasized in the revised report of the UN Decade of Women (1985), which stated that 'the ability of women to control their own fertility' is 'an important basis for the enjoyment of other rights' and that 'the implications for women of advances in medical technology are to be carefully examined'.

Justice and health rights for victims   In 1985 the Declaration of Basic Principles of Justice for Victims of Crime and Abuse of Power, with the contributions of several non-governmental organizations, was passed by the UN General Assembly (UN, 1985a). Abuse of power refers to oppression at the hands of one's own government, and victimization can include that at the hands of a nationally supported health care system. The striking aspect of this passage was its message that the principle of national sovereignty was no longer inviolate – matters which could have previously been sequestered from attention by the international community because they were defined as 'internal affairs' now became the legitimate concern of observers and interveners from other countries.

The Declaration, following advocacy by the World Federation for Mental Health, also recognized the importance of mental health impairment in consequence of victimization. It calls upon Member States 'to implement social, health, including mental health' and other policies to reduce victimization and encourage victim assistance including psychological and social measures. It implicitly acknowledges the therapeutic value of legal restitution by responsible 'offenders or third parties'. Compensation for 'injury or impairment of physical or mental health' should include that to dependants of 'persons who have died or become physically or mentally incapacitated as a result of such victimization'. Of particular importance, in respect to national sovereignty, it recommends international and regional measures to provide 'recourse for victims where national channels may be insufficient'.

Human Rights in Relation to Public Health and Biomedical Practice

Societal Values and Public Health Policy

Three general purposes of public health (that is, social) policy arising from the accelerating presence of biomedical technology have been summarized by Pellegrino (1985). All focus on society rather than the individual. The first is to control the social, cultural and economic impact of the unrestrained use of technology with individual patients; the second is to achieve its more equitable allocation; the third is 'to advance some deliberately established social ideal or goal for the collective good of present or future generations' (p. 11). In respect of the last Pellegrino notes the 'serious moral implications' of several mandatory limitations on individual freedom which might be future consequences of advancing biomedical science. These include prohibiting procreation for carriers of defective genes; organ harvesting of all accident victims; denying dialysis for older persons or life support for defective infants; involuntary control of aggressive behaviour; and genetic–eugenic manipulation. All these practices have already been employed in one form or another at various times in different parts of the world. They have not yet, however, been explicitly mandated by law. The seriousness of their 'moral implications' can be argued depending on socio-cultural context. To them we may add a panhuman threat to the subjective sense of individuals as beings with potentially unlimited horizons who are part of the natural order.

Individual Freedom and the Public Health

Individual claims to freedoms and entitlements are not always compatible with the community's obligation to preserve the general good. While this incompatibility is usually latent in the health field, it can surface in dramatic ways. One reflection, prominent in most civilizations before the present era, was infanticide; deformed or defective neonates who could become burdens to the community were usually left to die of exposure. Their rights to life or care were typically denied by not granting them fully human status.

New technologies inevitably influence the balance between individual freedoms and the power of the state to protect the public welfare. In the USA this is seen in successive interpretations of the protections offered to individuals by the Bill of Rights suggesting the likelihood of constitutional challenges as still newer ways of influencing or identifying a person's mind or body become available (Congress, 1988a). With advancing medical capacity to guarantee the survival and growth of defective newborns, for example, the idea of rights equality has been extended in Western societies to include severely impaired individuals who in an earlier era would have been left to die or consigned to institutional existence. This new population, burdensome to parents, the health care system and society at large, has given rise to discussions about quality of life, the meaning of personhood, the right to die, and the rights of anencephalic neonates. In some respects these are reminiscent of earlier discussions about whether or not members of non-European races had souls, or whether slaves or captives, in contrast to free men, had rights.

More recently, especially in the industrial democracies, limitation of the reproduction of persons deemed 'inferior' on grounds of intelligence, ethnicity or other criteria has been attempted under the rubric of 'eugenics'. While its intellectual basis is Darwinian the term was coined by Francis Galton and discussed in his book, *Hereditary Genius*, published in 1870. Its purpose was 'to give the more suitable races or strains of blood a better chance of prevailing speedily over the less suitable . . . than they otherwise would have had' (Galton, 1870, in Lappe, 1972/1977, p. 358). The genocidal horrors committed by the Nazis in pursuit of this policy indicate the enormous and socially maladaptive consequences which can flow from it. Sterilization without information or consent was performed upon sixty thousand, presumably mentally defective, women in the USA (with the socially disadvantaged at greatest risk); this practice, espoused by national scientific and progressive leaders, took place mainly in the 1920s and 1930s, but continued in one state hospital until at least 1960 (Reilly, 1991). One current emphasis with retarded or mentally ill patients is upon dialogue which may persuade them to voluntarily engage in family planning. While the World Health Organization's Mental Health Division has been reluctant, presumably on political grounds, to enter this field, other WHO offices have collaborated with NGOs. Thus WHO's European Office, in conjunction with the World Federation for Mental Health and the Danish Family Planning Association, was able to sponsor a seminar on 'Sexuality and Family

Planning for the Mentally Ill' (Osler and David, 1987). 'Genetic engineering' for disease prevention and treatment, and protection of the gene pool, will be discussed in Chapter 5.

In the late twentieth century research-based knowledge with public health significance has led to a number of measures experienced as restricting individual freedom. Prominent has been the linkage of cigarette smoking to pathogenic changes, not only for the smoker, but for onlookers 'passively' absorbing the smoke, and for foetuses carried by smoking pregnant women. This has been the basis of an active anti-smoking campaign by the US Public Health Service. Smoking has been prohibited on many, primarily US, airline flights, and many public places have smoke-free zones. A few who smoke only away from the workplace have also been placed at risk of losing their jobs since employers do not wish to cover them with health insurance. In the face of these restrictions the 'right' to smoke has acquired some supporters as a manifest of personal freedom. The tobacco industry, placed at financial risk by the campaign as well as by restrictions on television advertising and warnings on cigarette packaging, has intensified its advertising efforts and employed scientists to cast doubt on the consensus about smoking's harmful effects. The freedoms involved in this instance include those to use a toxic, addictive though legal and widely accepted, recreational substance; to advertise, that is, to promote the use of a substance demonstrably injurious to health; continuing state subsidization of tobacco production; and the freedom of scientific investigation. Similar issues are raised with regard to alcohol, which can be harmful not only to drinkers themselves, and potentially to foetuses if they are pregnant, but, because of its destructive behavioural effects, to their families, friends and communities. While law enforcement against drunken driving remains lax in the USA it is rigid and effective in many European nations. The morality of forcible restraint for one's own good was rejected by John Stuart Mill, another founder of utilitarian philosophy, but he agreed that it could coincide at times with the general good of the community.

Restrictions on individual behaviour have followed research on the value of seat-belts (mandatory in a number of countries) and helmets reducing traumatic injury to automobile drivers and cyclists. These remain sources of controversy in many US localities, although they have produced significant cost-saving in regard to hospital shock–trauma units and the incidence of disability requiring long-term rehabilitation.

An example of behavioural restriction which has been cited as interfering with the right to work is that on driving by persons with diagnosed epilepsy. Physicians are involved both as care providers for epileptic individuals and as society's designated protectors of community health; they are expected to report diseases in their patients which might be harmful to others, and also to act as consultants to regulatory agencies. However, administrative mechanisms for dealing with these issues are not well standardized. Krumholz et al. (1991) report that a one-year seizure-free interval is the most popular US criterion for judging the driving potential of people with epilepsy. But decisions about driving for particular individuals require a risk–benefit analysis, balancing the traffic safety risks of seizures against 'the dangers and hardships imposed by restricting driving' (p. 623).

A developing late twentieth-century conflict is between the consequences of advancing biomedical science and individual privacy rights. Basic in the USA has been the Bill of Rights' inclusion of a right of people 'to be secure in their persons, houses, property and effects'. This may have different significance in differing socio-cultural settings. Invasion of privacy, in the sense of making personal health-related information available to others, is a different issue in complex industrial than in agrarian village societies. In the former, with modern information technology, personal records go into data banks available to third parties other than patient or doctor. These include potential employers, educational institutions, agencies which pay medical bills or insure against death or disability, and various government offices. In the latter, privacy concerns are more important with regard to neighbours and members of extended kinship groups. Revelations about health or heredity, in particular, may interfere with marriage, reproductive, partnership or business plans.

Concern with privacy rights has also been stimulated by the availability of new screening techniques. Mandatory screening, whether for chemical substances, infectious agents, biological predispositions or genetic features, involves the same issues of due process, search and seizure. Objections to screening have been based on the Bill of Rights and the Fourth Amendment to the US Constitution which prohibits 'unreasonable searches and seizures', stating that 'no warrants shall issue but upon probable cause'. They permit personal invasion (through examination of obtained or excreted bodily materials) for the purpose of detecting transmissible disease or illicit drug use.

There is increasing pressure in the industrial world for random drug screening of low-risk populations, or those regarded as performing 'high risk' or sensitive tasks (physicians, soldiers, customs employees, or railroad workers). Some populations have been suggested for screening on the basis of age, such as high school students. While mandatory testing on the basis of occupation can be justified if the government can show a 'compelling interest' in its outcome, the demonstration of such interest may in itself be questioned. Medical privacy is an issue for persons on prescription drug regimens. Beyond these concerns there are more subtle rights issues. Supervisors may use testing as a way of intimidating employees. Efforts to reduce occupational hazards may be prematurely terminated if evidence of drug use is found. Drug use has not, in fact, beem demonstrated to be a major workplace safety hazard. Even when it has contributed to accidents, testing before or after the fact will not necessarily detect it. Alcohol, for which no mandatory screening is proposed, is, on the other hand, demonstrably a major cause of impairment, interpersonal difficulties and accidents, in and out of the workplace. However, the US Constitution has been found in general to permit compulsory testing in particular instances in which sufficient evidence of procedural regularity and other justifications are provided (Congress, 1988a). For example, compulsory breath and blood alcohol tests have been permitted without a warrant (*Schmerber* v. *California*, 1966).

Objections to testing are generally countered by the stated need to protect the public from injury from drug users or from transmissible disease, although it is not established that screening will achieve the desired goal. Efforts to achieve a balance between the individual and public goods take into account current scientific knowledge, economic factors and associated tax burdens, as well as ethical considerations. In testing for chemical substances or sexually transmitted diseases (STD), including AIDS, scientific–clinical issues include the validity and reliability of tests and the likelihood of false readings; economic factors include the high cost of mass testing. These, along with privacy rights considerations, could lead to a decision against mandatory mass screening with low-risk populations which would, in any event, yield few valid positives. However, mandatory testing, with physician reporting (as in the case of other infectious diseases), might be effective from a health standpoint, and would not be regarded as antithetical to individual rights when used with populations of persons who agree because they know that they are at risk. Community welfare as well as individual rights would be protected when persons at risk, and in the case of sexually transmitted disease their partners, themselves decide that their own health needs outweigh their privacy rights. Such personal decisions, however, may be unlikely in individuals who persist, against competent advice, in risky behaviour.

In traditional public health settings analogous questions have arisen in respect to immunization, and the quarantine or public reporting of intermittently impaired (as with epilepsy), as well as chemically intoxicated or infectious, individuals. While occasional objectors to immunization emerge, mainly on religious grounds, the

public in the main has accepted this violation of individual autonomy, understanding its justification in terms of personal prevention
of disease as well as the public health. The imposition of quarantine
on the contagiously ill is a classic instance in which individual
autonomy has been constrained in the interests of the community.
The community's 'right to the preservation of health' through
quarantine was regarded as 'inalienable' by Representative William
Lyman of Massachusetts in 1796, although he was opposed to giving
quarantine authority to the federal (rather than state) government in
order to control the spread of yellow fever introduced into the USA
by ships from other countries (Chapman and Talmadge, 1971/1977,
p. 555).

In general, the issue for many persons continues to be whether or
not the restraint involved is directly beneficial to them. While general
alcohol screening of motorists at routine checkpoints, for example,
has been questioned as not immediately beneficial to the motorists
who are stopped, it has been ruled constitutional in the USA (*State* v.
Superior Court, 1984). Helmets for motorcyclists and seat-belts for
automobile drivers are accepted by some as personal protection and
in some areas laws are being proposed for their mandatory use by
persons under the age of 18. In the case of epileptics who have had
their driving licence revoked, violations of a right to work have been
charged. Testing of food workers for communicable disease has not
raised objections. However, sequestral of the very few food-
handlers who are typhoid carriers raises the usual questions; it has
been attempted, but the handlers have escaped. Mandatory pre-
marital testing for syphilis has become routine, but should a sexually
promiscuous HIV-infected individual have his or her freedom
restrained? This remains a controversial question, complicated by the
possible stigmatization of persons so infected. However, as noted in
Chapter 2, the spread of AIDS is being accompanied by greater
willingness to consider both contact tracing and quarantine.

The freedom to bear arms, so intensely defended in the USA, has
only recently been systematically studied as a public health hazard. It
has been identified as a risk factor not only for physical injury and
death, but for postraumatic stress to victims and their families.
Comparisons between socio-economically similar populations in the
USA and in Canada, where handgun ownership is strictly controlled,
reveal significantly more assaults and homicides in the former (Sloan
et al., 1988). There is also a strong positive association in these
communities between the rates of handgun ownership and the rates
of suicide by firearms; although the correlation did not hold for
suicide in general (adults used other means) there was a small but
significant association of gun control with lower rates of suicide in the
15–24-year-old age group – that is, among the Canadians living in a

context in which handgun ownership is restricted (Sloan et al., 1990).

Another example of conflict between individual claims to health care and the community's claim to the general good concerns the possible obligation to provide abortions to women claiming such a procedure as their right. In this instance opposed physicians could, hypothetically, claim a right not to be forced to carry out a procedure violating their moral beliefs. An opposing argument could appeal to the general care-taking obligations of physicians, all of whom (even in capitalist societies) are educated in significant measure with the support of general taxes. Given the public educational support which they have accepted, physicians' personal conflicts might not be considered relevant to their obligation to provide (remunerated) publicly approved health care. This question is complicated because abortion is not considered a form of legitimate health care in all contexts. The right in question would, then, not be that to health care, but to the requesting woman's control over her own body. In this instance, leaving aside rights to health or privacy, the historical evidence indicates that when safe, legal abortion has not been available it has been sought extra-legally with a high toll of injury, infection and death. Under these circumstances it could be concluded that, even while excusing some reluctant care providers, community health would be enhanced by regarding abortion as a right.

A closely related question concerns the obligations of government to make safe and effective self-administered health care products publicly available – including those which can enhance a woman's right to manage her own body. The converse would be the government's obligation to justify depriving women of such products. Such withholding demands scrutiny of covert governmental/political motives other than the scientific/safety ones which are usually presented. A case in point is the drug Mifepristone (RU–486), which, in combination with a prostaglandin analogue, has resulted in a 96 per cent efficacy rate of pregnancy termination after 49 days of amenorrhoea or less (Silvestre et al., 1990). It was first used to terminate human pregnancies in 1982 and in France is used as a medical alternative to surgical procedures for voluntary interruption of pregnancy. It has not been available worldwide, however, because of unclear national or local abortion laws; manufacturers themselves, fearing boycotts from anti-abortion groups, have withheld its availability. This withholding, interpretable as violating the human rights of the women who need the drug, could be regarded as contributing to an increase in illegal abortions with a reduction in the level of public health. It also stifles freedom of enquiry and information. Regelson et al. (1990) (see Chapter 3) believe that cancer victims and others who might benefit from the drug are held hostage to the abortion issue, and urge physicians to join the public debate on the matter. In this respect it can be considered part of the same process which imposed a US ban on the use of federal funds for foetal tissue research (see Chapter 4). An 'alert' indicating that the drug is considered potentially harmful and insufficiently tested was imposed by the US Food and Drug Administration (FDA), allegedly in consequence of the hostile political climate associated with the administration's anti-abortion stance. This 'hostile political climate' was cited in a 1991 resolution of the American Association for the Advancement of Science (AAAS) encouraging pharmaceutical companies and the FDA to make RU–486 and related agents available for research and medical use. The resolution noted the other potential benefits of the drug, aside from its value as 'a safe, effective method for the termination of early pregnancy', and stressed the AAAS commitment to 'freedom of scientific enquiry and the advancement of modern technology'.

A more traditional expectation, only occasionally involving new technologies, is that of a right to reproduce. In many parts of the world this is regarded as a universal right. In others, such as Singapore and the People's Republic of China, it has been considered a privilege to be carefully allotted and controlled. In this instance the presumed right is violated in favour of maintaining what policy-makers regard as the general good of the community. More drastic in the context of an industrial democracy is the judicially imposed compulsion to contracept. While there are no data indicating this as a widespread practice, an example is a judge's decree that a woman convicted of excessively punishing her children either serve a prolonged prison sentence or accept an insertion of Norplant (levonorgestrel) (MacKenzie, 1991).

The idea that while reproduction may be a right its scope should be defined or in some way constrained implies a right–privilege continuum (Brody, 1976). Many of the issues regarding this continuum involve questions of distributive justice or equal access to life's goods. Thus, the presumed right of adults to have as many children as they wish may violate the rights of others – of the ensuing progeny for maximum life chances, or of other adults to share equally in scarce resources.

Universal and Particular Health Care Moralities: Towards International Consensus

The process of culture change accompanying biomedical research has been noted by the United Nations. Only twenty years after proclaiming that human beings have a right to 'the benefits of scientific advancement' (UN, 1948), it remarked on the possibility that all such 'advances' might not be beneficial for human well-being. The 1968 UN International Conference on Human Rights warned that 'while recent scientific discoveries and technological advances have opened vast prospects for economic, social and cultural progress, such developments may, nevertheless, endanger the rights and freedoms of individuals and will require continuing attention' (UN, 1968, para. 18). That conference also recommended that the agencies of the UN family undertake a study of the problems relating to human rights which arise from developments in science and technology.

These considerations emphasize the importance of developing an international and cross-cultural consensus about what can or cannot be considered desirable or permissible despite variations in society and culture. It is important that participants in the consensus should include clinicians and scientists (and if possible other community leaders and consumers) from the less developed countries in which research, advocacy or clinical and preventive programmes are to be carried out.

> The formulation of global, universal public policy on the basis of moral (or rights) standards embraced only by particular segments of the world population could be a source of continuing conflict. The purpose of public policy should be acknowledged to be limited and limiting – that is, to set consensual limits within which particular moralities can be practiced with respect and tolerance (Grobstein, 1988, p. 15).

At the same time there is general agreement that, while cultural appropriateness is important, there must be a minimum standard, applicable across political, social, cultural or economic boundaries, of dignified, humane professional treatment of persons who have become medical patients (Gostin, 1987b). This point of view is incorporated in the World Federation for Mental Health's *Declaration of Human Rights and Mental Health* (1989) (Appendix 3).

2 Human Rights in the Culture of Science and Technology

Science, Society and Culture

Scientific Advances, Human Perceptions and Self-concepts

Science has vastly extended human capacities, mental and physical, by technologies ranging from steam engines to computers. However, contemporary humans are not different in brain size or function from their biologically identical ancestors of the recent past. Their inborn characteristics have not changed to meet the new demands placed upon them by advancing knowledge and technology.

Nevertheless, they are psychologically and socially different. Science has transformed their perceptions of their universe, themselves, their societies and their values. It has given them new conceptions of animate and inanimate nature, of human life, of freedom, dignity and human rights. These new perceptions and concepts have made possible deliberate human use of the new technologies in ways which might change the evolutionary course of the species, and, perhaps, reverse the deterioration of the global environment. Perhaps the most important consequence of science is that human beings can conceive the possibility of doing so.

The Freedom of Biomedical Information

Modern societies attach high value to free access to politically or legally relevant information. Less certainty exists about the freedom of biomedical information: to generate (as through research), disseminate (through scientific journals and popular media), and have access to it (Brody, 1975a, 1975b). But it is recognized that information, including that about science and health, can be personally liberating at the same time that it threatens the *status quo*. There have been well-known moments in human history when scientific findings have aroused the ire of governmental or religious authorities. This happened when it was suggested that the earth was not the centre of the universe, or that *Homo sapiens* evolved from, or has features in common with, non-human creatures. A contemporary example concerns research on foetuses which embodies, for some, a potential threat to traditional concepts of humanhood. The US authorities, as of 1988–9, banned federal support of the research on the grounds that it could increase the incidence of induced abortion (see Chapter 4).

Contemporary controls on information about health and disease also reflect its potential commercial or military value. Access to data related to such areas as biological warfare, the medical care of casualties, or other aspects of military conquest has often been limited. This is not compatible with the understanding that health (as well as welfare) problems in one part of the human family inevitably place the rest of the family at risk. If funding health-related biological research of international significance is not to impair basic health services in particular nations, it must eventually be organized on an international basis. The moral value attributed to sharing versus exclusiveness contradicts the value accorded by the UN to the sovereignty of its Member States. The possibility that governments will, in time, become the major distributors as well as generators of medical information raises new questions as to its eventual freedom and control. 'Information is one of man's most precious possessions, but its actual "ownership" is often in doubt. Does it belong to its discoverer, the social powerholders who made the work possible, or the people whose lives it might affect?' (Brody 1975b, p. 73).

The difference between personal, intellectual, community and commercial property becomes even more blurred as biomedical scientists, in response to national security issues or in pursuit of patentable inventions or rewarding prizes, do not share data freely. The biomedical science community appears to agree that research secrecy in this field is not justified, and that the world public has a right to be informed about new advances in medical treatment and their possible human costs. At the same time it is aware that making all records available to the public could have an inhibiting effect on free scientific discussion.

Science and Consciousness, Engagement and Disengagement, in Modern and Traditional Societies

At the same time sharp differences exist between the modern societies of the industrialized world in which scientific knowledge, its technologies and associated values are incorporated into the consciousness and thinking of most persons, and the traditional societies of the less developed world. Mass education, industrialization and extension of the mass media lead to the structural modernization of societies as they provide bases for new types of individual learning and work experience, producing in turn new ways of thinking, feeling and acting (Miller and Inkeles, 1974). One of the essential features of this transformation is regular employment, which can contribute to the self-esteem and feeling of belonging necessary for identification as a member of a group which understands that power can be achieved through collective effort (Brody, 1973a). Literacy itself may be a consequence of employment, requiring the ability to read directions. With the development of modernization both the individual's organization of knowledge and cognitive style can change (Berger, Berger and Kellner, 1974). Education is the main factor producing Inkeles's (1969) psychological modernity syndrome, including openness to change, valuing equal rights for women, autonomy rather than subjection to kinship obligations, and acceptance of the findings of modern science (Inkeles and Smith, 1974). Other reflections of individual psychological modernity are attitudes and feelings favouring self-determination (beyond autonomy opposed to kinship linkages), activity rather than passivity in the face of external influence, and recourse to technology rather than religion (Brody, 1981a). It follows the ancient Greek image of civilized man who, like the gods, makes his own destiny.

In less developed or traditional societies scientific knowledge and values are not automatically trusted (although available technologies may be deliberately used in order to attain traditional goals); decisions are made significantly in accordance with rules and values handed down from past generations; the concept of human rights, so familiar in the industrial democracies, is still strange. This is true both for members of caste-ridden or mobility-blocked hierarchical societies, including those in which women, have subordinate status, and for subjects of authoritarian rulers with daily lives circumscribed by rituals requiring conformity rather than thought.

In some respects, as George Sarton remarked, 'The history of science is the history of mankind's unity.' This reflects the tendency of diverse societies to converge in consequence of science-based industrialization and modernization. As the process of modernization leads to the acceptance of science and technology as major bases for individual and group behaviour, newly acceptable information is incorporated into individual and group decision-making processes. It contributes to the formation of new, personal as well as collective, symbols, ideals and values. Thus, it tends to push dissimilar societies towards similar institutional solutions, and dissimilar individuals towards more similar world-views.

However, while many problems generated by modernization are, indeed, similar in different societies, their definition, the range of institutional solutions to them, and the consequent institutional dynamics differ (Eisenstadt, 1983). Cultural tradition influences not only the ability of different societies to modernize, but their modes of development and modernization. Cultural continuities are significantly reflected in family structure and responsibility (including the relations between the sexes and between generations), modes of childrearing, education, and specialization, 'the conception of authority and hierarchy, ruler and ruled, relations between God and man – all of which influence . . . the modes of coping with social problems'(Eisenstadt, 1983, p. 3).

Even in modern societies a strong undercurrent of belief in various supernatural forces and a surprisingly high prevalence of reported 'paranormal experiences' co-exists with suspicion and fear of science (Ross and Joshi, 1992; Hufford, 1992). However, the degree to which this undercurrent represents a residual from the past, or to which it reflects a way of dealing with the loss of traditional beliefs, is unclear. The issue has been obscured by psychiatric stigmatization of such experiences and beliefs, leading to a reluctance to respond to research enquiries about extraordinary experience. However, no human group has not constructed a cosmology couched in culturally acceptable religious terms in which an extra-human force is concerned with its behaviour and future.

Engagement in the traditionally comforting belief systems, despite their temptation, is discouraged for most modern persons by scientific knowledge and by uncertainty about the essence of what is human made possible by biomedical technology. This can promote a kind of general psychological disengagement which, while it may have defensive value, is uncomfortable for many. As Taylor points out, the disengaged mode of life, which becomes instrumental, can be attacked on the grounds that it 'empties life of meaning', promoting a utilitarian value outlook and, because it undermines self-regulation, a 'bureaucratic mode of existence'. The other view is that 'disengaged reason . . . powers the austere ethic of self-responsible freedom' (Taylor, 1989, p. 496). This perception of a needed 'self-responsible freedom', regularly confronted by threats not only to individual political but to biological freedom, must lead to a conception of human rights in biomedical practice. The advances of biomedical technology require a revitalized and immediately human, in contrast to an abstract analytic and technical, understanding of human rights in practice.

Science in Culture: the Socially Sanctioned and Facilitated Search for Meaning Through Knowledge

In the nineteenth century, Hegel (1807) called religion 'the sphere in which a nation gives itself a definition of that which it regards as the

True'. In modern twentieth-century society science has become a major definer of truth via the progressive illumination of the seemingly unintelligible. This is despite the fact that, like any human creation, it reflects only the workings of the human mind. As Nietzsche (1882, p. 336) put it, 'We cannot look around our own corner.' But the 'mind' does not exist within an isolated brain; it emerges in interaction with the environment (Brody, 1990c):

> All facts are . . . selected from a universal context by the activities of our mind. They are . . . interpreted . . . relevant to us either for carrying on our business of living or from the point of view of a body of accepted rules of procedure of thinking called the method of science (Schutz, 1962, p. 4).

Freud's psychoanalysis, a central twentieth-century truth definer for many, pursues intelligibility. For many scholars it is an interpretive rather than a biological discipline. But despite its power to convince and stimulate, it is an epistemological dead end in the sense that its clinical formulations about the unconscious can never be ultimately validated (Brody, 1990c). At the same time its theoretical structure allows a host of disparate observations to fit together in a coherent manner, and thus invests them with new, and sometimes therapeutically useful, meaning for the patient.

The illumination of what was once considered unintelligible influences the shared values and symbols which are at the heart of culture – the design for living which, with progressive inter-generationally transmitted modifications, is developed by every society (Kluckhohn, 1944). Culture affords the bridge through which the external, collective elements of social organization become individual, personal and internal. Cultural beliefs and values provide the collective meanings that form the context of individual experience (Levine, 1981, p. 64). A shared cultural form can become a 'personal symbol for representing and working out . . . earlier conflicts' (Kracke, 1976, p. 9). Personal meaning is invested in such shared symbols as language, works of art, patterns of action (for example, rituals), or the regularly encountered and rewarded pursuits of particular goals, such as science, knowledge or truth. All are involved in a human person's sense of identity as a being with particular goals and values *vis-à-vis* other humans and the universe – the unknowable as well as the possible. Scientific research itself is both a cultural phenomenon and one 'embedded' in the social–educational context which has formed the investigator, so that it attempts to force nature into the conceptual boxes which it supplies (Kuhn, 1975, p. 5). More generally, it is conducted in accordance with prevailing social norms and cultural values: 'At certain points in its history someone has to generate a new conceptual scheme and then persuade others that it makes more sense than the old' (Bowler, 1989, p. 8). 'To make a phenomenon intelligible is to make it accord or fit in with the standards of human rationality which prevail at a given time' (Graves, 1971, p. 14).

The standards of the research community regarding scientific acceptability at any given time also determine success in establishing a major line of investigation. 'Social constraints' are implicitly or covertly present in the kind of theorizing acceptable within a new discipline (Bowler, 1989, p. 9). But standards of intelligibility and the acceptability of particular focuses of study reflect relationships based on power as well as intellectual clarity. In the contemporary era of research requiring expensive equipment and highly trained staff, success in acquiring support for particular programmes can depend upon connections with high-status persons or groups in government or the scientific community. This may also be the case for less costly research perceived as threatening to established cultural values, including those defined as human rights.

It is abundantly clear that, personal convictions to the contrary, the scientific community is not involved in a disinterested search for a value-free reality. The debate about a hypothetically autonomous and value-free science has been formulated by Longino (1990) in terms of two questions, both relevant to the human rights aspects of research. One asks about the extent to which scientific theories do, or should, shape moral and social values. The other asks about the converse, the extent to which social and moral values shape scientific theories. The first 'has to do with the autonomy of questions of personal, social and cultural values from the revelations, discoveries and inventions of scientific inquiry'; the second concerns 'the autonomy of the content and practices of the sciences from personal, social, and cultural preferences' (Longino, 1990, pp. 4–5). With regard to contemporary biomedical research and its clinical applications it seems probable that 'evidential reasoning is always context-dependent', that 'social interactions determine what values remain encoded in the theories and propositions taken as expressing scientific knowledge at any given time', and that values are taken into account as 'objectivity is analyzed as a function of community practices rather than as an attitude of individual researchers' (Longino, 1990, pp. 215–16). As biomedical research is increasingly able to control the nature of human beings (threatening the political process as well as our conceptions of the essence of being human and of human rights) society will increasingly assert a right to control the search for new knowledge. The context of the search for meaning will become politicized.

Finally, the role of science in the human search for meaning may be formulated in terms of an adaptive function. Beyond striving for a sense of purpose and meaning in human existence, it is part of the struggle of humankind to cope with the conditions of its universe; this involves both mastery of and acknowledgement and acceptance, however reluctant, of the uncertainties and fragility of human life, with the inevitability of disease, disability and death. As Leslie White said, science 'is preeminently a way of dealing with experience' (1938). 'The novel stage in man's capacity for looking at himself objectively . . . has been reached in Western culture in so far as it has led to [his] continuing search . . . for more and more reliable knowledge about himself' (Hallowell, 1965).

Biomedicine, Values and Social Policy

The Universal and the Particular: Cultural Values, Justice and the Good

The medical communities of the world have become involved in two old conflicts which have gained new dimensions. One is the tension between the restrictive demands of particular moral systems and a universal concept of what is just and good. The first, the particular system, provides stability and certainty to its adherents while denying access to some biomedical advances which it defines as wrong or bad. The second, the universal concept, searches for commonalities between varying moral beliefs, and aims at equitable access to the benefits of available technologies. This is the sense of the United Nations statements fostering equal access to 'the benefits of science'. Such a universal concept, however, is difficult for many to accept since it implies the potential fallibility of their own particular moral system.

The other conflict is between the international standard of biomedical scientific research, accorded almost universal positive value, and the application of its results in accordance with national economic considerations, and the operation of international markets.

Justice recognizes national differences in health care associated both with unequal resources and with the demands of cultural appropriateness and moral acceptability; however, it requires a minimum standard of dignified, humane professional treatment applicable across cultural as well as political, social and economic boundaries (Gostin, 1987b). 'The purpose of public policy should be . . . to set consensual limits within which particular moralities can be practiced with respect and tolerance' (Grobstein, 1988, p. 15). These specific concerns have their counterpart in the more general problem of international policy-making. The increasingly interdependent, global economic–environmental and security system is almost completely influenced by local and national determinants (Trent, 1990, p. 9).

Examples of parochial (local, morally specific, culturally specific, legally constricted) permissibility or allocation of universally valued biomedicine are found in regard to high-technology life extension. Although this is virtually unobtainable by most of the world's peoples, its availability has given rise to anguished discussion by citizens of the industrial democracies about rights to live or die, and the quality of life (see Chapter 7). High value accorded to individual choice implies a right to die with appropriate counselling and consultation. Within nations this is in potential conflict with some moral systems, and with legal structures protecting the *status quo*. In Spain, for example, despite the approval by an overwhelming majority of physicians of passive euthanasia for victims of irreversible, incapacitating disease who urgently request it, they would not participate for fear of being accused of a crime – co-operating in an act of suicide (*El Periodico*, 1990). The practice of passive euthanasia can also impose an undesirable obligation upon morally disagreeing hospital staffs unwilling to disconnect life support systems.

Social Organization and Access to the Health Benefits of Science

Even in the absence of conflict between moral particularities and universal standards, actual access to the benefits of science is uneven. Contemporary social organization reflects the history of human beings forming themselves into groups in order to survive. In most societies power and prestige and economic statuses have become fused. The most desirable tasks and the largest share of goods and services (including medical care) go to the highest ranking individuals, their families and friends. This differential access is continued to the next generation as high-status parents expand the opportunities and resources open to their children. The privileged, in comparison with others, are best nourished, protected from exposure to injury, defect and disease, and (through education, social services and health care) have increased capacity to cope with them. In all societies they as individuals, measured by quality of life, are the primary beneficiaries of biomedical science. As subpopulations, however, measured by numerical increases on a global basis, the less privileged inhabitants of agrarian, non-industrialized societies are, arguably, the primary beneficiaries. The continuing value which they attribute to early fertility and large families, coupled with improved control of infant and child mortality, as well as access to emergency care for young adults, have increased their reproductive efficacy; the inhabitants of these less developed areas with traditional cultures are the world's most rapidly growing populations.

The International Context: UN Rights Declarations

The health and biomedical science concerns of the international community are major ingredients of the social context in which biomedical technology is used. They were formalized with the birth, after the Second World War, of the United Nations which has enshrined biomedicine as a fount of 'rights' basic to survival and the good life. Rights to the 'highest obtainable level of physical and mental health' (UN, 1948), to 'freely . . . share in scientific advancement and its benefits' (UN, 1948), and to 'enjoy the benefits of scientific progress and its application' (UN, 1966a), exclude little in the realm of human opportunity. However, human rights do not exist as independent entities in the natural world. The activity of formulating desirable opportunities, freedoms or material goods, and then claiming them as rights, reflects a particular set of values, that predominating in twentieth-century Western culture. It has not existed in every society at every moment of history, and it is not uniform throughout the late twentieth-century world, either in declaration or practice.

The National Contexts

In the industrialized world a clinical medicine firmly rooted in science reflects the nature of contemporary values as well as the ancient human search for meaning and purpose in life. Its power to transform the human condition in new and unexpected ways challenges traditional conceptions of the meaning of human life. Threats to formerly secure beliefs, and the anxiety which they engender, are met by attempts to protect whatever is seen as an immutable aspect of being human. Each country is evolving its own legal governmental structures to keep pace with scientific advances. In the United States this is significantly a process of reinterpreting the freedoms granted by the Constitution and Bill of Rights. The Bill of Rights includes elements immediately applicable to contemporary biomedical issues (Congress, US, 1988a). Their relevance, however, changes with progressive decisions by federal courts. Thus the Bill's indication of a sphere of personal autonomy safe from government intrusion (a 'right of privacy') has been challenged by decisions concerning reproductive health, for example in regard to contraception and abortion. However, its prohibition on 'unreasonable searches and seizures' has not yet influenced the Supreme Court to prohibit the taking of bodily airs (breath), such fluids as urine, semen and blood, or other tissues for evidence. Public health practice, in particular, is influenced by potential conflict between the State's police power and a constitutional right to due process. As technology increases the power of the medical profession or the State to identify or modify human biological status, the basic tension between the general welfare and individual rights will define new constitutional issues – 'the testing of the terms of the social contract' (Congress, 1988a, p. 17). The United Nations has approached the matter much less specifically, understanding that its enforcement powers in this sphere lie mainly in the laws of specific nations. Thus, it has limited itself mainly to noting the potential hazards of biomedical advances (UN, 1968) and the hope that biomedical science will not increase the economic and other disparities between social groups (UNESCO, 1985).

Unintended Consequences of Biomedical Science

The Nature of New Knowledge

Unpredictability stems in part from the interlinked and interactive nature of contemporary searches after new knowledge. Some traditional disciplinary boundaries have dissolved, reformed, expanded or further splintered. A salient characteristic of the new biology is the degree to which work in one field overlaps with that in another: 'discoveries in one area almost inevitably generate ideas or techniques applicable to a widely different area' (Koshland, 1986, p. ix). Overlap also exists as industrial, agricultural and ecological endeavours interact with those of medicine. 'We must show ourselves capable of thinking through the possible consequences of future lines of research and of making funding choices accordingly, not just of "advancing" in any direction' (Berkowitz, 1989, p. 874).

Conflicting Rights and Values

The specific UN emphasis on rights to health stemming from scientific advance is complicated by the social and cultural consequences of new biomedical information and technologies. Many of these consequences involve the values attributed to justice (freedom from inequitable restraint on medical grounds, as well as equitable access) and beneficence–autonomy.

The beneficence of human research is classically a matter of whether or not the patient receives some direct benefit from the medicine or procedure applied. With adequately informed consent it is a matter of how it is conducted and its results applied, when, by whom, in what context, and to what end. In every instance the local judgement of beneficence rests on the values of the particular culture involved. In the industrial democracies, for example, research-based methods of detecting narcotic substances in urine are necessary to the treatment of accident victims in urban hospital emergency rooms. As part of a random screening of low-risk populations, however, they have been regarded as violating the civil rights of unwilling subjects through unreasonable search and seizure, invading personal privacy, and forcing self-incrimination. As the testing involves compulsory production of a urine specimen under direct personal observation, it has been described by a US court as a 'gross invasion of privacy and a degrading procedure that "detracts from human dignity and self-respect" ' (Curran, 1987, p. 320). Clearly, these values emphasizing personal privacy and autonomy would not carry equal weight in other countries more oriented to the presumed well-being of state or society. This is true for many lineage-oriented traditional societies. It is also true for some modernizing authoritarian societies, although the issues can be debated. In Cuba, for example, with mass HIV testing to enforce relative quarantine of persons testing positive, the effectiveness and human rights significance of personal responsibility for behavioural change versus externally imposed regulations remains unsettled (Perez-Stable, 1991). It is only the Western individual citizen of an industrialized democracy who is so convinced of the value of knowledge gained by looking into and reflecting upon him or herself that it is considered self-evident that such knowledge constitutes a claim upon others to be respected as an individual (Brody, 1990c).

Approaches to the AIDS epidemic offer another view of the changing social context of biomedicine and its technologies. In this instance the context concerns public and professional attitudes toward disease and screening and treatment technologies. As Angell notes, AIDS tends to afflict people who are 'for one reason or another objects of discrimination' (1991, p. 1498). Because their identification as HIV carriers could lead to further stigmatization with severe social consequences, these sufferers and their representatives have argued successfully for confidentiality and against screening and efforts to trace sexual partners. Now, with the growth of the epidemic, the infection of health care providers, and increasing numbers of AIDS-infected infants, there is growing opposition to the policy of strict confidentiality (Bayer, 1991) with an emphasis on tracing exposed contacts and screening all pregnant women. Angell (1991) recommends a dual approach, distinguishing social from epidemiological problems. This would require protective measures for jobs, housing and insurance benefits, and a nationally funded programme analogous to the end-stage renal disease programme for the medical care of HIV-infected persons. Only if socio-economic discrimination against persons identified by screening is countered by statute, she believes, can the basic elements of infection control be effectively pursued.

Another unintended threat is to values which recognize the limitations of human ability to promote optimal function or to delay death. This extends to the social infrastructures in which expectable security in the face of serious illness and disability are embedded. Diagnostic and therapeutic procedures aimed at helping patients are not equitably available; their administration, despite the best of intentions, is not always wholly beneficial, and can and does impair individual autonomy. The very technology aimed at ensuring more humane survival or dying for the sick, defective and disabled has, paradoxically, led to less humane circumstances for those whose lives are endangered and constricted, and for their families. The existence in developed societies of such 'prisoners' of medical technology (Angell, 1990) has reached the status of a social problem (see Chapter 7).

Actual and Possible Conflicts Regarding the Goal of Beneficent Prevention

Research aimed at preventing disease or deficit, especially in children, tends to be regarded in all cultures as unequivocally beneficial. However, this shared value may not be reflected in the allocation of resources to preventive or developmental research. Nutritional research, for example, bears directly on rights to freedom from hunger and for optimal development. But the application of existing knowledge may conflict with the goals of entrenched sources of political and economic power. The likelihood of conflict is predictable from the premises set forth for effective action regarding hunger:

> The outstanding situation . . . is the inequitable economic relationship between the North and the South, which withdraws net capital from the South, diverts agriculture in developing countries from producing food to meet local needs, creates contentious food trade barriers, underprices food commodities, and often encourages capital investment that undermines rather than advances sustainable uses of agriculture and resources (Bellagio Declaration, 1989).

Major US programmes have aimed at identifying and eradicating lead in the old paint of dwellings inhabited by the urban poor. This should reduce the likelihood of lead ingestion by children reared in these dwellings, and reduce the future incidence of lead-induced developmental central nervous system damage. Similarly, research continues to identify previously unknown health hazards at home, at school or in the workplace, as for example asbestos. These support the right to live in a healthy environment. However, it has been asserted (although argument persists) that the content of asbestos fibres in the air of buildings containing asbestos is essentially the same as in outdoor air, and does not pose a hazard until the removal process releases asbestos fibres. US federal legislation and regulations of disparate minerals, some dangerous and some not (as indicated by ignored epidemiological data), have been lumped together under the label of 'asbestos' (Abelson, 1990).

More troubling has been the possibility that elements of preventive research can lead to unintended threats to the rights of particular groups, especially minorities, including women. The US Pregnancy Discrimination Act of 1978, for example, includes distinctions based on 'pregnancy, childbirth, or related medical conditions' among those which must not be used for gender-linked discrimination. However, the identification of workplace threats to foetal well-being led some US employers, hoping to prevent later lawsuits for foetal damage, to attempt exclusion of female workers of reproductive age. This pre-employment screening for sensitivity to potential workplace hazards has attracted the attention of civil rights advocates as it could interfere with the right to work. Civil rights activists and women's groups objected to this as gender-linked discrimination violating a US federal statute applicable to employment. Reviews of available data, including the reproductive impact upon both men and women of exposure to a number of physico-chemical agents, did not support the differential treatment of workers according to gender in regard to reproductive function in general or to the hazards specified in employers' foetal-protection policies (Becker, 1990). Despite this scientific finding, judges as well as employers and other (predominantly male) decision-makers appeared at first to behave in terms of cultural stereotypes and values, perceiving the traditional and desirable role of women to be the reproductive one, and ignoring the biological role of men in favour of their instrumental–economic one. They seemed to be influenced, further, by the technology-based concept of the foetus as 'a second patient' (see Chapter 4), forgetting the primary rights of the pregnant woman upon whom foetal existence depends. Later, however, US judicial rulings in these cases did not support the employers' gender discrimination. In keeping with an emphasis on personal autonomy and self-determination it seems likely that personal, practical solutions to this question will be determined by the individual concerned. Under these circumstances the future of possible litigation for foetal damage still remains unclear.

Socio-cultural Change: the Anxiety Associated with New Forms of Social Organization, New Values and New Choices

Contemporary societies, driven by science and technology, are engaged in a continuing process of rethinking what they consider desirable, preferred, valued or merely acceptable. Changing values reflect the increasing prevalence of literacy, public knowledge and acceptance of the findings of science as a basis for action. People no longer depend on the behavioural rules and standards of their forebears, which may have been adaptive in an earlier era. Development itself has become suspect. Nations are beginning to confront the hazards of uncontrolled population growth and industrial–agricultural pollution upon the earth's fragile biosphere, and to weigh these against the presumed benefits of continued economic growth and development. However, the change process is uneven. Attempts by industrial nations, for example, to control deforestation, may be resented at home by threatened industries based on logging, and in the societies of the less industrialized agrarian world as blocking their development. Science and technology still remain foreign to the bulk of the world's population; the values and belief systems based upon them have not been assimilated into everyday thinking, feeling and acting. Crucial decisions in most societies, especially those around life cycle milestones, are still strongly influenced by ancestral rules of conduct. Their prevailing values which strongly influence perceptions of human rights, tend not to be those of personal autonomy and independence but of responsibility to family and lineage. In other groups, especially those controlled by strong authoritarian leaders, the security of food, shelter, employment, and medical care, even at the level of basic necessity, is often granted higher value than personal privacy and autonomy. In the medical sphere most people continue to prefer local, familiar pharmaceuticals and devices from familiar sources, which they themselves can control; they feel that drugs and technologies manufactured abroad place them at risk of being controlled by foreign influences (Brody, 1981a). At the same time, even the most traditional and poverty-stricken societies contain small numbers of affluent persons of upper-socio-economic status with access to scarce amenities, including travel and expensive, high-technology, medical care. Their wealth differentiates them more decisively from the poverty-stricken masses of their own country than from the rich of the industrialized nations.

In the industrialized world biomedical science has given physicians, patients and their families a vastly expanded range of options, not all of them welcome. The new options, demanding new decisions, have emphasized the values of self-determination and change over those of authority and the *status quo*. But as Jean-Paul Sartre has pointed out, freedom can generate anguish; human ability to tolerate uncertainty is limited. Advancing technology raises questions about previously stable beliefs, once considered timeless. It creates new uncertainties about the essential nature and meaning of life – its creation, purpose, prolongation, and termination. The inequitable distribution of life-sustaining goods in general, dramatized by differential access to scarce medical resources, emphasizes a seeming disparity in the value accorded to the lives of the poor and deprived in contrast to the affluent and privileged.

These changes have evoked responses in both the professional and larger communities. Health consumer organizations act as mechanisms for reducing anxiety and dependence upon paternalistic medical authority, more powerful as it commands increasingly esoteric technology, and is more remote from individual human concerns. Patient-advocates articulate the new expectations of cure, protection from the threats of strange technologies, and equitable access to beneficent treatment. They also force awareness of the fact that an effective exercise of choice requires a minimal level of competence and personal security. This reinforces John Rawls's view (1971) that public policy should consider the interests of the least-advantaged members of society, aiming towards an equitable distribution of self-esteem.

The medical community has also responded to the new options. It devotes increased attention to its responsibility to respect the help-seeking patient as, in Kantian terms, a self-legislating moral agent. It has also responded in its role as an agent of society which values social control and cost-effectiveness over individual autonomy. In this role it has considered health care rationing and produced boards and committees which institutionalize the practice of ethics as part of medical due process.

Biomedical Technology Transfer and Unintended Socio-cultural Change

The health care systems of the developing world contain a mix of traditional and modern elements. Modern hospitals, research laboratories and Western-trained practitioners co-exist with traditional healers and healing systems as well as with total neglect. Areas of conflict, co-operation, or mutual rejection of Western and traditional health systems vary from locality to locality.

'Despite an idealization of scientific medical knowledge and technology in the developing world, barriers exist that often prevent their direct applications' (Zeichner, 1988, p. v). Colonialism and colonial attitudes continue to influence the interrelated health and economics of the developing world, including the new nations which emerged after the Second World War (Brody, 1973a, 1981a; Zeichner, 1988). The ability to use any resource, including biomedical technology, for personal health management requires the ability as well as the opportunity to discriminate between health care choices; effective discrimination is difficult for patients unfamiliar with or made anxious by manufactured drugs and devices. In Jamaica, for example, rural women in traditional settings were more comfortable with contraceptives, despite their lack of effectiveness, based on local familiar botanicals (Brody, 1981a). Many procedures, drugs and devices, including those exported from industrial to developing nations, are not relevant to or may even be contraindicated for disorders with cultural roots. Or they may have negative consequences, as was the case with baby food which, marketed with an appeal to modernity (and freeing women to enter the labour force), reduced breast feeding with subsequently increased infant morbidity. Some Third World scientists have denounced the application of concepts from the professional culture to the village culture as harmful in the sense of destroying local initiatives, naturally occurring therapeutic modalities, and innovations appropriate to the context. Their emphasis has been on empowering local peoples to use local low-technology methods to gain more control over their own environments, and hence over their own health.

In a sense these people have become victims of technology, as it has widened the economic and social gulf between them and the developed world. Multinational corporations, often with the aid of governments, have concentrated scientific–technological information, personnel and production capacity in the industrial nations. The accompanying hierarchical technological elite makes access to wealth and knowledge increasingly difficult in the non-industrialized areas. Further, these corporations have acquired 'a free hand to shop internationally for the cheapest resources and labour', a move which has threatened the earlier social advances of the labour force in industrial nations, and blocks the accumulation of resources by Third World workers (Trent, 1990, pp. 8–9).

At the same time access to technology has facilitated changing self-concepts. New awareness of the importance of access to health care has encouraged socially submerged groups to apply concepts of human rights to themselves. Women, in particular, are becoming self-aware as gender has become recognized as a factor in access to opportunity. The revised report of the United Nations Decade for Women (1985) regards 'the ability of women to control their own fertility . . . [as] . . . an important basis for the enjoyment of other rights'. It also states that 'the implications for women of advances in medical technology are to be carefully examined'.

The Impact of Science as Commercial Property on the Subculture of Medicine

Equitable access to medical diagnosis and treatment is threatened by the increasing commercialization of biomedicine. The aggressive development and competitive marketing of new biomedical products are reflected in the rising costs and ethical complexities of medical service (see Chapter 8). This reflects the fact that the biomedical research enterprise has become a major factor in the economies and reward systems of the industrialized world. It offers support, gratification and social power to a growing elite of clinicians and scientists. They participate in the design and manufacture of high-technology medical equipment and the development of new pharma-cological and genetically engineered products. They also work in, and sometimes manage or own, for-profit laboratories, diagnostic centres or hospitals which employ physicians to produce medical care. One consequence is that in the industrialized world private solo practice is increasingly out of the reach of individual practitioners as equipment costs mount and are multiplied by the need for technically trained teams to operate them. At the same time high-technology diagnosis or treatment may be mandated in major hospitals, or in technology centres such as those for radiology, owned by groups of practitioners, on non-clinical grounds for reasons ranging from the need to make a profit to defensive coverage in the face of potential lawsuits. Some institutions have sufficient venture capital to support highly publicized, sometimes still experimental, surgical procedures such as implantation of artificial heart pumps on their patients. But loyalty to shareholders is not compatible with loyalty to the welfare of patients or other potential beneficiaries of advancing bioscience (see Chapter 8).

This point of view has been disputed, and there are many examples of productive, non-coercive relationships between industry and academic medical research groups. It seems likely, however, that university investigators, often working in publicly supported laboratories and hospitals, do have a conflict of interest which may not be consciously acknowledged even to themselves as they engage in research with eventual commercial rewards. The older conflict between the desire to know (to do research) and the desire to help is now complicated by the desire for personal profit in terms of money, power and prestige: 'There is anguished ethical study of the dangers to academic research of the new practicality of biological research' (Koshland, 1986, p. x). An obvious consequence is a restriction in the flow of freely available information about scientific fields with potential commercial application. The pursuit of basic knowledge is limited both by secrecy about such information and by the easier availability of support for short-term commercially useful than for long-term basic research.

The Power of Medicine and Biological Information

The Social Power of Biological Information and the Medicalization of Modern Life

In 'primitive' or pre-industrial cultures the institutions evolved to manage human suffering dealt broadly with individual and group behaviour and served to enforce social conformity. Conformity was effected in part by the healers' presumed magical power over natural objects and persons. This view is embodied in the title of John Cawte's volume on Australian tribal societies, *Medicine is the Law* (1974), which refers to 'divine law' observed and enforced by institutionalized tribal religious belief. In this last respect it is self-evident that, even in the modern era, medical and priestly functions continue to overlap – especially since medicine retains its effective monopoly over the definition and treatment of illness which spills over into the management of social deviation (see Chapter 6). However, the direct correspondence between current and earlier medical–priestly functions is less impressive than the widespread professional and public acceptance of the value of biological science. It seems that such acceptance is moving towards overevaluation, and that for some a type of 'belief in science', analogous to religious belief, is beginning to supplant rational scrutiny. In Western culture the social power of biological information with its aura of scientific validity and inevitability is immense (Nelkin and Tancredi, 1989). At the level of social philosophy it is illustrated by the impact of the hereditarian ideas of the early twentieth century, which represented 'an ideological transformation because they centered on the claim that one could not stimulate individuals to greater efforts' (Bowler, 1989, p. 11). It is true that 'the social consequences of hereditarianism have been less visible than the effects of the Darwinian revolution because the new interpretation . . . was challenged from the start by opponents determined to show that human nature can be improved by reformed social conditions' (Cravens, 1978, in Bowler, 1989, p. 11). Yet it is possible to minimize issues leading to questions about social reform by redefining them in biological terms (Nelkin and Tancredi, 1989).

The Medicalization of Behaviour

At the level of clinical practice and popular labelling the expression of advancing biomedicine extends to the medicalization of regularly encountered life cycle changes, responses to stress, and deviation from social norms. The most extreme instances of medicalizing apparent social deviation in recent history were efforts in the USSR and other totalitarian states to deprive political dissidents of credibility and responsibility by defining their behaviour as mental illness (see Chapter 6).

The idea of medicalization refers to the broadening social in contrast to the more limited clinical use of medical diagnostic categories or classifications. In the latter sense, diagnoses (most apparently psychiatric syndromes) are conceptual, man-made, 'cultural objects' which designate 'ideal conditions of illness'(Fabrega, 1987). As they are applied to particular patterns of naturally occurring behaviour these come to be regarded as diagnosable syndromes; in so far as they are perceived as diseases they are removed from the responsibilities of families or other community groups and add to the purview and power of physicians expected not only to diagnose, but to 'treat' or otherwise modify them.

A few of the new diagnostic categories, constructed from probabilistic conclusions about the prevalence of observable behaviours, are thought by some to discriminate against minority groups: thus we find a detailed analysis of value concerns in research on sexual differences (Longino, 1990). At the more narrowly clinical level, defining the discomfort and tension preceding the menses as Premenstrual Syndrome has evoked charges of anti-female discrimination. Another controversial proposal has been to establish a diagnosis of Late Luteal Phase Dysphoric Disorder (Frances et al., 1990). The view of infertility as a disorder to be medically treated, rather than a naturally occurring though often undesired state, is debated by some. The expansion of medical indications for *in vitro* fertilization to include infertility in the male member of a couple has aroused charges of anti-female discrimination since the woman rather than the couple is regarded as the unit for diagnosis and treatment; she, rather than the couple or the male partner, is subjected to potentially hazardous and emotionally taxing surgical 'therapy' (Laborie, 1987).

A particularly troubling possibility, as noted above, is that the social and moral questions involved in decisions about treatment or education can be minimized by redefining the issue in biological terms (Nelkin and Tancredi, 1989). When a condition is medicalized by identifying it as a disease, especially of a genetic or constitutional nature, and the way is open to control or eliminate the problem by some form of medical treatment, needed social reforms or programmes will not be introduced; medicine may be inappropriately called upon to solve problems that should be dealt with by social measures. The new techniques of genetic diagnosis and therapeutic gene manipulation, for example, have reduced interest in the social and environmental contributors to disease and malfunction.

In the past psychiatrists have been among the advocates of social reform as a way of reducing the frequency of aberrant behaviour, especially of an anti-social nature. This reflected a view of social context as an important determinant of how an individual thinks, feels and acts. However, under the influence of advancing bio-medical science, particularly genetics and pharmacology, the psychiatric subculture has changed. In pursuit of an unequivocally medical identity, psychiatry (with many individual exceptions) has largely abandoned its earlier emphasis on past personal history as a determinant of adult behaviour in favour of a view of mental illness as a function of a largely de-contextualized biological system. The significance of the 'person' in the system is becoming obscured. One reflection of this is the absence of the term 'culture' in the basic Diagnostic and Statistical Manual (DSM-III) of the American Psychiatric Association, and its mention only in passing in its revised version (DSM-III-R). Ways of including a more adequate reference to culture are being debated in preparation for the next version of this evolving nomenclature (DSM-IV.) The use of discrete behaviours, largely taken out of social context, as diagnostic criteria encourages a tendency to view many phenomena as reflecting the nature of the organism (the individual human being) itself, rather than organism–environment interaction. While popular or folk diagnoses in traditional societies include stresses such as frights and bereavement, or externally imposed spells, those in modern societies tend now to focus on the popular understanding of biomedical science expressed in terms of heredity, brain damage or constitutional and inborn problems. One reflection of this is a de-stigmatization of mental illness as it comes to be viewed as comparable with any other disease of biological rather than psychosocial or demonic origin.

Illness, Deviance and Technology in Cultural Context

As patterns of illness, defined in terms of surface manifestations or hidden aetiologies, acquire shared and socially transmitted meaning they become symbolic, value-laden aspects of a particular culture. Diseases presumably of psychosocial origin such as mental illness, or those related to stress such as peptic ulcer, coronary heart disease and hypertension, have had such meaning in late twentieth-century industrial society. Their prevalence and the importance accorded to them stimulated the development of pharmacological and surgical treatments and high-technology diagnostic devices. The most value-burdened disease to have emerged in this period is AIDS. It is unique in having had an international consultation on human rights devoted to it (26–28 July 1989), organized by the UN Centre for Human Rights.

Biomedical science also interacts with a culture's conceptions of crime and punishment, conformity and deviance. Physicians are employees in the world's forensic and penal establishments using their expertise to help states pursue the varied targets of their justice systems. The use of genetic and early behavioural screens to predict the later possibility of anti-social behaviour has already raised fears about violating the civil rights of the subjects of these predictions.

Beyond these factors are the societal functions of medical diagnosis, increasingly complicated by the emergence of biomedical technology. A particular diagnosis, depending upon the country in which it is applied to a patient, may permit compensation by government insurance, qualify one for release from work, permit dismissal or exclusion from school or certain kinds of employment, or excuse one from military service. It may put someone on a waiting list for a scarce resource such as haemodialysis or renal transplant or, conversely, may exclude them. Some of the social functions of diagnosis, now increasingly dependent upon technology, can be clarified by attention to the concept of the sick role (Parsons, 1951) and the benefits and excuses from responsibility which it provides. There are also new variations brought by advancing technology. The stigmatizing effects of laboratory diagnoses of conditions with variable and sometimes unrecognized clinical manifestations for which no treatment exists have already been demonstrated. One example, with usually non-disabling symptoms, is sickle-cell anaemia. Another is HIV infection in clinically healthy people.

Biomedical Technology and Medical Morality

Healers are significant shapers and enforcers of values in all societies and cultures. Advancing biomedical science has clearly enhanced the role of organized Western medicine and its individual practitioners in this respect. It has reinforced their share of the social power and sacrosanct status which led sociologist Elliot Freidson to describe medicine as akin to the state religions of yesterday, with what amounts to an official monopoly on the definition and treatment of disease (1970). This is seen both in the participation of physicians in formulating and promoting ethical codes, and in their clinical role with the patients to whom the newer technologies are applied.

The preservation of human status in the face of illness and medical intervention has traditionally been in the hands of individual physicians, the essential intermediaries between available technologies and the patient. They, as well as the folk healers who retain their ancient status in much of the world, have had enormous powers of discretion to make life and death decisions, alone or with consultation from their peers, on a case-by-case basis, dependent on the patient's trust within the doctor–patient relationship. One corollary of doctors' awareness of their special status was the growth of ethical codes or maxims supporting the concept of the physician as bound by a special morality. Many of these emphasized, although not always explicitly, the idea of patients as ends in themselves rather than means to ends. Yet, as physicians, indoctrinated into paternalistic attitudes, were increasingly trained in scientific thinking, they began to test their ideas and newest helping agents by administering them to uninformed or unduly persuaded patients, some of whom were incompetent to understand or protest because of age, disease or differences in cultural or socio-economic status between them and their doctors. In every instance the practice was justified on utilitarian grounds – advances in science and clinical knowledge would help humanity. To this justification was added the glorification of medical knowledge as an end superseding all others, and, in the USA, as part of the national mood of the Second World War, a sense of urgency. However, the transforming potential of advancing biomedical technology had a growing impact on public consciousness. Rothman (1991) has traced the growing awareness of this potential, and the essential conflict between the research and helping tasks of physicians in the United States. During senatorial investigation into possible abuses, 'the senators . . . consistently confused experimentation with therapy and the investigator with the physician' (p. 65), as did leaders of the premier national health research institutions, the National Institutes of Health; they assumed that 'the physician and the investigator were one and the same, and that the trust patients afforded to doctors should be extended to researchers' (p. 82). A major impetus towards undermining these assumptions, and circumscribing medical decision-making prerogatives, was Henry Becker's (1966) exposure of the prevalence by leading US physicians in prestigious institutions of medical research upon non-informed and non-consenting patients. This was a 'devastating indictment of research ethics' (Rothman, 1991, p. 15), as every example offered by Becker was one in which the 'health and well-being of subjects' were endangered 'without their knowledge or approval' (p. 75). It became clear that the research environments of both national institutes and academic schools of medicine 'nullified a concept of identity of interest between researcher and subject' (p. 83). Becker's exposés had an especially critical impact on the US National Institutes of Health and the US Food and Drug Administration:

> The fact that authority was centralized in bodies that were at once subordinate to Congress and superordinate to the research community assured that the scandals would alter practice. Indeed, this circumstance explains why the regulation of human experimentation came

first and most extensively to the United States rather than other industrialized countries (Rothman, 1991, p. 86).

One aspect of this regulation was the attraction into the field of a host of concerned non-physicians, theologians, philosophers, lawyers, social scientists and others. The ideal of the doctor alone with the trusting patient 'gave way to the image of an examining room with hospital committee members, lawyers, bioethicists, and accountants virtually crowding out the doctor' (Rothman, 1991, p. 107).

Many physicians harbour doubts about the need for and outcome of much high-technology medicine. Yet they feel the very availability of the new technologies, from CAT scans to artificial reproduction, to endarterectomy, to life-sustaining technology, as a moral imperative to use them (Brody, 1987b, 1989a). The conflict between the desire to use newly available power, and recognition of its hazards with resulting uncertainty, reflects the fact that doctors, for all their increased capacity, remain in the position of the Sorcerer's Apprentice. They are amateurs with uncertain goals, not fully aware of how to manage their new powers with their ultimately unpredictable consequences for individual patients and the human community at large.

At the same time this condition of uncertainty, demanding case-by-case rather than categorical decisions regarding the use or withholding of high-technology treatment, is preferred by many to the rigidity and adversarial decision-making of the legal–judicial system or the abstractions of ethical codes (see Chapter 7). Some professional ethicists have stated their preference for the medical profession as the monitor of human rights-related issues through its own codes of practice. This is true even though many observers doubt physicians' consistent adherence to the principle of beneficence, that treatment must be carried out solely for the welfare of the patients and not the family, the state, or the medical profession. Further, there is great variability in the use of medical procedures and devices between individual physicians, hospitals and regions, sometimes correlated with market supply and demand factors. Idiosyncratic motivations are always potentially present in medical decisions. Thus physicians, subscribing to an ideal of achievable self-improvement, have often tried, not always consciously, to make their patients into 'better' persons while ostensibly trying to make them into healthier persons. In the West this last tendency has been reinforced by research indicating the importance of personal habits in the aetiology of illness: smoking, overeating, ingesting too much fat or salt, and lack of exercise are all understood as self-indulgence. Being virtuous in terms of health habits has cultural roots in the value accorded to abstinence and self-discipline. Physicians may become unwitting upholders of such virtues in so far as they are creatures of their own cultures.

The new cultural phenomenon, consequent on the new biomedical technologies, has been the emergence of ethics boards, commissions or committees. While their overt aim is to protect the rights of patients and the public they also function as devices for diffusing responsibility. Beyond this they might be understood as having the covert aim of protecting and perpetuating traditional values considered essential to the integrity of the particular social fabric to which they belong. At the national level commission membership has often been based on particular proportions of scientists, physicians, other health professionals, lawyers, jurists, ethicists, theologians and the general public, including representatives of differently defined lobbying groups. The political aspects of foetal tissue transplant in the USA, for example, revolve mainly around the presumed status of pre-embryo, embryo, and foetus as human persons killed by abortion (see Chapter 4); anti-abortionists were, therefore, represented on the US Human Fetal Transplantation Panel. The composition of commissions considering this and other issues, and their reports, appear to reflect a competition between secular and religious, liberal and conservative–reactionary groups for control of public morality. This may appear discouraging. However, while, as Annas and Elias (1989, p. 1079) point out: 'Ethical issues cannot be resolved by a vote of experts . . . they can help to define and clarify issues publicly and to build a consensus.' Further, the decisions required by the new biomedical technologies are too sensitive and too drastic in terms of individual human lives to be left to representatives solely of philosophy/ethics or the law. The interaction of the individual patient and family, with the responsible, socially sanctioned caretaker, the physician who has worked intimately with the case, must remain central in the decision-making process. But the physician should have the best consultative assistance available.

3 Human Rights Aspects of Reproductive Technology

Human Rights and Reproduction: General Considerations

The United Nations and its specialized agencies, especially UNFPA, the UN Fund for Population Activities, have promulgated 'rights' relevant to both the older reproductive (essentially contraceptive) technologies for child-spacing and limiting family size, and the newer ones intended to enhance the fertility of women unable or unwilling to conceive through sexual intercourse. The impact of these proclaimed rights has been limited by gross national disparities in educational level and resources, as well as in prevailing values and beliefs. Thus, Jamaican women did not use the contraceptive methods distributed by international agencies even though none lived more than six miles from a family planning agency (Brody, 1981a). It has also been established by UNESCO and UNFPA that the largest families and the smallest intervals between births, typically associated with the highest infant mortality, are in countries with the lowest rates of female literacy. At the same time, women in the less developed world have shared with those in the industrial democracies a belief in 'reproductive freedom', that is, from 'compulsory pregnancy', and 'reproductive rights', the knowledge and means to manage their own fertility (Brody, 1976).

Contraceptive technologies are discussed briefly below in so far as they enhance women's opportunities for careers other than motherhood, their quality of life in general, and their children's opportunities to realize their own latent potential by making it easier for them to manage their own fertility. Contraceptive devices and substances are used, with major variations, throughout the world.

The newer technologies concerned with facilitating reproduction are practically relevant mainly to a minority of the inhabitants of the industrial democracies and the political–economic elite of the less developed and totalitarian states. The countries of the European Parliament have discussed the desirability of regional compacts for regulating not only technological reproductive practice, but research related both to reproductive functioning and foetal physiology. Concordance has been reached about a number of issues. However, cultural and historical differences between the European states have prevented comprehensive agreements. Rights issues associated with abortion, with particular reference to the transplant of foetal cells, tissues and organs, are discussed in Chapter 4.

In the developed world the human rights issues raised by aids to or substitutes for coital reproduction and vaginal delivery of offspring have stimulated intense debate and attention by national governments as well as regional legislative bodies. This is partly, as noted below, an aspect of the historical attention paid by human societies to matters of sex and reproduction. It also reflects the continuing tension between a right to at least a minimum level of competent, dignified, humane health care (in this instance reproductive health care), and the strictures of particular moral systems, as well as the continuing dominance over women (and children) by males in most of the world. In addition, both non-coital reproductive methods and the use of surrogate mothers raise questions of lineage and legal identity, the rights of children so produced, and the granting of reproductive privileges to persons who have typically been celibate or regarded as sexually deviant and in the past would not have reproduced coitally; the fact that they can now have children through artificial insemination or other technological means has sparked discussion about their qualifications to be parents.

Beyond these issues the debates stimulated by these technologies, especially surrogate motherhood, have emphasized the everyday roots of a personal concept of 'rights' which is seemingly distant from, but still relevant to, the formal analyses of professional ethicists. These roots are in the concerns of persons attached to each other by affective bonds who are motivated to promote and preserve each other's lives and well-being. In pursuit of the survival of those to whom they are attached the conventional or legal dicta of acceptable behaviour pale beside their personal convictions about what is morally right under the circumstances. This is also true for the sometimes 'desperate' wish of non-fertile couples to reproduce; this raises questions not only about the 'best interest' of the couple (most often the woman) involved, but the responsibility of the state to underwrite a desired, but not necessarily needed, technology. The major emphasis should be on human relationships rather than judicial–legal considerations as a basis for human rights determinations: 'What matters most is how these techniques can be used to enrich people and their relationships rather than diminish them' (Glover, 1989, p. 84).

The definition of need and its distinction from desire has not yet become a focus of major interest for the world's health establishments. Scrutiny of this issue would include the relative advantages to physicians of applying complex expensive technologies in response to patient's desires or fears, versus the relative hazards to the patients or the society which supports their care.

Experience to date has already made it clear that using the newer reproductive technologies can give rise to significant conflicts between participants in the process. Responsibility and authority in these instances, ranging from the wish of surrogate mothers to keep their babies to battles for the custody of cryopreserved embryos, have usually been assigned to the legal–judicial systems of the countries involved. Greater understanding of the human needs and feelings activated by the new reproductive opportunities should lead to their emphasis and a reduced focus on legal–judicial issues. This could bring about a new appreciation of counselling, negotiation, and conflict resolution between quarrelling parents (however defined) mediated by health care personnel, rather than final dependence upon judicial decision. This new emphasis should be reflected in the accumulating international, primarily UN, documents meant as guidelines for the UN's Member States.

Finally, media reports of individual experiences with the new reproductive technologies have led to increased public knowledge and a firmer base for consensus about what privileges or opportunities should, in fact, be considered as 'rights'. These reports, as well as other documents and programmes, also educate the public about the scientific aspects of the new technologies, their uncertainties, and potential unintended effects. In the late twentieth century, as never before, a worldwide informed and reflective public will be essential to the survival and well-being of the human species.

The Social Control of Fertility-related Behaviour and Women's Rights

Social and Cultural Reproductive Rules

Contemporary societal attention to the concerns raised by advancing reproductive technology continues a central theme in human history: in matters of sexual relations and reproduction human beings have never been content to let nature take its course. Fertility-related acts, contributory to continuity and membership in society, have, throughout recorded time, been identified by tribe, village, State and Church as too important, too powerful, and too vulnerable to nonconformity, to exist without control and limitation. Sometimes, as in the twentieth century, limitation has been formal and imposed by local or national governments. Cultural limitation has been structural, as in the intergenerationally transmitted rituals of traditional societies, or codified and specific, as in the directives of particular religious spokesmen or Churches. Limitation has also been imposed by males whose self-esteem and economic status have been linked to the possession of fertile women and the production of large numbers of offspring. Many attempts at regulation have aimed at restricting sexual intercourse to child-producing, and prohibiting the use of contraceptive devices or pregnancy termination (abortion). Under these circumstances women have had to defend themselves against the hazards and burdens of excessive child-bearing on the one hand, and infertility and consequent abandonment by their male protectors on the other. In non-industrialized settings they have defended themselves by recourse to indigenous fertility-regulating substances and procedures, both abortifacient and contraceptive, sometimes of doubtful efficacy, and by consulting folk healers or shamans (Brody, 1981a; Newman, 1985); and by infanticide and child abandonment. In order to protect their lives and health it has some-times been necessary for women to conceal their fertility-regulating activities from their mates or other dominant males in the family.

Since the advent of advanced reproductive technologies, especially those procedures permitting procreation without copulation, societies have recognized a new multiplicity of definitions of just what constitutes a parent. Non-coital reproduction separates issues of genetic, gestational-birthing and child-rearing parenthood. These are in the domain of family law, which in the USA is a matter for the states rather than the federal government. Parenthood for both men and women can be functionally defined on the basis of a genetic relationship to the child, or whether one has assumed responsibility for and has engaged in the activity of rearing the child, or both. For women, parenthood can now be defined on the basis only of having gestated and given birth to the child, with or without having made a genetic contribution to it. Parenthood now also extends to relation-ships with gametes or embryos preserved outside the body. The actual production of embryos *in vitro* raises questions not previously encountered of transactions concerning them. They may, hypo-thetically, be stored for short or long periods, sold or given away, have their custody transferred under other circumstances, be implanted in the uterus of genetically or non-genetically related women, or killed or allowed to die. In every instance legal decisions, compatible with some human rights or ethical code, and perhaps incompatible with others, must be made. These require, among other factors, determinations of the legal status of the extra-corporeal embryo, and of the property rights of the genetic 'parents' who produced them. The urgent desires of some of these parents to preserve an embryo, sperm or eggs may be driven by irrational motives, but the rationality of motives has not been the concern of the courts. The judicial approach to resolving disagreements between sexual partners regarding custody would be, conventionally, through legal determinations both of property rights and the status of the embryos. A procedure more in keeping with developing international concepts of human rights would be an approach through counselling and conflict resolution. There is no reason why recommendations for this kind of approach could not be formalized in international documents.

Surrogate motherhood, a social arrangement for producing children which depends on the technology of artificial insemination (see below), will be discussed later in this chapter; many of the issues which it raises are the same as those involved in non-coital reproduction. It has stimulated legislative action in much of Europe, especially since it became well known in the USA in 1987 with media coverage of the Baby M case.

These concerns, however, are realistic only for a tiny fraction of the world's economic and political elite, mainly in the industrial democracies, to whom the advantages of biomedical technology are available. In most of the world parenthood is defined on the basis of child-rearing, sometimes of children carrying the genes of neither the particular female nor male parent, in the context of an extended family. Informal adoption of children without officially designated caretakers is the rule. Even in the industrial nations which continue to consider complex regulations for the protection of both parent and child, it seems unlikely that caretaking of genetically unrelated or remotely related children, or even surrogate motherhood within families, will ever be effectively controlled by the State. Even the production of a foetus or an infant to yield tissues or cells for an already living and loved family member can be (and is being) carried out discretely through the collaboration of physicians without being subject to formal control either by the State or hospital ethics committees (see Chapter 4). In all of these instances formal analysis of the human rights issues involved takes second place after consideration of the affective and intuitive concerns of the parents or other family members. In the relative balance of rights, the thinking, self-reflective adult, already belonging to a community context, related to other individuals, takes precedence over the unborn (and sometimes never to be born) foetus, or the infant whose cells may be useful to a sick family member, but is, none the less, an integral and highly valued member of that family.

The Intergovernmental System: Women's Rights in United Nations Declarations

The UN, in its various declarations on women's rights (see Chapter 1), and the UNESCO 1985 Symposium (see Appendix 1), officially embraces the individualistic values of the West which emphasize women's personal autonomy in reproductive matters. The UN identifies the freedom of personal fertility control as 'basic to the enjoyment of other rights'. At the same time, the UNESCO Symposium in its references to the importance of the family suggests that a collective value is also taken into account. This collective value in many cultures is that of the male patriarchal leadership of the family in both its nuclear and extended forms. It was noted, for example, that the impact of reproductive technologies on women's rights, and the social, clinical and ethical issues surrounding them, 'most closely touch families and individuals'. With this in mind it was recommended that 'concerning genetic manipulations and artificial procreation, the responsibility for final decisions should be left to the individual and family and their chosen advisers, rather than to governmental agencies' (UNESCO, 1985, p. 3). There is no reference to the relative primacy of adult or child or maternal or foetal rights, and state or collective regulations are, by implication, dismissed in favour of the individual's or the family's 'chosen' advisers.

However, the power of particular cultures usually outweighs the universal, internationally aimed declarations of the UN. While representatives of traditional, patriarchal communities, often with autocratic governments, endorsed the 1948 UN Universal Declaration and the 1985 Nairobi document ending the UN Decade of Women, their actual intent to promote changes in the status of women is uncertain. The degree to which the values promoted by the UN clash with those of a patriarchal family in a traditional culture, and the possible ensuing conflict between a woman, her male family members, and local custom has not been fully confronted. Women in traditional societies, mainly in the developing world, where their access to methods of personal fertility control is resisted by the force of traditional culture, are generally subordinate to men. They are also less literate and less educated than those in societies in which gender relations are more egalitarian. Still, it is clear that, despite resistance, increased literacy, modernization and awareness of technological possibilities are contributing to a gradual increase in their freedom of choice and movement. Paradoxically, it is in the officially secular United States that the trend towards increased women's freedom of choice regarding control over their own reproductive processes has been interrupted by a mixture of political, religious and metaphysical objectors.

There is more general acceptance within individual countries of a right to procreate than of a right to general reproductive freedom, to manage one's own fertility, by methods which may include pregnancy termination (abortion) (Brody, 1976). The US Constitution contains no specific statement of a right to procreate. A review of

US Supreme Court decisions (Congress, 1988a, p. 1; 1988b) yields neither a certain right to procreate, nor a prohibition against doing so either by coital or non-coital means, or for homosexual or heterosexual couples, or for single individuals – all of whom are now able to do so by artificial means.

Internationally, disagreement continues, in and out of the UN, as to how to balance a claim to reproduce against other needs or 'rights'. There appears to be no disagreement, however, that forcible, involuntary abortion (alleged, for example, in media reports in the People's Republic of China, and in Tibet at the hands of the PRC government) or involuntary sterilization (which has, in the past, been carried out with persons labelled as mentally defective in the USA – see Chapters 1 and 2, and Reilly, 1991) do constitute human rights violations. The crucial issue is not the procedure itself, but the fact that it is coerced and constitutes a direct assault on the involved woman, and an indirect assault on her family, community and culture. However, the international condemnation of the practices may not recognize their cultural acceptability, for example, in China. The Gansu Province law of 1988, aimed at improving the calibre of the population by sterilizing persons with an IQ less than 49, has aroused virtually no opposition in China, where a high value is placed on collective rather than individual interests (Kristof, 1991). Several other provinces have similar laws, including the sterilization of married persons with 'serious hereditary disease', including mental retardation.

Modern Social Control of Reproductive Technology: Ethics Committees, the Law and an Informed Public

As noted elsewhere in this volume, representative committees of professionals and other citizens may be convened to protect the values of the State and its professionals, as well as those of the patient. Among these are the values attached to child-bearing, motherhood and the family. The likelihood that any ethics committee will be concerned with these issues, considered to promote societal stability and the *status quo*, is greatest when its members are appointed by representatives of government or institutions with a stake in maintaining public and conventional standards of morality. A number of observers, however, have expressed their distrust of empowering an appointed 'priesthood' to regulate research into reproduction and the clinical applications of that research. Rather than depend exclusively on presumed experts to determine propriety or policy, they recommend increasing 'the level of expertise in the community' so as to broaden participation in the debate over ethical issues (Singer and Wells, 1985, p. 180).

There is also another, but not incompatible, viewpoint which does not agree with the easy assumption that rights questions can be adequately answered by a focus on ethical theory alone or by possibly politicized committees of ethics 'specialists'. This view takes psycho-social and interpersonal factors into account, but would also enlist scientific and clinical–biomedical experts to contribute by focusing on quality assurance in research and clinical care. Ethics committees created by hospitals and research institutes as well as professional societies do, in fact, often concentrate on issues related to quality assurance. But without expert knowledge about the scientific nature, limits and possible elaborations and applications of a particular technological intervention it is impossible to intelligently address questions bearing on its human rights significance. More specifically, the determination of rights significance, requiring a grasp of the scientific–clinical aspects of the technology being considered, also requires knowledge of its psychological and social impact. With regard to the Western ethic, these are essential to understanding the significance of any biomedical application for just or beneficent dealing with any individual patient, or for the preservation of that patient's autonomy. In the USA such professional organizations as the American Association of Tissue Banks, the American College of Obstetricians and Gynecologists, and the American Fertility Society have offered physician training and clinic staffing as well as guide-lines for gamete and participant screening in medically assisted conception.

Modern and Traditional Orientations

Feminism in Relation to Reproductive Technology and the Special Rights of Women

The burdens of reproduction fall disproportionately on women. The social importance of this fact is heightened by the prominence of feminism as a political force, especially in the Western world. A major strain of feminist thought asserts that the reproductive technologies, primarily contraceptive, but including newer non-coital reproductive techniques, provide broader role options and support a variety of lifestyles for men as well as women. The more militant feminist approach views reproductive technologies as enhancing the dominance of men over women through the patriarchal systems of medicine and politics by which the technologies are created and controlled. Manipulation of natural reproductive processes is also perceived by militant feminist groups as threatening the uniqueness of the female capacity to reproduce (Corea, 1985).

A more constructive approach has come from FINRRAGE, the Feminist International Network of Resistance to Reproductive and Genetic Engineering. It has made its views known to the European Parliament and other comparable bodies. It urgently recommends increased research into the causes of sterility, the risks of IVF, a ban on pharmaceuticals with possible harmful effects, and women's freedom of self-determination with regard to many issues such as access to antenatal examinations, pregnancy termination, and new research information (Congress, 1988b). These recommendations fit a view of human (including women's) rights informed by a preventive (rather than solely reparative) public health viewpoint. It expresses a widespread concern about the exploitation, not only of inhabitants of the less developed world, but of the industrialized democracies by the pharmaceutical industry with insufficient regulatory attention from governments; these last, in some instances, may be unwitting collaborators in activities antithetical to health in the name of economic development. These recommendations have general applicability as they reinforce the position of the health consumer movement, and the importance for human rights, in an era of advancing dominance of the biomedical technology industry, of an informed, reflective world public.

Justice and the Basic Concerns of Poor and Disadvantaged Women

The basic issues for poor and disadvantaged women everywhere have not been changed by the newer technological advances. They continue to be access to safe, effective family planning, including contraception and abortion; access to reproductive and other health care; and safety at home and in the workplace (UNESCO/ISSC/WFMH, 1987). Poverty means exclusion from satisfaction of these basic needs, that is to say, from just and equitable access to health care.

In industrial nations concern with safety in the workplace has given rise to two related sets of women's rights issues. One is the right to work in an environment free of reproductive health hazards. The other is the right to freedom from gender-related discrimination based on an employer's assessment of the woman's vulnerability to such hazards. This area has been systematically reviewed by the US Congress Office of Technology Assessment (Congress, 1985). More recently advances in knowledge of foetal physiology have led some employers to exclude pregnant women (and those unwilling to state that they would never become pregnant) from the workplace on grounds of potential exposure to chemicals which might harm foetal development. Challenges to this exclusion, interpretable as a denial of rights on grounds of gender, were initially supported in US courts, but later denied. This issue has been discussed at greater length in Chapter 2.

The spectrum of issues concerning reproductive technologies is tied together by the question of equitable resource allocation. Lack of resources, and lack of leadership interest, necessary to developing family planning education or services for the poor, are ultimately linked to national and professional investments in the development of artificial reproductive technologies available mainly to the affluent. A focus on *in vitro* fertilization, for example, deflects resources and the public policy focus from research into causes and prevention of infertility that would benefit the largest proportion of the world's infertile population. Among the preventable causes of infertility are pelvic inflammatory disease, often due to sexually transmitted infections, malnutrition, untreated injury and illness. Campaigns to deal with these do not require expensive technologies.

For poor Third World women rights may also involve some special issues depending upon their cultural membership. For many this raises the question of a woman's right to consider life careers or roles alternative to reproduction, which may not be usual in the traditional culture. For some they include the capacity to avoid such reproductive mutilations as clitoridectomy or female circumcision. These have been demonstrated to contribute to infection and thus infertility in societies where a woman's position is predicated on reproductive capacity. For most, reproductive decision-making power within the family represents a significant gain in autonomy. However, it has been reported that in some traditional patriarchal societies, especially in Asia, the newly available ability to identify foetal gender has already been used in a manner fitting traditional male dominance. Thus, a disproportionate termination of pregnancies with female foetuses has been reported – a contemporary version of what was once female infanticide. The degree to which the pregnant women concerned have agreed with pregnancy termination on these grounds has not been reported.

In the middle class of many countries, especially those of the industrialized world, exclusionary and cultural differences are less easy to define than among the poverty-stricken women of the developing world. The basic rights issues, as everywhere, begin with participation in reproductive decision-making and access to the means of family planning and personal fertility management. But they also include avoidance of unnecessary medical–technical intervention in pregnancy and delivery, and attention to such technological aids to adequate reproductive health care as amniocentesis. Upper-class and professional women are more concerned than others with the 'new eugenics' and a search for the 'perfect' child. They are most likely to seek prenatal diagnosis, *in vitro* fertilization, artificial insemination, surrogacy and medical support for these desires.

Another technology-based issue in the developed world concerns the comparative rights of pregnant women in relation to those of the foetuses which live, totally dependent, within them. This concern follows the new medical definition of the foetus as a 'second patient' (Spallone, 1989) in direct consequence of IVF and foetal research. These issues in relation to induced abortion are discussed in the section of Chapter 4 dealing with foetal tissue transplants. It includes a discussion of pre-embryonic, embryonic and foetal development with special reference to whether or not these transitional developmental stages deserve to be treated with respect as possessing a humanity with accompanying rights equal to or surpassing those of the women within whose bodies they exist.

Women's Rights in the Clinical Interaction

The Emotional Vulnerability of Pregnant and Infertile Women

The nature of the interaction of doctor and patient is relevant to all clinical uses of biomedical technology. Women, often facing male obstetrician–gynaecologists, are particularly vulnerable to institutionalized condescension and paternalism when they are concerned with their reproductive functions. Those who are poor and uneducated are at a particular disadvantage in dealing with physicians separated by the gulf not only of specialized knowledge, but social status and power. As one Jamaican woman said, she could not speak with her doctor 'because he so high' (Brody, 1981a). The vulnerability of a woman's rights in the clinical encounter stems in part from her longings and fears as a help-seeker, a supplicant, in relation to the healer who, besides possessing greater knowledge and social power, is by comparison free from pain and fear. The physician is also a socio-culturally sanctioned moral arbiter in relation to health matters, a role which may influence his behaviour as a gatekeeper to technologies of contraception, pregnancy termination, and the more esoteric ways of dealing with infertility medicalized into the status of an illness. Susceptibility to emotional discomfort is greatest when the patient is insufficiently informed about her situation. Even in developed nations general knowledge about reproductive physiology and how to manage it appears to be seriously lacking. A study commissioned by the American College of Obstetricians and Gynecologists (Gallup, 1985) suggested that a large majority of American women were seriously misinformed about the safety and effectiveness of currently available contraceptive methods, especially the pill.

Women labelled as 'infertile' or 'barren', and trying with difficulty to become pregnant, are especially dependent and can feel abandoned at the hands of unsupportive physicians who may possess the key to their future happiness via motherhood. This can be especially marked in the less developed world where women's perceived worth, as well as their self-esteem, is often linked to their production of children. Because of the emotional as well as financial stress involved in IVF with its small positive return, it has become apparent that adequate evaluation of the psychological state of the would-be parents and provision for counselling are essential to respecting their human rights. The US Congress Office of Technology and Assessment officially recognizes that 'counseling is an important and often underutilized component of infertility treatment' (Congress, 1988b, p. 7). The most explicit recognition of the stress imposed by *in vitro* fertilization upon women and their mates was earlier published by the Australian government (National Women's Consultative Council, 1986). It recommended that psychological counselling be offered when infertility is first diagnosed as well as at times of crisis. Counsellors should be professionally trained and independent of the programmes which the woman or couple are considering.

The need for counselling has become particularly evident to the general public in relation to surrogate mothering. Medical and legal counselling is also indicated in these situations. This has become increasingly apparent with the increase of highly publicized cases in which the surrogate mother has not wished to give up the baby she has carried, even in cases of a transferred embryo to which she has made no genetic contribution. Carrying the embryo, and later foetus, inside one's body, feeling it move, fantasizing about it, and undergoing the physiological changes of pregnancy and the experience of birth can result in an emotional attachment which is sufficiently strong to outweigh the more abstract contractual commitment to supply a womb in which someone else's fertilized egg can develop. 'The use of reproductive technologies raises questions about the minimum requirements for bonding and the meaning of parent–child relationships – and what they ought to be' (Congress, 1988b, p. 11).

Physicians as Gatekeepers

In most of the industrial democracies modern contraceptives have become freely available in pharmacies, but in many countries they require interaction with a health professional. Access to the newest reproductive technologies is always through specialized clinics and hospital departments. Social policy here, as in the case of other biomedical technologies, is mediated at the personal level for the individual woman through her interaction with individual physicians, nurses, social workers, psychologists or others working in a medical setting. The physician is the leader, the gatekeeper for most reproductive technology, and prescribes or advises when the woman is uncertain about what to use. Even in cases of surrogate motherhood in which legal–contractual and property-rights rather than technological issues are primary, the physician is involved as the guardian of the surrogate's health during the prenatal period, and the interpreter and predictor of possible outcomes to the contracting would-be parents.

Medical Responsibility for Protecting the Woman's Best Interests

The discovery of the patient's best interests can suffer when the physician acts blindly as an agent of culture, society or in the interests of his or her own self-esteem. Decisions made ostensibly on medical grounds may in fact be based on unacknowledged moral or social grounds. The physician carries the worldwide biomedical ethos, co-existing with folk medical systems in the developing regions, which routinely equates variations in function with disease or abnormality. The conceptualization of infertility as chronic illness (Becker and Nachtigall, 1986) reflects the physician's socialization into the values and belief systems of medicine, and the tendency to medicalize variations from the norm. The physician who deliberately or inadvertently ignores the possible contribution of the male partner to infertility contributes to a potentially harmful loss of social support for the woman who may increasingly feel herself stigmatized and inadequate. Related is the physician's desire to give patients the full range of technically feasible services. This reflects the value attributed to technology, often perceived as a mark of 'objectivity'. The incorporation of advanced technology into a clinical practice may be deliberately or unconsciously undertaken to instil new excitement into a professional life which is becoming repetitive and dull, or in order to be at the cutting edge of new research-oriented medicine. The best interests of the woman patient, for example, are not protected by medical reinforcement of her socially constructed and possibly irrational desire to become a mother at any cost. This can be true even when the doctor is consciously motivated by a wish to relieve the desperate longing of a woman for a child. The doctor who accepts such 'desperation' as normal and justifying extreme measures to gratify it may be acting as an unwitting defender of a set of values which requires re-examination. In so doing he or she may miss an opportunity to help the patient discover her own actual best interests (Brody, 1987b).

Epidemics of enthusiasm for new and unproven technologies are shared by both practitioners and clients. Some, like that for the efficacy of diethylstilboestrol (DES), a new technology of two generations ago, rise, do their damage, and fall (Fisher and Apfel, 1985). At their peak they lead to a suspension of critical judgement by doctors and patients alike; unrecognized therapeutic ambition contributes to the belief that all available technology should be used not only to ameliorate disorder or postpone death, but to gratify desire, a belief often rationalized on ethical grounds. This leads to failures in empathy, missed diagnoses, and the dismissal of iatrogenic pathology as irrelevant or the patient's own fault.

The DES story also illustrates scientific–technical problems with human rights significance. One concerns the unpredicted long-term or delayed untoward effects of drug or hormone treatment. If such effects are regarded as impossible by the scientific community the clinician's failure to consider them in dialogue with the patient would be regarded as within the limits of customary practice. If, however, the possibility has been considered, informed consent should include the existing uncertainty about undesired consequences, even in the remote future. Some drugs have short-term undesirable effects which have not been identified at the time of prescribing. Some which appear to have no side-effects will produce them when a third factor becomes active. DES was widely used for many years to prevent miscarriages during pregnancy, and, to a limited degree, as therapy for psychotic depressions with onset of the post-menopausal years. It was not until a generation later that it was blamed for cancer of the uterus and cervix in adult daughters of women who had used it (Fisher and Apfel, 1985). Enthusiasm and uncritical optimism for a particular treatment may simply be wish-fulfilment garbed in a scientific cloak. In 1989 US courts opened the way for manufacturers to be sued for damages resulting from the use of this product, although they, presumably, had no reason at the time of manufacture to suspect its toxicity, and were not directly involved in prescribing it to patients.

The case of *in vitro* fertilization provides another illustration of how medical enthusiasm may override the best interests of the patient. It is a procedure which is socially approved and publicized, and regarding which the physician's own unacknowledged desires, professional and perhaps financial, may take precedence. In this instance a woman's right to equal access to a scarce resource may conflict with her right to beneficent treatment at the hands of her physician. The possibly destructive effect upon patients of untrue claims for the efficacy of IVF has been raised within the medical profession itself. A central question is whether or not non-coital methods of reproduction should be considered a legitimate part of publicly supported health care.

Personal Fertility Control

Contraceptive Technology

As noted in Chapter 1, the report of the UN Decade of Women (1985b) stated that 'the ability of women to control their own fertility' is 'an important basis for the enjoyment of other rights'. Historically, women have defended themselves against the hazards and burdens of excessive child-bearing by recourse to indigenous fertility-regulating substances and procedures. While these may often have been of doubtful efficacy they have had the major value of giving them the immediate experience of control, however limited, over their own bodies and persons. Major obstacles continue to be illiteracy and the opposition of men in cultures in which status is correlated with the number of children. In Rwanda, for example, where more than half of the female population is illiterate and the fertility rate is among the world's highest, the male attitude has been described by a nurse at a contraceptive clinic as 'a cult of egoism' (Perlez, 1992).

The advent of modern female-controlled contraceptive technologies introduced a change in family functioning as it permitted them to leave the home for the labour force. The consequent change in their traditional child-rearing and family-building roles has initiated, depending upon family and community, a shift in paternal and institutional responsibilities.

But even in the industrialized world there is some evidence that contraceptive efficacy is not improving, and in fact may be declining (Jones and Forrest, 1992). In the USA the pill is the most effective reversible method, with only 8 per cent of users becoming accidentally pregnant, and the condom second, with 15 per cent failures. Periodic abstinence and spermicides have a 25 per cent failure rate. The highest failure rates are found in younger women who are unmarried, poor and from minority racial or ethnic groups.

An apparent contemporary violation of the UN-supported right of access to the benefits of science, and women's right to control their own fertility, concerns the 'morning-after' pill, RU–486 (Mifepristone), described in Chapter 1. It can be used without the involvement of a physician or other socially designated gatekeeper. Since it is totally under her own personal control it even raises the possibility that a woman wishing to produce a foetus for donation can time her abortion to fit the needed level of foetal development. 'For the first time, the medical needs of patients are being thwarted by a political and economic battle involving the "unborn"' (Regelson et al., 1990). Further, the issue of physician versus non-professional control of pharmaceutical availability is confronted. The drug in question, in combination with a prostaglandin analogue, has interfered with adequate implantation of the fertilized ovum yielding a 96 per cent efficacy rate of pregnancy termination after 49 days of amenorrhoea or less (Silvestre et al., 1990). It has not been available worldwide because it is regarded in some quarters as an abortifacient. Manufacturers, fearing boycotts from anti-abortion groups, have withheld it from the world market, although the French government has compelled its use in that country. Legislative moves to permit its use elsewhere are under way. The UN and its health arm, WHO, have taken no position on it. However, this withholding is interpreted by many as violating the human rights of women who need it, and could be regarded as contributing to the high prevalence of non-medically produced or illegal abortions with subsequent infection, sterility or death, reducing the worldwide level of public health.

Beyond the issue of abortion is the fact that this is a drug 'of proven or potential value' in Cushing's disease, meningioma, and breast cancer.

> As RU–486 poses no religious or moral issue in patients who are not pregnant, have no intention of getting pregnant, or are incapable of pregnancy, it may be concluded that the drug ban self-imposed by [the manufacturer] because of the issue of abortion and contraception should be lifted from studies of its medical application. . . . Mifepristone must be made available for study in the 'crisis constituency', those patients with limited life expectancy or serious compromise of quality of life whose medical needs have nothing to do with abortion or contraception. The value of Mifepristone must be decided by physicians in the clinical area. It is time to join the public debate on the ethics of denying drugs to the living because of political activism regarding the unborn (Regelson et al., 1990, pp. 1026–7).

The factors contributing to the description of the USA as a 'hostile environment' for contraceptive research have also led to a delay of several years in the approval for medical use of the injectable long-lasting contraceptive Depo-Provera, while it has been widely used in the rest of the world (Charo, 1991).

Technological Interventions in Pregnancy, Labour and Delivery

Prenatal Diagnosis and Abortion

Many of the new reproductive technologies such as ultrasound are aimed at the detection of embryonic or foetal anomalies. Some of these may be corrected before birth or soon thereafter, though often to a limited degree. In every instance the question of pregnancy termination may be raised in consequence of diagnosed foetal pathology. Parental rights issues involve access to the desired intervention, the information essential to participating with the physician in a decision regarding it, and the circumstances which facilitate such participation (exercising the right of personal autonomy). The question of a foetal right to life is also raised when the almost certain outcome of a negative prenatal test is abortion. This question has been raised mainly in the industrialized nations with a sufficiently affluent population to warrant such tests. The report to the European Commission (Glover, 1989), for example, formulates it in familiar terms: the possible elimination of a right to life by a severe handicap; whether being born with certain conditions is in the child's best interests; whether the right to life is eliminated by the effect of a severely handicapped child on the family (p. 127). The Glover committee, recognizing that most parents would not wish to produce a child suffering from severe handicap, did not, however, arrive at a consensus view in this area. In the USA some 'wrongful life' lawsuits, with both parents and children as plaintiffs, have been brought against laboratories for missed diagnoses, or by children against parents for not having opted for abortion. In these instances life has been thought to be not worth living. The metaphysical issues involved in discussing non-existence versus existence with unpleasant and limited features make this an almost insoluble issue when it is couched in terms of a foetal right to life. However, a complaint of technical negligence can imply that the potential parent has not been supplied with the data needed for autonomous decision-making.

Access to abortion varies among countries, as it does between US states, and its denial typically reflects political as well as religious concerns. The 1991 US Supreme Court decision upholding a federal right to withdraw funds from services which even mention abortion as a possibility for women in need is an example. Since it clearly discriminates against poor women, often members of ethnic minority groups who cannot afford private or non-federally funded care, it has elicited major congressional efforts to pass legislation which does not prohibit physicians from discussing all necessary forms of reproductive health care with their patients. A number of US professional associations have adopted strong positions in favour of the right to abortion. The American Public Health Association in its *amicus curiae* brief submitted to the Supreme Court emphasized 'the right of every individual to the possession and control of his own person as a common law notion of bodily integrity underlying the requirement of informed consent for medical treatment'. Respect for bodily integrity is a basis for refusing 'to order individuals to put their own health at risk or otherwise to suffer a bodily invasion (such as an operation) even when such an effort is necessary to save the life of another person' (*APHA*, 1992, p. 12).

Sometimes laws are ambiguously phrased. Abortion in France, for example, may be permitted if the foetal disease is 'incurable' or 'severe'. Medical pressure to have a corrective procedure with a problematic chance of success can reflect an ethical conflict within the physician. Conflict between spouses can occur. One Swedish study noted that 'pregnant women and their spouses often decided about prenatal diagnosis jointly, but the women have the final decision' (Sjogren, 1989, p. 223).

Prenatal Visualization Techniques

Ultrasonography, in which high-energy sound waves are reflected from pelvic structures, is considered the preferred imaging modality for the female pelvis (Council on Scientific Affairs, 1991) because it is non-ionizing. Its clinical use, widespread for detecting gynaecologic pathology, requires a thorough understanding of normal anatomy and cyclic changes and the limitation of the technique. Despite its accepted status for gynaecologic disease detection, however, controversy persists regarding its use in foetal monitoring. In this instance the sound waves are reflected from the foetal figure *in utero*. It has been used for these purposes for at least 18 years with 28 identified diagnostic indications for its use (Thacker, 1986). These include establishment of gestational age, identification of placenta praevia, multiple pregnancy, foetal abnormalities and non-viable pregnancies. An intravaginal transducer enables visualization of details as small as one or two millimetres, and permits diagnosis of complications within a day or two of the onset of pregnancy. Initially welcomed as a way to avoid undue radiation from abdominal X-rays during pregnancy, it has, over time, become acceptable practice without a major clinical trial; while it has immediate usefulness in verifying suspected abnormalities, no large-scale testing has been done on potential long-term hazards. Some question remains, therefore, about its use for universal routine screening. This is not because it has been demonstrated to have adverse effects, but because some observers feel that it has not been appropriately tested for such effects. While no data are available regarding the women with whom it has been used, some long-term follow-up studies in Canada and England have shown no untoward effects on children born to them (Brody, J., *New York Times*, 1 November 1990, p. B 12).

This technology has political–religious human rights significance as it is used to support the view of the foetus as a patient separate from the mother. Even when it is viewed simply as a technique for ensuring maternal health, as well as normal pregnancy, its human rights significance is interpretable from different viewpoints. Thus, some women's rights advocates regard sonography as another way of enhancing the status of physicians. They perceive it as part of the medicalization of childbirth which strengthens the role and increases the income of obstetricians to the possible detriment of the parturient woman. Some women undergoing ultrasound and electronic foetal monitoring feel that their own reports have been replaced by reliance on fallible mechanical signals. With a machine rather than a human helper the need for counselling support may actually be intensified. When the techniques do detect anomalies considerable anxiety is aroused. If the woman and her mate are to participate in the choices which must be made regarding pregnancy interruption or elective surgery they will require both information and emotional support.

These concerns have, in fact, been matched by segments of the medical profession. A 1984 Consensus Statement of the US National Institutes of Health (National Institutes of Health, 1984) concluded that universal routine ultrasound screening could not be justified on the basis of the then available evidence. In the same year, however, in the UK, the Royal College of Obstetricians and Gynaecologists concluded that routine ultrasonography at 16 to 18 weeks was justified (Royal College of Obstetricians and Gynaecologists, 1984; Nielson, 1986). Since then (Saau-Kemppainen et al., 1990) a Helsinki study compared half of a group of 9300 pregnant women given routine sonography from the sixteenth to the twentieth weeks of gestation with the other half who did not receive this routine screening. In the systematically screened group only half as many foetuses died near the time of birth. Current confidence in the procedure is such that one group (Nadel et al., 1990) has suggested that there is no need for amniocentesis to diagnose possible spina bifida in patients who have both a normal untrasonographic examination and an elevated serum alpha-fetoprotein level. This assumes that false positive results do not occur. However, small defects can be missed (Nyberg et al., 1990). Further, a review of the literature reveals an overall false positive rate of 1.2 per cent, which could result both in abortions of unaffected foetuses and missed diagnoses in affected ones (Wald et al., 1991). Most diagnostic errors could be recognized by examining the amniotic fluid for alpha-fetoprotein and acetylcholinesterase levels which together yield a 97 per cent rate of detection and 0.4 per cent false positives in women whose alpha-fetoprotein levels are elevated (Wald et al., 1990). This is an instance in which protecting the rights of patients requires expert knowledge of advancing biomedical technology.

Electronic Foetal Monitoring

This is a continuous recording of foetal heart-rate and status, used particularly during labour. In order to maintain its regular signal the woman must be stationary, imposing a degree of discomfort during labour. Highly sensitive to any movement, it can yield false indications of foetal distress mandating unnecessary emergency delivery procedures such as Caesarean section. Early randomized clinical trials between its introduction in the USA in 1968 and its expanded use to cover nearly half of US deliveries demonstrated a statistically significant increase in Caesarean delivery without significant benefit (Banta and Thacker, 1979). A review of later reassessments (Banta and Thacker, 1990) indicates that it carries risks sufficient to warrant clinical concern: 'Its association with operative delivery is serious'. In general, its expenses and potential risks appear to outweigh its benefits. None the less, while in 1989 the American College of Obstetricians and Gynecologists indicated that monitoring through auscultation is acceptable in high-risk as well as low-risk pregnancies, there is no evidence that the use of electronic monitoring has decreased. It seems likely that the reasons for retaining the technique include continuing patient demand for available technologies, and physician's needs to protect themselves from lawsuits for negligence.

Caesarean Section

Caesarean section rates vary internationally, constituting from 5 per cent of all hospital births in Czechoslovakia to 18 per cent in the USA. The higher US rate seems to be largely due to reliance on the procedure for first births and for pregnant women considered at high risk because of being older than 35 years. However, while American and Canadian (16 per cent) rates are up to 200 per cent higher than those of some other countries in Europe and the Pacific (Notzon et al., 1987), the overall international rate seems to be increasing evenly. These wide individual disparities reflect differences in practice and attitudes towards the use of technological interventions, and, probably, differences in available resources. The largest proportion of these disparities is accounted for by the relative frequency of vaginal delivery in subsequent pregnancies after a Caesarean section, that is to say, differences in repeat Caesareans. In the USA and Canada, for instance, less than 5 per cent of women with previous Caesarean sections deliver subsequent pregnancies vaginally. The high US rate also reflects the routine use of Caesareans for possible, although not always proven, complications, often indicated by electronic foetal monitoring and ultrasound visualization. Actual complications, but of varying severity, include plural births, maternal genito-urinary infections, and hypertension. Each of these has a 50 per cent rate of Caesarean delivery in the USA compared with rates in other countries of 10–20 per cent. Thus, in Scotland, foetal distress leads to Caesarean section in 19 per cent of the cases compared with 69 per cent in the USA; 93 per cent of breech presentations are delivered by Caesarean in the USA, compared with 39 per cent in Hungary.

This procedure has proved unequivocally necessary in some cases, such as foeto-pelvic disproportion. However, the frequency of its use in the USA cannot be justified by reductions in maternal or infant morbidity or mortality. Further, it incurs substantially greater financial costs for patients and hospitals, as well as physiological trauma for patients. In fee-for-service systems, motivation to use the procedure may include increased profit and certainty of the time and outcome of delivery. Its financial, physiological and emotional costs justify its being regarded as an example of the excessive and unnecessary medicalization of childbirth at the expense of patients and their families (UNESCO/ISSC/WFMH, 1987).

Infertility and Non-coital Reproduction

General Considerations

Infertility is widely recognized as both a personal problem for which medical assistance may be sought and a social construct. Its significance in terms of the latter varies between countries, and has become less clear in the industrial democracies as the age of marriage has increased and more women and couples have opted not to have children. In the USA infertility, defined as the inability to conceive after 12 months of unprotected intercourse, affected an estimated 2.4 million married couples in 1982. That resulting from sexually transmitted disease, an estimated 20 per cent of the US cases (Congress, 1988b), is generally considered the most preventable. Tubal occlusion, from whatever cause, accounts for 25–30 per cent of female infertility. It has been dealt with by microsurgical tubal anastomosis with an optimistic 44 per cent probability of conception within a year thereafter (Patton et al., 1987). Transcervical balloon tuboplasty, a non-invasive technique to treat proximal tubal occlusion, has demonstrated its effectiveness; for some patients it represents an alternative to IVF and microsurgical anastomosis of the Fallopian tubes (Confino et al., 1990).

As previously noted, artificial reproduction is not an issue for the bulk of the world's population. In industrialized countries which offer technologically supported health care, for a fee or as part of governmentally supported services, the non-coital reproductive technologies, IVF and gamete intrafallopian transfer (GIFT), are used with increasing frequency in the treatment of infertility, although in

public health terms the recipients still constitute an almost infini-
tesimal minority of the population. It is still, however, difficult to
evaluate the skills and efficacy of various groups offering the
treatments, and in the USA regulation of the procedure is largely in
the hands of individual states with federal efforts focused on study
commissions.

Artificial insemination by husband or donor (AID) is carried out
with increasing frequency and relatively few legal or cultural
objections. If a married woman is the recipient her husband's consent
is usually required and under these circumstances he is regarded as
the legitimate father of the child. In most countries the desire of an
unmarried woman to be impregnated by AID remains controversial.

The situation regarding surrogate motherhood, ovum donation,
and research on human embryos is inconsistent and controversial.
Major national efforts resulting in publications and guidelines
regarding non-coital reproduction have been made in Australia,
Canada, the Federal Republic of Germany, France, Israel, South
Africa, Sweden and the United Kingdom. At least 35 other countries
have devoted national attention to the matter, as have the Council of
Europe, the European Parliament, and the World Health Organization. A summary review of these trends has been carried out by the
US Congress Office of Technology Assessment (Congress, 1988b).
While they bear on human rights (for example, the informed consent
of all parties involved), most focus on legal issues aimed at protecting
all parties from exploitation, and on the moral status of the embryo
(see Chapter 4). Some reflect the varying political and religious views
of participants, and many of these proposals have not been adopted
by the legislative bodies to which they were made.

Artificial Insemination by Donor

This practice, long entrenched in clinical medicine, continues to draw
ethical discussion. Some of the considerations regarding payment for
one's body parts, or services such as those involved in surrogacy, are
discussed elsewhere in this volume. A frequently raised issue,
discussed in the chapter on genetic technologies (Chapter 5),
concerns unacceptable socially based eugenic determination of the
source of the sperm which is used. Another is the matter of payment
versus voluntary donation. In the USA the use of anonymous
medical students as paid semen donors, accepted without question
in earlier periods, has been criticized on a variety of grounds,
including its status as a type of social eugenics, the risk of marriage
between genetically linked AID children, the possibility of masked
coercion of the donor due to the request from a senior faculty
member, and the potential later discomfort of the donor (Annas,

1979). While the European Commission has taken no general position on the matter, the French federation of sperm banks asks recipients themselves to look for donors (to be used for other anonymous recipients), tries to diversify the donor population by appeals for donors through the media, and prefers that no payment be made; some countries such as West Germany discourage AID altogether because of concerns about anonymity, and its eugenic aspects (Glover, 1989, pp. 32–3).

Donor anonymity is the rule worldwide, although the legal position tends to be unclear in most countries. The major human rights issue concerns the child's right to know his lineage versus the adult's right to privacy. In this respect Elias and Annas (1986) have noted that AID potentially places the private contractual agreement between adult participants regarding parental rights and responsibilities above the best interests of the child. The traditional cultural relevance of legitimacy, lineage and individual identity linked to kinship, and of fatherhood in the life of the family and child, are ignored (Kass, 1985). However, there are no national policies on family integrity in this respect. Nor is there a body of data-based thought concerning the impact of reproductive techniques which involve contracts between adults upon child-rearing or child development, though some information is beginning to accumulate. Although the donor remains unknown to the child-rearing (social) parents, Swedish law now grants the AID-produced child upon reaching the age of 18 a right to knowledge of the donor's identity and of his or her genetic origins. On the one hand there is some evidence that this has temporarily decreased the donor supply, and that the donors now tend to be older and married. On the other, the 18-year lapse after the Swedish child's birth should provide adequate time for the development of strong family bonds with the social (that is, rearing) parents (Glover, 1989, p. 35). The human rights concern, again, weighs the child's claim to knowledge against the donor's claim to the protection of anonymity, with the child's interests creating 'a strong presumption in favour of openness, but with protection for the various parties involved' (p. 38). Since this is a presumption rather than an absolute right, it is suggested that a Swedish-type law might be adopted for Europe for an experimental period.

Insemination of a married woman with her husband's sperm is generally considered ethically acceptable, with mutual agreement and informed consent. Legislation in several countries states that children issuing from AID are the legitimate offspring of the woman and her consenting husband. However, uncertainty persists about a donor other than the husband, anonymous or not. Much hesitation also persists by physicians and, perhaps, the public, regarding artificial insemination of single women or members of lesbian couples. The rights to adequate parenting of a child artificially conceived by a single woman or a lesbian couple continue to be debated. However, there are no compelling data to support the contention that a child is necessarily placed at developmental or emotional risk by these circumstances. There is also a tendency to politicize the issue with regard to the gay rights movement. In the USA, for example, the New York Court of Appeals has ruled that a lesbian cannot seek visiting rights to the child (produced by AID) of her former partner. Her designation by the court as a 'biological stranger' (despite earlier rulings that a homosexual couple could fit the legal definition of a family for housing purposes) has been denounced as a setback for the lesbian and gay rights movement (Sack, K., *New York Times*, 3 May 1991, p. B1).

Surrogacy with a Gestational-birth Mother Inseminated by Donor

This is a social arrangement utilizing the technology of artificial insemination by donor. The surrogate is a woman who is hired or volunteers without pay (in this case typically a family member) to be artificially inseminated with a would-be father's sperm. She functions, thus, as a substitute (surrogate) for the would-be father's mate, usually his wife, when the latter is unable to become pregnant. A voluntary, non-commercial arrangement should theoretically fit the values of a modern society regarding freedom of choice as a human right. This approach allows persons to make any agreements among themselves with which they feel comfortable. Many cultural objections are, of course, possible. Catholicism rejects interference with the natural processes of reproduction as interference with the process of creation itself. Orthodox Judaism may be concerned with such issues as adultery, illegitimacy, incest and lineage blurring (Shalev, 1992).

Although the surrogate is inseminated artificially rather than by copulation, she is in every respect the biological mother of the child she will produce, that is to say, she is both its genetic mother and the gestational-birth mother who carries it during the pregnancy and undergoes the birth process in order to deliver it. However, she has agreed to forgo the usual rewards of parenthood. She gestates and gives birth to the infant with no expressed intent to rear it. This procedure has been used by would-be parents as an alternative to adoption, and a way to have a child genetically related, at least, to the male member of the rearing couple. It thus permits continuity of the male, but not of the female, genetic line in a manner congruent with the culture of traditional patriarchal societies. Since physicians are always involved in performing the artificial insemination, with or without a commercial surrogacy transaction, their responsibilities to both sides in the arrangement may be greater than they realize. These should, clearly, include mandatory screening for transmissible disease from both father and surrogate, as well as investigating and counselling, or providing counselling for the issues noted above. Many physicians are uneasy about any kind of involvement in the process. In West Germany doctors have been prohibited by their professional associations from such involvement (Benda Report, 1985).

A major point of controversy is the use of a potentially enforceable contract paying a hired surrogate for her service (the surrogate could not be legally forced to perform the service). By 1992 the USA was the world's only country permitting commercial surrogacy; a review of the practice highlights its vulnerabilities. The hiring is usually done by a couple, the female member of which is infertile. While the commercial transaction may involve only the principals the hired surrogate is often found through an agency which includes lawyers, physicians and sometimes clinical psychologists concerned with her mental health and stability. The surrogate voluntarily enters into a legal contract binding her, in return for a fee, to give the baby to the father and his wife after birth. The contract typically calls for the major part of the payment to be made when the mission is completed, that is, when the woman gives up the child (and her parental rights) to its genetic father who will rear it, usually along with his wife.

If commercially institutionalized this practice could clearly contribute to the creation of a class of lower socio-economic status female breeders, in a manner reminiscent of such women employed as wet-nurses for the infants of the affluent in the nineteenth century, especially in England. In all available accounts of commercial surrogacy the employing couple is in a more advantaged socio-economic stratum than the surrogate. This impression is supported by the US Congress Office of Technology Assessment review of a number of studies including surrogate matching service reports (Congress, 1988b). The data 'demonstrate that women who have volunteered to be surrogates are distinctly less well educated and less well off than those who hire them'. While their self-reported motivations for offering to be surrogates include non-commercial considerations, for example the desire to experience pregnancy, it should be noted that 'without financial remuneration few say that they would offer to participate as surrogates' (p. 268).

The question of payment raises issues of altruism, or a gift relationship, perhaps analogous to that of organ, blood, semen or egg donors. Payment for donating semen or eggs for surrogacy, and even payment for the surrogacy act itself, diminishes the altruistic significance of what could be a gift. This aspect is emphasized when the surrogacy arrangements are made by a commercial agency. The European Commission (Glover, 1989) is opposed to permitting the involvement of commercial agencies in surrogacy. As many observers have stated, it carries the danger of exploiting poor women. A market approach to surrogacy also introduces the problem of justice – equal access to a scarce service. Parenthood without gestation or delivery becomes yet another commodity, available mainly to the affluent.

By early 1988 approximately 600 surrogate mother arrangements had been concluded in the USA; there were about 15 surrogate mother matching services, some multidisciplinary including psychiatrically trained physicians, and others primarily law firms. These matching services arranged contracts for paying the surrogate mother, typically in the $10 000 range, in addition to her living and medical expenses, and attorney's fees. The total cost to the employing would-be parents may be as high as $60 000 or more.

Contracts often specify surrogate behaviours aimed at ensuring the well-being of the foetus and child-to-be, such as restrictions on smoking and alcohol, and regular prenatal care including mandatory amniocentesis (Congress, 1988b) (but, apparently, no mandatory abortion in case of foetal abnormality). According to most surrogacy contracts the father will take custody even if the child is not healthy as expected, and in the event of his death custody will pass to the wife. Yet an unclear area remains if the child is born with a health problem which can be attributed to the surrogate mother's failure to conform to the contractual agreement. Similarly, attempts to control the psychological and physical health of the hiring family, clearly relevant to the rights of the surrogate as well as of the child she will bear, appear to be inconsistent. The surrogate's informed consent for the broad medico-social aspects of the procedure, for example, might include its impact upon her relationship with her husband (if she is married) and an estimate of her ability to conform to the behaviour recommended in order to produce a healthy infant. (The matter of a surrogate's husband's informed consent to the procedure has not been systematically dealt with although most matching services do obtain it.) There is a trend, but no routine requirement, for psychological evaluation and counselling of the hiring couple, or physical examination of the sperm donor and testing his semen for sexually transmitted disease.

As noted, a number of surrogates, emotionally attached to their infants which grew inside them, and to which they gave birth, have refused to honour their contracts. These infants are biologically 'theirs', as much as if they had been impregnated by AID without a paid contract requiring them to give them up. The question is whether or not a person's biological child can be legally assigned to another person or couple on the basis of a financial contract executed prior to conception. Since the child is not to be adopted by the others involved, and has no voice in making the arrangements, the transaction has some elements in common with baby selling; hypothetically, and extremely, it might be compared with selling the baby into slavery (understanding that the child is to be cared for as a member of the family rather than raised to be an unpaid worker).

Some critics have also regarded the contract as analogous to the surrogate mother selling herself into temporary slavery. This raises the familiar question, relevant to selling one's own organs, of the legitimacy of state intervention to protect persons from their own self-destructive decisions. A psychosocially oriented human rights approach would recognize the surrogate's own feelings in relation to the infant which has been part of her body during a prolonged period of gestation. It would avoid the pitfall of dehumanizing her in the sense of some observers who speak of a 'rented womb' as though no human person is involved. This is among the major reasons why all the world's countries which have considered the problem (and many have not) have outlawed commercial surrogacy, with the exception of the USA. In the USA legislation addressing the problem has been introduced in more than half the state legislatures, but with uneven outcomes. Most state court decisions have ruled surrogacy contracts to be unenforceable, even when they have split on their legality (Congress, 1988b, p. 13). However, the legal outcome remains uncertain. A UNESCO/ISSC/WFMH Working Group (1987), focusing on the international context and after considering all the factors involved, including the surrogate mother's tendency to bond with her foetus, recommended that any commercialization of the procedure be banned. This fits the concept of human rights embodied in the present volume. It also recognizes that surrogacy cannot be definitively prohibited as an informal, non-commercial arrangement between relatives.

The European Parliament's Ad Hoc Committee of Experts on Bioethics (CAHBI) (Council of Europe (CAHBI), 1986) has recommended that surrogate motherhood should be allowed only if the surrogate does not receive material compensation and that contracts for the procedure should not be enforceable. The recommendations of the Warnock Commission in the UK (1984) would probably prohibit commercial surrogacy, since they included laws (which have already been enacted) banning sales of human tissues, including sperm, ova and embryos.

A more permissive attitude, recognizing some apparent hazards of commercial surrogacy (for example, surrogate behaviour which might harm the foetus, and refusal of a contracting couple to accept a handicapped baby), recommends regulation by a non-profit state surrogacy board (Singer and Wells, 1985). It does not object to IVF with donor sperm, ova or embryos, but favours informing the child of the circumstances of its conception and birth, and recommends record-keeping that would enable data (but not donor identification) to be given to the child if requested.

An official West German Commission (Benda Report, 1985) has considered a total ban on surrogacy except for that between relatives. In the UK (Warnock, 1984) a committee concluded that there was a central conflict between the interests of the childless couple and the surrogate mother. They therefore, as noted above, supported restrictions which would greatly reduce the frequency of surrogacy, while recommending that surrogacy should not, in itself, be illegal. The UK Surrogacy Arrangements Act makes commercial surrogacy a criminal offence. The European Commission (Glover, 1989) recommended that a contract should not be enforceable against a surrogate mother who changes her mind in any phase of the pregnancy or after delivery. This would maintain her autonomy and support her claims against those of the biological father. It suggests, as indicated above, that such a contract if enforceable could be considered analogous to selling one's self into slavery. If surrogacy were illegal it could emotionally damage or stigmatize an ensuing child.

'In Vitro' Fertilization with Implantation of the Embryo in the Genetic Mother or a Surrogate

Some of the considerations raised by surrogacy are applicable to IVF children if the rearing parents are not the biological ones. Fertilization outside the body (*in vitro*) vastly increases the possible outcomes of a human reproductive effort in terms of genetic endowment, lineage, intra-uterine environment, and parenting. It was first accomplished successfully in 1978 as a method of treating infertility caused by a block in the oviducts (Steptoe and Edwards, 1978). Since then more than 20 000 children are reported to have been born in consequence of this method (Angell, 1990b). Even with increased efficacy and reduced costs, however, it is unlikely that the procedure will account for a sufficient number of births worldwide to constitute a public health issue. The attention paid to it by the medical profession and international agencies cannot be justified on public health grounds.

IVF and embryo transfer are biologically unnatural forms of conception which require repeated overstimulation and multiple puncture of the ovaries in order to create an abnormal pre- and post-conception status. Although there is no evidence to that effect, it cannot yet be definitively stated whether or not repeated interventions will have unfavourable effects on the anatomy and functioning of the reproductive organs. Prior hormonal stimulation of the woman's ovaries is required in order to obtain the highest possible number of mature ova in one cycle. This is followed by surgical removal (follicle puncture) of ova for extracorporeal fertilization with sperm. The resulting blastocysts (pre-embryos, generally referred to as embryos – see Chapter 4) are transferred to a uterus through the vagina. The particular uterus can be that of a surrogate other than the genetic mother, or the genetic mother herself.

While the chance of fertilization is relatively high with IVF, about 70 per cent, the likelihood of successful embryo transfer is only about 20 per cent per treated cycle. With the increasing chance of foetal loss as pregnancy continues, the probability of the birth of a live child (the 'take-home-baby rate') has been widely estimated as between 10 and 15 per cent per cycle. Some hospitals, on religious or 'pro-life' grounds, require that all fertilized ova or pre-embryos be implanted in the birth mother's uterus. This practice has been criticized as a violation of the woman's rights since it incurs an increased risk both of spontaneous abortion and of multiple pregnancy. The pregnancy rate does appear to be improved by transferring two rather than one embryo. The refinement of ultrasound techniques has made it possible to visualize the foetus at an increasingly early stage. This allows a comparative estimate of the health and intactness of the embryos present in multiple pregnancy, and may be used to determine the selective abortion of one or more embryos in the interests of promoting the health and survival of those which remain.

The most commonly used instrumentation in IVF has been laparoscopy which requires hospital admission and general anaesthesia. This is being replaced by an echoscopic transvaginal follicle puncture technique that can be performed on an out-patient basis and, therefore, repeated more often. It is possible that with increasing time, practice and technological improvements the overall IVF success rate may rise to 30 or 40 per cent. It may be noted that, despite no indication of increased foetal distress, a higher than normal rate of delivery by Caesarean section has been reported among IVF pregnancies (Andrews et al., 1986). This may reflect the anxiety of obstetricians regarding the fate of IVF infants.

The available variants of artificial insemination and *in vitro* fertilization can enable a couple or an individual to predetermine the paternal and maternal genetic contributions to the new individual; decide in whose uterus the blastocyst will be implanted, with implications for a non-genetic contribution and for the impact of the delivery experience on both pregnant woman and infant (ultrasonography has been shown to increase maternal bonding to the foetus); and determine the gender of the new individual. This availability has been extended beyond the usual child-bearing years. Since the endometrium has been shown to retain its ability to respond to gonadal steroids and provide a receptive environment for embryo implantation even in women over 40 years of age, a new extension of IVF has been introduced. This involves the use of oocytes provided by younger women (who according to the report of results were paid US$1500 per cycle by the recipients), with oocyte recovery, fertilization, embryo culture, and subsequent transfer of the embryo performed by standard IVF methods. Five out of seven women, aged 40 to 44 years, who (after psychological consultation, including their husbands) received the embryos, had viable pregnancies (Sauer et al., 1990).

Cryopreservation of Ova and Embryos, Storage, and Parental and Children's Rights

Preserving ova, human eggs, for later use could be clinically indicated when pelvic disease, surgery, radiation or chemotherapy are likely to result in infertility. The development of an effective technique for freezing unfertilized ova obtained from ovarian stimulation, with preservation of function, would make it possible to apply IVF during later cycles, obtaining a closer approximation of the natural conception mechanism.

Three births have been recorded in Australia and West Germany from ova that were frozen and then thawed. However, the possibility of developmental anomalies in offspring conceived from frozen eggs is sufficient to require chromosomal analysis of such embryos before regularizing the procedure (Congress, 1988b). It is believed that, with improved technology, egg freezing could become as effective as embryo freezing and be used in the same manner as the cryopreservation of sperm (Al-Hasani et al., 1987).

Hyperstimulation of the ovaries in the IVF process typically results in more ova than are required for return to the uterus after fertilization. Cryopreservation of human embryos, although it significantly reduces their capacity for implantation (Levran et al., 1990), has become a routine procedure for conserving embryos. It also makes it unnecessary to repeat the egg retrieval procedures, and by preserving and storing them reduces the pressure to transplant several embryos when they are available, thus reducing the risk of multiple pregnancy. Later they can be transferred in a subsequent cycle if treatment fails, or, if it is successful, used when another pregnancy is desired. Preserved embryos can also be implanted in another 'birth' or 'wish' mother (Van Hall, 1985), or in a surrogate.

Major legal problems have arisen when the desires and circumstances of the parents (the producers of the stored embryos) have changed and they disagree about their fate and engage in custody battles over their control. In these situations the ignorance of judges

and sometimes juries about embryonic development, and uncertainty about whether or not an embryo should be legally regarded
as a 'child', have created confused and potentially untenable
verdicts. A recent verdict of a US state court ruled that frozen
embryos are neither ' "persons" or "property" but occupy an interim
category that entitles them to special respect because of their
potential for human life' (Smothers, 1992). It ruled that the divorced
father could prevent his former wife from implanting or donating the
embryos which had been fertilized with his sperm and then frozen
for future use, saying that his 'procreational autonomy would be
defeated'. In a certain sense he was protected from having
compulsory fatherhood imposed upon him.

Surrogate Embryo Transplantation

This procedure involves the removal by uterine lavage of the
fertilized egg a few days after artificial insemination of a surrogate
mother, and its transfer to the uterus of the 'wish mother'. Perhaps a
dozen viable pregnancies have been reported with the use of this
method since 1983 (Congress, 1988b). Although an advantage would
appear to be that conception takes place *in vivo*, this procedure poses
the risk of infection to the surrogate mother, of unplanned continuation of the pregnancy by failed lavage, and damage to the embryo.
Risks to the fertile donor include ectopic pregnancy, multiple
pregnancy as a result of supranormal ovulatory stimulation, and
transmission of disease from the donor semen. Further, the indication for embryo transplantation is questionable. If the infertility is
caused by the absence of oocytes in the 'wish mother', the desired
pregnancy could be more easily attained by IVF with donor eggs. If it
is caused by tubal pathology (not responsive to new methods of
inflating the tubes), IVF is even more strongly recommended to
preserve genetic motherhood. In neither situation is it necessary to
use a surrogate mother.

Gamete Intrafallopian Transfer

This procedure, transferring ova and sperm by catheter to the
Fallopian tubes where fertilization may take place, can be carried out
with both donor sperm and donor eggs. It has the advantage of not
involving an extracorporeal embryo. Since its first description (Asch
et al., 1984) it has been widely used in the industrialized nations as a
treatment for unexplained infertility, endometriosis, and male factor
infertility (Congress, 1988b). While it is unlikely that it will replace
IVF, since it is not an option in the presence of damaged oviducts, it
may become increasingly popular for many cases of unexplained

infertility or those for which other treatments have failed. Among its disadvantages are that it provides no diagnostic information about the status of the oocytes in response to sperm, and it usually requires general anaesthesia.

A Summary of Human Rights Issues with Non-coital Reproduction

Human rights issues in IVF and other forms of non-coital reproduction concern: overly optimistic, misleading advertising by IVF practitioners for an expensive, emotionally distressing and low-yield procedure; the need to provide counselling at every step; expansion of IVF indications to include male infertility (Becker and Nachtigall, 1986); ignoring the couple as the unit of infertility treatment in favour of procedures performed upon the female partner; the implantation of multiple embryos with potential compulsory multiple pregnancy; and the basic concerns of equitable access and public funding for high-technology procedures of an elective nature (see below). Strong medical interest in research and practice in the field, and the tendency to feel a moral imperative to use new technologies, mean that 'the doctor's role as an unwitting agent of social control in the reproductive arena' (Brody, 1987b, p. 155) remains a fundamental issue bearing on individual rights to beneficent treatment, autonomy and self-determination.

The technologies of non-coital reproduction also carry certain social and cultural hazards for the ensuing offspring and for families as agencies of socialization and enculturation. These, too, may be regarded as human rights issues. They include possible interference with a community's perception of the continuity of its lineage. In much of the world a major problem would be impairment of the sense of lineality. The pool of children available for adoption in most traditional societies is usually confined to that group's characteristic lineage, patrilineal or matrilineal. In the Sudan and Micronesia, for example, all adoptions are along kinship lines. This lineage group could, presumably, provide partners who might become surrogate parents. Related issues concern the offspring's rights to knowledge of social and genetic lineage and identity; parental rights to custody, including the possible right of officially recognized parentage, if desired, of a surrogate mother in whose uterus the foetus grew; and the development of institutional forums for considering these concerns.

IVF and Embryo Transfer: Health Necessity, Personal Desire, or Commercial Undertaking

Although it was originally devised as an alternative to the surgical treatment of tubal infertility, there is a tendency to extend the application of IVF to forms of sub-fertility in which traditional treatments, perhaps in combination with watchful waiting, are sometimes known to lead to pregnancy. Examples of these include ovulation disorders, endometriosis and male sub-fertility. As the indications for IVF are broadened beyond couples with untreatable tubal-factor infertility an increasing number of conceptions which cannot be regarded as due to 'treatment' may be expected (Haney et al., 1987). A basic question concerns the relationship between the demand for IVF, including both specific medical indications and sub-fertility, as well as a simple wish to have a child, and public (governmental) responsibility for its availability. Should it be regarded merely as a method for the treatment of certain forms of infertility, or should it be considered a new reproductive technique to which anyone who asks for it has a right? Public financial support for the procedure varies between countries, and appears to reflect the significance of pronatal values. Israel, for example, with the needed personnel and technology, and strong pronatal values, offers government support for couples wishing to undergo IVF. In the USA, where no government support is available, a number of states have mandated limited insurance coverage for it. In the USA in 1992, with 165 private clinics and an estimated $2 billion yearly IVF business, the demand for the procedure has been fuelled by advertising and the profit motive. The increasing commercialization of the procedure is reflected by the formation of chains of clinics with stock offered on the public market.

From this viewpoint IVF has the hypothetical potential of becoming the primary means of reproductive control, reducing the likelihood of unexpected results in terms of the gender and genetic make-up of the foetus. It is essentially a laboratory technique which lends itself to privatization and commercialization, including the establishment of banks of spermatozoa, ova and embryos, and data banks for surrogate mothers; this is already beginning to occur in several industrialized countries. At first glance its control would seem to be assigned to the medical profession, but through their payment for services consumers would ultimately be in charge. This trend if continued could promote situations in which a couple or individual not achieving a pregnancy as quickly as expected or desired would opt for IVF, that is, it would be available on demand. If surrogate mothers were readily available a couple able to pay for the service could (even if they were biologically capable of carrying through the process themselves) decide to produce an infant carrying their genetic material without undergoing the discomfort and hazards of pregnancy.

It could be argued (as it has been in cases of poor people selling their kidneys, or women selling foetal tissue which they themselves have produced) that this procedure dehumanizes the surrogate mothers. As suggested above, they could become, in essence, a socio-economically disadvantaged group of breeders for the benefit of the affluent. On the other hand, as in the case of organ and foetal tissue sales, an argument might be made for the woman's right to earn her living in any way she desires. Finally, without regard to the surrogate, the UN-defined right to 'benefit from scientific advancement' may be invoked. It could be said that, if a child is desired at a given time, and the technique to fulfil the wish is available, there should be no objection to using it. Questioning the indications for IVF and its use could even be regarded as a paternalistic attempt to limit the freedom of the 'wish parents' (Van Hall, 1985). IVF should, in principle, continue to be reserved for cases in which there is an organic inability to conceive, with restraint exercised in cases with unexplained or otherwise treatable infertility (UNESCO/ISSC/ WFMH, 1987). On therapeutic grounds it would be undesirable for couples who have made progress in working through and accepting their infertility, since offering them IVF could seriously disturb and even refuel their mourning process.

There have been emotional negative responses to proposals that women who are single or lesbian (or both) should be considered for IVF. However, the conditions for the well-balanced development of a child are not yet fully known, and it is likely that they include much more complex factors than simply the gender or sexual orientation of the parents. There are no good data about the psychosocial and sexual development of children born after AID or IVF to single or lesbian women, and none to suggest that they are more difficulty-prone than others. Single women who request AID appear to have seriously considered the social, financial and child-rearing consequences of parenthood. The peremptory rejection of single or lesbian women as candidates for IVF, therefore, must at this time be regarded as unjust and discriminatory.

4 Transplantation of Adult and Foetal Organs and Tissues

The Socio-cultural and Scientific Context of Traffic in Organs and Tissues

Scientific and Technological Development

The concept of transplanting human organs and the subsequent long history of clinical experimentation under public scrutiny constitute a remarkable chapter in the history of medicine. The clinical usefulness of organ transplants is beyond dispute. All major medical centres in North America and Europe, with few if any exceptions, carry out transplants on a routine basis. Traffic in human organs and tissues, existing for many years, has typically been regarded by Western authorities as contributing positively to human health and welfare. The most familiar organic materials donated or sold by persons from their own bodies have been renewable, that is, blood and sperm. The first organ widely used for transplantation from a living subject was paired or bilateral, the kidney; the donor could survive with only the remaining kidney.

The demand for donated organs continues to grow. As the expense of the various procedures involved also grows, so does the international debate about the justice of major publicly supported investment in transplants while a more significant public health result would be yielded by investing in disease prevention, health promotion, and supplying basic care for large populations. However, the emotional and symbolic impact of saving a single life remains an important influence in decisions about spending health care funds.

US data indicate that more than 60 000 people die annually or are maintained on suboptimal therapy who could probably be helped by a transplanted kidney, heart, liver, heart–lung, or pancreas (Evans et al., 1992). Preservation techniques have made it possible to establish banks for skin, bone marrow, and bone and related products as well as corneas and eyes from cadavers. Continuing research on organ preservation technologies will someday permit long-term organ banking which will further transform the field. These techniques and

97

the advent of new threats to human life have allowed public health officials as well as clinicians and medical ethicists to consider the possibility of dramatically more widespread needs for organ transplantation. Thus, radiation sickness has posed the possibility of a massive, catastrophic need for such human body products. The advent of AIDS has also intensified world public awareness of the need to regulate organ and tissue transactions with special reference to quality control in order to protect the public health. (The AIDS epidemic has led, at a conservative estimate, to at least a 10 per cent reduction in the number of potential donors (Evans et al., 1992).) These and other considerations make it evident that any understanding of the human rights or ethical aspects of organ transplantation must be firmly based on an understanding of the scientific–clinical status of such work, as well as ways, through prevention and health promotion, of reducing the demand for it.

The prime mechanical alternative to organ transplantation is haemodialysis for kidney failure. Ventilators may be regarded, within limits, as substitutes for failing lungs. An artificial heart programme exists in the US National Heart, Lung and Blood Institute, but controversy persists about the social–public health value (more precisely, the benefit in relation to the cost) of the immense investment necessary for its development, which, in any event, will require an extended period of time. This is significant in the light of US law requiring that devices constructed with public funds must ultimately be equitably available to all. The US Institute of Medicine has concluded that the costs of artificial heart development would be greater and its benefits less than for any medical procedure now in use, and wonders if insurers can support its wide use, estimating the potential demand as up to 200 000 yearly by the year 2020. None the less (in keeping with a national commitment to technological advance and furthering the possibility of at least some benefit to individuals) it recommends continued research (Hogness and Van Antwerp, 1991). In the light of the public ordeals suffered by recipients of an early model of artificial heart in the 1980s it seems likely that progress on a new model will take place very slowly through the selective support of a few contracts with physiologically limited goals (Marshall, 1991).

The most promising development to supplant organ transplantation in some instances is the likelihood that specific cells may be transplanted. The only ones which have been regularly used are those from bone marrow. The most immediate new prospects are pancreatic islet cells for diabetes, liver and adrenal cells. While many technical problems remain to be resolved the new probabilities for therapy have not stimulated new concerns for human rights.

Culture and Human Rights in Relation to Transplantation

Beyond scientific–clinical issues human rights considerations are embedded in the varying values and laws of countries in which the procedures are carried out, and from which organ donors are recruited. They concern every step of the process from donor recruitment to recipient selection and involve issues of justice (equitable treatment), beneficence (for whose good is the procedure carried out?) and autonomy (the preservation of free choice for all concerned). An often unidentified element of the overall cultural matrix is the almost automatic assumption of Western scientist–clinicians, supported by a public consensus, that it is desirable to maximize the supply of organs for transplantation. This is not universally shared in all cultures. As Lock and Honde (1990) suggest, perhaps it should be asked why the industrial democracies of the West, in contrast to others, notably Japan, 'have arrived, apparently so quickly, at the position of accepting organ transplants as routine' (p. 99). It is the routinization of such a vital matter, rather than a sensitive, thorough, intimate analysis of the single case of the affected individual in his or her family setting, which is at issue. This includes the cultural definition of death, the significance of body mutilation and dismemberment after death, of giving up one's body part to another, and the relevance of such procedures for family and lineage.

Organ and tissue donors have been recently dead adult or (aborted) foetal cadavers, ·or living adults, or recently alive anencephalic neonates. However, in no country or society is the body of the recently dead person regarded merely as a source of tissues or organs for removal at will to be utilized elsewhere. Every society expresses respect for and protects the bodies of the recently dead by means including appropriate ritual treatment and the elaboration of legal standards. Cultural considerations can override the presence of an industrial economy and technological mastery. In the USA racial minorities have been reluctant to donate organs even though they are among the major groups in need of transplantation (see the section on recruitment, below). In Japan, even with available technology, routinization of organ transplants has not taken place. The crucial argument concerns the definition of death, and transplants have been limited almost entirely to those which do not require a brain-dead donor. The concept of *kokoro* or spirit, understood as a core of the particular human individual, which cannot be taken away and given to another, is involved (Lock and Honde, 1990). No public or professional consensus has been reached on the acceptability of brain death as a criterion for the removal of organs for transplant, or on the idea of transplantation itself.

In many countries ignorance and apathy, or simple lack of confrontation with the problem, have resulted in uneven legal protection of exploitable potential donors. Even where such protection exists human needs and greed conspire to circumvent legal standards. Countries and cultures with religious or other cultural taboos on disturbing the deceased in any way, sometimes reinforced by law, appear especially susceptible to black markets in organs, particularly kidneys which can be taken from living donors. But in the less developed world, aside from cultural and legal considerations, extreme poverty and lack of education, sometimes associated with minority status, create the greatest vulnerability to exploitation. In countries without legal prohibition of organ selling, recruitment campaigns have used selling techniques which effectively negate informed consent among the poorest citizens for whom the possibility of a one-time financial gain of previously unimaginable proportions is so irresistible as to obviate rational judgement. Financial incentives in these circumstances are tantamount to coercion. This assumption is born out by press and television reports of recruitment for organ sales in the slum neighbourhoods of India. Interviews with donors have revealed both satisfaction at having acquired more money through the transaction than they might otherwise have expected in a lifetime, as well as instances of sadness and resentment at lost health and increased vulnerability to illness. The practice can spread to other family members, whose consent may be uncertain. Thus, a Uruguayan labourer reportedly sold his kidney to 'a wealthy merchant', his daughter's kidney to 'an ailing millionaire', and his son-in-law's kidney to 'a retired school teacher' (*Baltimore Sun*, 2 December 1991). For these people transplantation is significant mainly as it suggests a way in which they might exploit their own bodies for commercial gain, facilitating their economic survival (while, conceivably, putting their bodily survival at risk). While the surgeons involved justify their work on the basis both of financial aid to the poverty-stricken donors and saving the lives of affluent recipients, it is reasonable to assume that they also have personal financial motives. This issue will be further discussed with regard to the commercialization of organ recruitment.

Personal and Emotional Issues

Finally, the actual transactions involved in organ transplantation have roots in the personal concerns both of those controlling the technology and those subjected to it. The surgeon–scientists who do the research and carry out the complex procedures are motivated not only by a wish to help others (including, at times, recipients who may not fit established standards), but by the excitement of being innovators in a field which has transformed the horizons of medicine. Potential donors, even motivated by the feeling that they are giving themselves to humanity, may be made anxious by the recruitment process and fear 'premature harvesting' of their organs. Many potential recipients also have mixed feelings about the procedure itself, especially its possibly constrained and anguished sequelae, with some deciding against it in favour of an earlier, but more rapid, and possibly less tormented death (for their families as well as themselves). In this highly emotional interactive context the observance of formally defined individual and community rights can assume the dimensions of a set of rules intended to impose order on potential chaos. However, they may be irrelevant to the actual practices of organ recruitment and donation, and the selection of willing recipients.

All these matters have been the subject of intense public interest. In the contemporary era of mass communications public opinion, rarely confined to a single country, influences what is considered right or wrong, acceptable or unacceptable. Media coverage of transplant issues combines the emotional leverage of public appeals for organs with the anxiety attached to speculation about maintaining brain-dead or comatose individuals as organ sources. The possibilities of 'bioemporiums' to maintain adult brain-dead bodies, or of artificially produced foetuses or anencephalic neonates as 'organ farms', have received a share of lurid press coverage. Public interest is also reflected in the emergence of advocacy groups. Thus, the 'Parkinson's Support Groups of America' lobby to make foetal tissue transplant more easily and generally available. Despite the tensions involved, and the interest in gaining new knowledge as well as helping others, most involved professionals express a concern with dignity and respect for persons. These include 'both their autonomous wishes and their bodies . . . benefiting patients . . . not harming them' and 'other ethical considerations, which may derive from these principles . . . including truthfulness, fidelity, privacy and confidentiality' (Childress, 1987, p. 87).

General Human Rights Issues

Autonomy Rights

In terms of practical autonomy rights, (self-determination, personal liberty and freedom of choice) neither the recently dead adult organ donor, nor the aborted foetus, has a personal voice; the next of kin or the recently pregnant woman who has produced the foetus are the only ones for whom autonomy rights, in the sense of making their own decisions free of undue persuasion or coercion, can be invoked. US courts do grant families limited property rights in the cadaver of a relative, but none have extended them to include the cadaver for commercial purposes – for example, to sell its organs for transplantation or research. The US national standard permitting individuals to decide the disposition of their own organs after their deaths, or, without such expression, permitting families to decide, is embodied in the Uniform Anatomical Gift Act. However, the fact that kidneys are taken from living donors (and this may become true on a wide scale for liver transplants) raises the question of commercial exploitation. This will be treated below with special reference to what might be termed the international market in organs.

Some countries (and some US states with regard to corneas) have enacted 'presumed' consent or donation laws permitting organ extraction in the absence of explicit objection. Veatch (1989, p. 213), making the controversial suggestion that these tend to be countries 'without a long history of respect for human rights', questions the desirability of 'a society that conceives of body parts as essentially property of the state to be taken by eminent domain'. He states that 'if the body is essential to the individual's identity, in a society that values personal integrity and freedom, it must be the individual's first of all to control after . . . life is gone as well. If it is to be made available to others . . . it must be a gift.' Childress, on the other hand, believes that one should consider 'tacit consent as well as express consent' with regard to the transfer of human body parts (1989, p. 97). A more extreme opinion favours extracting organs even against the will of the decedent or family since the protective purposes of consent do not apply to cadavers which cannot be considered autonomous beings, and the benefit to others accruing from such organ salvaging may override other considerations (Jonsen, 1988). This again raises the question of emergency conditions which might be comparable, regarding transplantable organs or tissues, to those leading to a wartime policy of conscription. Massive radioactive injury, for example, treatable with foetal tissue, might require at least the temporary adoption of social utilitarian principles in order to save the social fabric upon which individual existence depends.

Justice Rights

The right of equitable or just access to organs or tissue (adult or foetal) needed to sustain life, and equal freedom from coercion in obtaining them, are aspects of the overall question of the equitable distribution of scarce resources. For most of the world's population, high-technology life extension via organ transplantation is not even a discussable option. In the USA, organ transplant operations, including the associated hospital care, are so expensive as to be far beyond the reach of most individuals; this situation will probably continue even though technology improves and organs and surgeons become more available. However, US transplant surgery is financed by the US Veterans' Administration, Medicare (a federal insurance programme for the elderly and disabled), to a limited and variable degree by Medicaid insurance for people on welfare, and, variably, by private insurance companies. It has been supported by private donations and public appeals, sometimes with the partici-pation of public figures either naive about the ethics of going beyond procedures established to promote equitable resource sharing, or sensitive of the public relations value and symbolism of their act.

Community needs and responsibilities have also been invoked. The communitarian argument asserts that 'as members of the community' everyone begins with an equal moral claim to the organ, just as they have an equal obligation to support (presumably through taxes) 'the like claims of others' (Schuck, 1989, p. 180). In its most common form the argument claims that all individuals should have an equal opportunity to extend their lives. There is no place in the world, however, in which this is true: access to health and life extension varies with power, money and personal connections. It may also vary with the judgements of physicians or community about the moral or social worth of a candidate for transplant. Such a judgement can be linked to one regarding the patient's likelihood of survival because of his or her own behaviour. Thus, it has been proposed that patients with end-stage liver disease due to alcoholism should have a lower priority for liver transplant than those not responsible for contracting their disease. The proposal is based on considerations of fairness and the possibility of diminished public support if alcoholics with diseased livers were to receive more than half the available organs (Moss and Siegler, 1991). Implicit, although not articulated, is the punitive idea that they were, after all, responsible for (and, therefore, deserve) their own plight, which could have been prevented by greater restraint and self-discipline.

From a public health viewpoint organ transplantation policy is 'a subset of a broader, generic health policy issue – the problem of coping with the costs of catastrophic disease' (Blumstein, 1989, p. 6). Earlier work suggested that 'viewing catastrophic illness as an independent policy problem calling for independent financing appears to presuppose that government's obligation to assure the provision of medical services is not unlimited' (Blumstein, 1989, p. 9). At the same time, the exigencies of politics and public opinion (international as well as national) require agreement with the view that government coverage of catastrophic illnesses 'plays to the highly symbolic character of life-threatening disease. . . . Because they confront government with basic questions of society's humanitarian self-image, individual episodes of illness are likely to elicit public sympathy and to secure public support' (Blumstein, 1989, pp. 9–11). It seems likely, given continued research and development, that, as 'transplant procedures become less constrained by organ supply and more routinely performed, they will lose the privileged political position that they now enjoy and will instead be obliged to compete for scarce governmental resources with other social goods on more equal terms' (Schuck, 1989, p. 169).

Beneficence Rights

Beneficence rights (ensuring that the procedure is carried out solely for the benefit of the patient) might sometimes be questioned if it appears that performing the transplant was motivated more by investigative, economic or public relations interests than concern for the patient's welfare. Even with transplants with which there has been wide experience, such as kidneys, questions continue to arise about the quality of life of recipients (Sensky, 1988). Experimental transplant procedures, for example for a composite allograft (or homograft) consisting of *en bloc* liver, stomach, duodenum, pancreas, jejunum and ileum, have been carried out in infants who died not long afterwards (Williams et al., 1989). The surgeons, while optimistic about long-term gain if the technical problems could be resolved, acknowledge 'the futility' of 'short-term gain in a child hopelessly consigned to an existence dependent on parenteral nutrition' (p. 1458). Concern has also been expressed regarding the impact of multiple transplant procedures on children and their families when the child's psychosocial status has begun to deteriorate (Reinhart and Kemph, 1988).

   Beneficence and equal access are related to variations in personal respect accorded to different human groups, especially those at the ethnic or socio-economic margins of the world's societies. As noted below, for example, Kolder and associates (1987) showed that in the USA low socio-economic status, unmarried, ethnic minority women have been at greatest risk of being involuntarily subjected via court order to medical interventions for the good of the foetus with which they were pregnant. The issue of beneficence has been raised in the case of an infant conceived in order to produce bone marrow cells for transplant (see below).

Organs for Transplant from Anencephalic Newborns

This issue touches on a range of human rights concerns in biomedicine. A major reason for considering anencephalic newborns, with no cerebral mantle but with a functioning brainstem, as organ sources is the lack of transplantable organs for infants. A protocol developed by Loma Linda University (California, USA) in this respect also suggests the emotional value to parents of having their anencephalic offspring (95 per cent of which die within the first postnatal week) contribute to sustaining the life of another. Despite an increase in the number of anencephalic foetuses aborted after prenatal testing, and despite the fact that a majority are stillborn, it seems probable that 'if access to ongoing programmes were more widely available, many couples might choose organ donation over abortion, to create some benefit from their otherwise tragic pregnancies . . . organs obtained from these anencephalic newborns could make a substantial contribution to the supply of infant organs' (Truog and Fletcher, 1989, p. 388). This view, however, is challenged by data suggesting that the relatively low frequency of anencephaly and a relatively high frequency of other organ anomalies in these infants make it unlikely that, even with changes in the law, they would provide a significant proportion of transplantable organs (Medearis and Holmes, 1989). The law in question is the US Uniform Determination of Death Act (1980) which requires that anencephalics (like all organ donors) meet established criteria for brain death, including cessation of brainstem activity, before they are used as donors. The technical problem posed by this requirement is that the solid organs of such infants receiving customary care usually undergo sufficient hypoxic injury in the process so that they are not suitable for transplantation by the time of death. With this in mind, six such infants were given intensive care from birth and six only when signs of imminent death developed. When intensive care was provided from birth, organ function was maintained, and brainstem activity ceased in only one infant within the first week (Peabody et al., 1989). This led the authors to conclude that under current law anencephalic infants are not a feasible source of solid organs for transplantation.

The Loma Linda protocol was suspended in mid-1988 after a 7-month trial, only in part for these reasons. Another reason was decreasing conviction by the participants of the moral desirability of the project. This included concern about the possible expansion of the effort to include infants with less drastic defects, that is, the 'slippery slope' argument. This last was expressed most drastically by Shewmon et al. (1989):

> Either homicide should be lawful if it is motivated by saving the life of another whose life is not threatened by the person killed, or homicide should be lawful if the victim is about to die anyway. But if these are valid principles for anencephalics, then they are also valid for a whole

host of other patients, when, in fact, the law makes no exceptions. This logical inconsistency might then be used to justify subsequent expansion of the exceptions to include incompetent patients in the final stages of a terminal illness or even prisoners on death row, whose organs would be much more suitable for transplantation than those of anencephalics and whose execution could be timed according to the availability of an optimally matched recipient (p. 1775).

Walters (1989), a medical leader of the Loma Linda effort, responded that the basic issue 'is not whether . . . anencephalics . . . have differing moral status' but 'what constitutes valuable human life. . . . The question about the moral standing of anencephalics and other such marginal individuals is essentially a philosophical issue, and it is one that society must decide' (Walters, 1989, p. 2093). Oberman, a lawyer, noted:

If the concept of brain death is valid, then the only real reason for not defining anencephalics as dead by virtue of brain absence is that there is a risk of misdiagnosis. If this risk could be eliminated, then the fear that society may devalue the lives of severely handicapped individuals in the future and seek to use them as donors should not justify banning donations from anencephalic infants any more than it justifies banning all withholding of treatment (Oberman, 1989, p. 2093).

However, Medearis and Holmes (1989, p. 393) believed that anencephalics could not be distinguished well enough from infants with other severe intracranial disorders to justify legal changes.

The related question is whether or not a pregnant woman, knowing that her foetus is anencephalic, should carry it to term 'solely to provide organs for donation' (Shapiro, 1988). In favour of this Cefalo and Engelhardt (1989) argue that women do have a right to forgo abortion, in which case 'there is no legitimate ground for opposing women's seeking meaning in their pregnancy through maximizing the opportunity of others to use the organs of their anencephalic newborn once death has been declared' (p. 25). On the other hand, it is possible that changes in the Uniform Determination of Death Act or the Uniform Anatomical Gift Act facilitating the donation of an anencephalic's organs would bring 'intense and possibly economic pressure' to carry such foetuses to term. Those who counsel women carrying anencephalic foetuses

must be disinterested and dispassionate about the need for organs for transplantation or the termination of pregnancies that might be thought undesirable. They must be committed to keeping the mothers fully informed and ensuring them freedom to decide about the subsequent course of their pregnancies (Medearis and Holmes, 1989, p. 392).

The debate surrounding these questions may be rephrased in terms of whether the usual standards for protecting human life should apply to anencephalics. The United Network for Organ Sharing (1989), after reviewing the positions of a number of medical groups, including that of the Conference of Royal Medical Colleges in London, opposed the application of any special standards to anencephalic infants, either for excluding them as organ donors, or applying unique brain death criteria to them. The two sides of the question are, perhaps, most forcefully couched in terms of the 'personhood' of the anencephalic. Cefalo and Engelhardt (1989) argue that a minimal condition for personhood is capacity for sentience, and that since that capacity has never been (and never can be) realized by an anencephalic it may be considered as never having been alive as a person. They support revising definitions of death 'so that individuals can be recognized as having died when the destruction of the brain is so extensive as to preclude any further sentient presence in the world' (p. 38). It follows that 'there should be no opposition . . . after proper declaration to making their [anencephalics'] organs available as one would after whole-brain death, despite the continued functioning of the brainstem' (p. 25). Truog and Fletcher (1989) also favour change, proposing as a standard of death: 'a distinct and precisely definable condition characterized by the absence of integrative brain function, such that somatic death is uniformly imminent' (p. 389). This standard is met both by anencephalic and brain-dead patients, but excludes all those in a persistent vegetative state since they do not face uniformly imminent deaths. It also excludes all others endangered by the 'slippery slope'.

The opposing view (Arras and Shinnar, 1988) declares that maintaining an anencephalic's life only to benefit another is a violation of moral law. Shewmon et al. (1989) imply an intuitive and emotional distaste for the procedure, stating: 'The possibility of defining a logically consistent neurological boundary between persons and non-persons is why even people who ascribe privately to the non-personhood theory mostly do not advocate its practical application in law' (p. 1776).

The debate incident to the Loma Linda experiment suggests that the possible social costs of continuing the project might outweigh the benefits to be achieved. These costs could include moral confusion with a loosening of cultural–legal restrictions on the manipulation of human life, beginning with an expansion of the criteria under which defective neonates might be considered as organ sources. On the other hand, the work of Engelhardt and colleagues, and of Truog and Fletcher, suggests that increased conceptual clarity in the area may, in time, make the use of anencephalic neonates for donor purposes possible with less social cost than at present. This would be facilitated by increased scientific work to ensure the viability of their fragile tissues.

More immediately, a perception of human rights rooted in relationships would argue for the use of an anencephalic's organs for another neonate who might be able to survive with them. The right to life of the infant who needs the transplant can be based on its status as an already loved and loving entity, already tied by affective bonds to the parents who are searching for a means to keep it alive. In contrast the anencephalic neonate will never become a sentient, reflective organism capable of independent existence and relationships. From the clinical standpoint there is no question as to whether or not an anencephalic neonate, or one with another type of severely damaged or defective brain, will ever have the capacity to survive to personhood with any imaginable technology. Under these circumstances the 'slippery slope' argument seems legalistic and, as it may deprive parents and salvageable neonates of the essentials for life, not supportive of human rights.

Interspecies Transplantation

A possible alternative is the use of organs from other species for implant into humans. In 1984 the heart of a 7-month-old baboon was transplanted into a 14-day-old dying infant who survived for 20 days. Specially bred pigs and other animals have been considered as donors. The morality of such interspecies transplants (xenografts or heterografts) has been analysed from the viewpoint of the major religions, just allocation of resources, and unfair subject recruitment, without identifying overwhelming reasons to reject them (Veatch, 1989).

Transplantation of Adult Organs

Technology and Logistics in Relation to Human Rights

Even in the West with its acceptance of routinized procedures, issues related to human rights continue to arise at every step of the process: procuring organs, finding recipients, and implanting the organs into them. Partial answers to these human rights questions are found in the state of scientific knowledge and the organizational systems aimed at logistical efficiency as well as moral validity. Practical ways of attempting a just distribution of this scarce resource had to be devised along with technical methods for ensuring quality control. In 1969 US physicians and interested others, many belonging to the still new American Society of Transplant Surgeons, formed an alliance of transplant centres which, in 1982, with organ transplantation already part of the medical mainstream, developed the first computer program for matching donors and recipients. This became the US-based United Network for Organ Sharing (UNOS). When in 1982 a donor liver for a child was found through the family's public appeal this focused general attention on the scarcity of transplantable organs. In 1983 UNOS was formally organized into a national organization.

Organ Donation and Recruitment of Organ Donors

In all the US states organ donations are regulated by the Uniform Anatomical Gift Act (1983), a revised version of which may ban the commercialization of human organs. It specifies that physicians certifying death shall not participate in the extraction or transplantation of body parts. This is an apparent attempt to reduce the likelihood of their premature 'harvesting' (which might technically be designated as murder) by doctors who want them for their patients or for research. The next of kin can make the decision to donate organs if the decedent has expressed no wishes regarding medical use.

Under present technical limitations all donors must have died in a hospital where they could be maintained on a respirator after brain death was established. Identifying criteria for establishing brain death is a domain of biomedical research relevant to human rights and related to the public trust of physicians. A decline of organ donations in the USA, accompanying the increase in publicity given to transplantation, might have been fuelled in part by worry that if they sign a donor card 'physicians might take premature action to obtain their organs before they are really dead, or even hasten their death' (Childress, 1989, p. 91). Between 1986 and 1989 the number of annually available donors in the USA remained essentially unchanged, although in 1990 the supply increased by 9.1 per cent (Evans et al., 1992).

Success at organ procurement through donations depends significantly on the voluntary co-operation of medical professionals, often in relation to the families of potential organ donors (Prottas, 1989). Families may be reluctant or require discussion and persuasion before deciding to donate. The possibility of coercion, however mild, is an issue. It is now widely regarded as an ethical breach to go outside the system for an appeal which will inevitably diminish the chances of a patient already on the waiting-list for an organ.

Given the hospital location, nurses inevitably play a major role in the organ-recruitment process, not only in their contacts with families, but, in many instances, in co-ordinating donors, surgeons and recipients (Dowie, 1988). The nature of medical co-operation with the process may be influenced by local circumstances regardless of state or regional agreements. Thus, a nearby patient surviving at home could, despite prior agreements, have a better chance of receiving a heart or other scarce organ than a more distant hospital-ized patient who, in terms of established criteria, should have priority (Edmunds, 1989). Such factors as the surgeon's personal knowledge of the patient's family and a tendency to make triage decisions favouring someone less intensely ill with a greater chance of survival can play a part. Competition between surgeons and transplant centres, intense and sometimes ethically disturbing as the field developed, has diminished in the USA since the advent of UNOS, but has probably not completely disappeared. Given the fact that transplantation requires highly trained specialists and their teams, it is unlikely that the elements of personal and professional narcissism can ever be totally eliminated.

As indicated above, local value systems and subculturally based fears often interfere with the willingness to donate organs for transplantation. By the late 1980s there was some evidence that in the USA willingness to become donors was lowest among members of minority groups and others perceiving themselves 'to be on the margins of the system and to have even less reason to trust it' (Childress, 1987, p. 92). In this respect abstract human rights issues are secondary to the religious and cultural beliefs of families. A case in point is the 'Hispanic–American' population (not a single com-munity, but an aggregate of groups from different cultural and national backgrounds); because of a high prevalence of diabetes-related end-stage renal disease, members of these groups use a disproportionately higher number of kidneys than the white community. At the same time they donate a disproportionately lower number of organs (Randall, 1991). It is particularly important to rectify this situation because histo-compatible donors are most likely to come from other Hispanic–Americans with similar genotypic diversity.

This problem was studied by the Patient Care and Education Committee of the American Society of Transplant Physicians (Kasiske et al., 1991) which reached several conclusions with regard to recruitment and transplantation among US minorities. These may have cross-national relevance. Despite a higher prevalence of end-stage renal disease in racial minorities than in whites, fewer blacks than whites in the USA undergo kidney transplantation; further, the rate of survival of renal allografts is lower among blacks than whites. The reasons for this last finding may include greater disparities in antigens as well as patient noncompliance, and socio-economic factors. Allograft survival among Hispanic and Asian minorities appears similar to non-Hispanic whites, but both groups have low rates of organ donation. The problems of racial and ethnic inequality regarding kidney transplantation are at least as great, and perhaps greater, with regard to other organs.

A report focusing on the US African–American community (Callender et al., 1991) identified five principal reasons, as at 1978, for the reluctance of blacks to grant permission for organ donations. First, they were not aware of the current scientific–clinical status of organ transplantation and of the urgent need for organs by members of their community. Second were religious beliefs and mis-perceptions. After this came three reasons which might be attribu-table to their sensitivity to their minority status and a mistrust of the majority. These were: distrust of the medical establishment; fear of premature declaration of death if a donor card has been signed; and a wish for assurance that their organs would be given preferentially to black recipients. On the basis of these findings a programme of education and trust building, involving the creation of several coalitions between government agencies, universities and com-munity groups, was initiated. Reported results, beginning in 1982, suggest that the programme has been effective.

The problem for recruiters in all cases is to acquire sufficient cultural awareness to develop trust through dialogue, to know who in the family structure can give permission (for example, a parent rather than a spouse, a female rather than a male), and to increase public education on the topic in local communities. At the same time, respect for individual self-esteem, and for human rights, requires avoiding the use of authority symbols, such as priests or other religious leaders, whose influence would constitute undue per-suasion in many contexts and make informed consent impossible. In circumstances where financial urgency does not override all other considerations requests for organ donation must be made in a way which recognizes differences in the locus of familial and community power and ability to answer requests authoritatively. It is important to be certain that commitments for a family member, perhaps a female, to give up an organ are not made, without her full participation, by a male head of family. In other situations it is important to make sure that a matriarchal figure has been sufficiently involved in the dialogue.

Transplantation from Live Donors

An alternative to transplanting organs from cadavers is the transfer of whole organs (kidneys) or organ materials (liver or bone marrow) from live donors. This practice seems likely to expand, especially with the accumulation of successful attempts to transplant sections of liver from parent to child. Among the advantages, besides the availability of a new organ source, is the ability to carry out the transplant while the child is still healthy, that is, before the congenital liver defect (the most widely publicized basis of the need for a new organ) has resulted in severe physiological damage. A human rights hazard is the possibility that a parent, perhaps under social pressure to donate a kidney, or part of his or her liver, will suffer adverse effects from the transplant surgery. Psychologically adverse effects could stem from the parent's sense that the donation was coerced, with a possible impairment of the integrity of the parent-child relationship.

The ambiguity of ethical judgements based on general principles sometimes emerges in circumstances where human feelings are intense. The US press has featured a story of a middle-aged couple who conceived a child solely in the hope that the baby's bone marrow cells would save the life of a teenage daughter dying of leukemia. (The chance of the infant having the necessary compatible cell type was one in four.) As the parents said, they had been searching unsuccessfully for a donor and could not 'just stand idly by and do nothing' waiting for their daughter to die (*New York Times*, 16 February 1990). Criticism from professional ethicists centred on the fundamental principle that each person is an end in herself or himself and is never to be used solely as a means to another person's ends without the agreement of the person being used. The critics, however, refrained from outright condemnation of the parents, expressing only their discomfort with the situation. The parents for their part asserted their love not only for their teenage daughter but for the newly produced infant. While the oncologist involved thought it a 'peculiar' reason to have the baby, she had no question about carrying out the necessary procedures. It was noted that the transplant could be made unnecessary by obtaining the necessary stem cells from the infant's umbilical cord blood at the time of birth. Physicians also noted that bone marrow can be obtained with little risk to an infant who is at least six months old. In 1991 an apparently successful marrow transplant was accomplished. While formal ethical (human rights) criticism has continued, the parents insisted that their love for their new child was unconditional; the public appeared to regard their actions as justified on emotional and intuitive grounds and to be more concerned with the teenage daughter's right to health than the possibility that the infant's rights were violated. At the same time, the insistence of at least 40 other parents on maintaining silence about their having conceived infants as tissue (and in one case organ) sources suggests possible discomfort about having done so (Kolata, 1991).

Another case in which the compatible bone marrow of one of twins was requested by the father of their half-brother in the face of their mother's objection has been reviewed by Curran (1991). After lengthy examination the court denied the claim, noting that there was no sense of family relationship, that the three-and-a-half-year-old twins were incapable of a competent opinion of their own, that in the event the procedure were carried out they would need the close support of their mother, and of her own opposition, feeling that the procedures were too dangerous for her young children. Curran made the point 'that law alone cannot provide all of the answers to matters of human relations' (p. 1819).

Commercialization of Organ Transactions

The US National Organ Transplantation Act, enacted in 1984, prohibits the sale, purchase or brokerage of certain human organs for transplantation. It makes it illegal to export organs on a commercial basis, and prohibits transactions with a list of human organs and tissues (which may be expanded by the Secretary of the Department of Health and Human Services) 'for valuable consideration for use in human transplantation if the transfer affects interstate commerce'. It does not, however, prohibit sales of parts of their own bodies from living persons unless 'the removal of the part is intended to occur after the death of the decedent'. Arguments in favour of the commercial marketing approach to organ transactions continue to emerge. Some note that transplant surgeons and hospitals do garner substantial gains from the procedure; in that case, why should the original owners of the organs not share in such gains? The issue of property rights of persons over their own organs and bodies, those of relatives, and those of foetuses which they produce, requires additional clarification.

Ethical opinion in the United States is mixed, although it is evident that profound uneasiness persists regarding the possible commercialization of organs for transplantation. Thus, Childress (1989) argues that non-commercial means of increasing the supply of organs for transplantation are at least as effective, probably safer in terms of quality, and more politically as well as ethically acceptable than commercial ones. While a trial of transfer by sales might become necessary if the supply diminishes 'it would not express the value of altruism that leads many to favor the gift relationship' (p. 101). Veatch (1989) is also concerned about undermining the existing altruistic donation system, with a possible reduction in the quality of organs. He notes that vendors of their own organs subject themselves to risk; a market in a fundamental life-saving good such as organs 'makes the poor the suppliers of life-saving human tissue' at the cost of 'pain, suffering and inconvenience. The organs procured primarily from the poor would go to the highest bidder' (p. 218). Annas, in a similar vein, believes that, while individuals should have the liberty to use their bodies as they see fit, 'sale is an act of such desperation that voluntary consent is impossible' (1988, p. 381). He regards 'the strongest argument against a market in non-vital organs' as 'society's instinctive reaction against permitting individuals to directly sacrifice themselves and their health for monetary rewards' (p. 382). However, Veatch opens the way to considering commercializing organs when he comments that 'in a liberal society persons are routinely permitted to take risks. The only requirement in the medical context is that they be informed of the degree of uncertainty' (p. 218). More significantly:

> If life and death ought to be beyond monetary considerations then it is not only human organs that should be beyond commercialization . . . a policy that prohibits the poor from selling their organs to provide food for their starving children ought to ensure that those children have enough food to eat . . . a prohibition on marketing organs should carry with it a right to universal access to a decent minimum of health care as well as the other necessities of life (p. 219).

The alternative might, after all, be acceptance of 'the free-market ideology with all its implications' (p. 219). At the extreme of the range of opinions is Engelhardt's (1989) belief that there is no *a priori* reason 'to hold that commercialization of human body parts is any more or less exploitative or morally opprobrious' than drafting individuals into armies, and that the focus should be on regulations diminishing the likelihood of exploitation and avoidable health risks.

From the universal human rights viewpoint it would appear that the crucial issues are whether or not coercion, direct or subtle, takes place, and the thoroughness of informed consent before a person gives up an organ for sale. It seems impossible to conclude that a person driven by extreme poverty is not the victim of implicit coercion, and that for such an individual, especially one suffering from chronic low self-esteem and a sense of powerlessness, 'informed consent' can ever be a reality. This is another instance, as in the case of surrogate mothers, in which socio-economically disadvantaged persons become biological service suppliers to the elite. Under these circumstances legal permission to sell one's own organs represents governmental collusion in the process of exploitation. The only constructive approach is to supply an alternative means of earning a livelihood.

Commercial Exploitation of Organs for Transplant with Particular Reference to the International Market

As reviewed by Fluss (1991), an Italian law of 1967 was the first to prohibit any award or compensation for kidney donors, and in 1970 the Transplantation Society, an international body, declared that the sale of organs from living or dead donors was indefensible. By 1987 the World Medical Association condemned the purchase and sale of human organs for transplantation, and in the same year adopted a Declaration on Human Organ Transplantation affirming this view. A series of other resolutions and declarations from international sources culminated in a WHO set of Guiding Principles on human organ transplantation endorsed by the World Health Assembly in 1991. They prohibit giving and receiving money as well as other commercial dealings in human organs, but do not affect payment of expenses incurred in organ recovery, preservation and supply. They also specifically prohibit organ removal from the body of a living minor for purposes of transplantation (except under national law for regenerative tissues), and emphasize the importance of freedom from coercion and informed consent for all others. These rules do not apply to reproductive tissues (ova, spermatozoa, ovaries, and testicles) or to embryos and blood and blood constituents for transfusion purposes.

Despite these injunctions the sale of their own kidneys by poor Third World individuals for use by more advantaged people, either their own more affluent compatriots or those from other nations, continues to receive wide public attention. It seems likely, as noted above, that a personal decision to sell one's body part under conditions of extreme poverty can be regarded as an expression of exploitation rather than of autonomy. The medical profession is involved since kidneys have been surgically extracted and implanted for a fee. As one Bombay surgeon argued: 'What if it was your relative who needed a kidney, and one couldn't be found from a family member or altruistic donor? . . . We discourage paid donors, but . . . when all avenues are exhausted . . . we consider one' (*Boston Globe*, 9 December 1985). It is possible that an international black market in kidneys from living donors may develop further, as religious taboos in a number of countries forbid disturbing the deceased in any way. This has begun to concern those industrial democracies which had not previously banned commercial organ transactions. The British Parliament in mid-1989 enacted a law prohibiting commercial dealings in human organs after public allegations that British surgeons were transplanting kidneys of Turkish peasants, flown to London for the purpose, into wealthy Indian and Pakistani patients. In 1991 press reports indicated that Hong Kong doctors have been offered kidney transplants at a People's Republic of China military hospital from living donors for a substantial fee. The possibility that the donors, who could be prisoners, are coerced has been recognized. This is only one of the offers to provide kidney transplants that are attracting growing numbers of Asian patients (Basler, 1991).

Countries with laws in this respect are listed by Fluss (1991). A review of the international free enterprise market in organs (Lillich, 1990) has noted its one-time legality in Brazil, both in terms of buying organs of abandoned children and medical sales of organs from young fatally injured patients, without anyone's permission, to hospitals and private clinics. This situation ended in late 1988 when that country amended its constitution to prohibit the buying or selling of human organs. However, such buying and selling was not prohibited, up to 1990, by Indian or West German law. In fact, only a small percentage of the Member States of the UN forbid the buying and selling of organs taken from living donors (Lillich, 1990). Since 1969, according to a preliminary study by the Procedural Aspects of International Law Institute (PAIL), 22 states have adopted laws prohibiting commercial transactions in human organs: Argentina, Australia, Bolivia, Brazil, Canada, Czechoslovakia, Finland, the former German Democratic Republic, Greece, Hungary, Iraq, Kuwait, Lebanon, Mexico, Panama, Romania, Spain, Syria, Turkey, United Kingdom, Venezuela and Yugoslavia (Lillich, 1990). To these states, according to a recent report of the Council of Europe, may be added Austria, Belgium, France, Ireland, Luxembourg, the Netherlands, and Switzerland. The European Health Ministers have unanimously endorsed the principle of non-commercialization (Council of Europe, 1988).

A review of Latin American legislation regarding organ transplantation (Fuenzalida-Palma, 1990) surveys laws in 16 countries up to 1989. Most such laws call for written consent from the donor or next of kin for use from a cadaver, indicating concern that any living person from whom organs are extracted should be mentally competent and over the age of majority. Bolivia and Mexico specifically prohibit prisoners and pregnant women as well as minors and mental incompetents from donating organs. This is related to the possibility that prisoners 'might be induced to donate organs for early parole, a situation that has reportedly occurred in the Philippines' (p. 431). Laws regarding organ recipients refer variably to 'medical necessity', the nature of their relationship to the donor (with matching in mind) and to the procedures required by the health ministry of the particular country. The pronouncement of death typically requires certification by two physicians, but brain death is listed among the criteria in Bolivia, Chile, Colombia, Ecuador, Panama and Peru. 'Commerce' in organs is prohibited except, in the case of Bolivia, 'when authorized for charitable purposes' and (in the case of Colombia) 'for reasons of grave public disaster or human solidarity'. The author recognizes the expense to volunteer donors and stresses the 'lack of distinction between commerce in organs and compensation of donors for related costs' and the 'absence of a legal basis for donor compensation' as impeding both the encouragement of donations and the collection of data (pp. 433–4). Costa Rica's procedure of donation by will incurs such delays that organ retrieval is virtually impossible.

The interpersonal and human rights ramifications of organ transplantation have been recognized by most world bodies. The World Medical Association has gone on record in a declaration (1987) calling for protection of the rights of both donors and recipients. Fuenzalida-Palma (1990) suggests that uniform or at least coherent legislation involving the Latin American states is necessary to ensure useful clinically motivated traffic in organs between those countries. The World Health Organization's annual Assembly has passed a resolution (Resolution 40.13, 1987 'Development of guiding principles for Human Organ Transplants') calling for further legal and ethical study of issues related to organ transplant. Lillich (1990) proposes an international convention with three articles: Article 1 'would forbid the buying and selling of human organs, at least when living donors are involved. Article 2 would require States Parties to enact national legislation making such buying and selling a crime, with serious penalties attached. Article 3 would establish mechanisms for bringing the convention into force' (p. 11). The UN Sub-Commission on the Prevention of Discrimination and Protection of Minorities has had an item in the purview of its Working Group on Contemporary Forms of Slavery under which initiatives in this direction might be taken.

Medical Responsibility for Organ Transplantation

The US Organ Transplantation Task Force Report (1986) contained a series of recommendations aimed at all facets of the medical profession, its institutions, and regulatory bodies. Although most recommendations focused on logistical, quality-control and technical concerns, they were also intended to safeguard the rights not only of donors and their families, and recipients and their families, but of the medical profession and society at large. Among the Task Force recommendations were: improved determination of death; granting broader permission, for example to medical examiners, for organ and tissue procurement; increased voluntary responsibility by all health care professionals for identifying and referring potential donors; adoption by hospitals (to be carried out by staff) of routine enquiry and required request policies and procedures; education relevant to organ transplants in medical and nursing curricula, and specialist education in the field; certification of both physician and non-physician procurement specialists; and required affiliation with an organ procurement agency by all acute hospitals. The Task Force did not devote systematic attention to the alleged rush by hospitals to gain the prestige and financial rewards of entering the 'transplant market' and 'doing high-visibility, state-of-the-art medicine' (Winslow, 1989). The seeds of an ethical problem appear to lie in the competition between low-volume centres which have entered the field to get their 'fair share' of patients and prestige and established high-volume centres where patient morbidity and mortality rates appear to be lower.

Foetal Tissue Transplantation

Foetal Transplantation and Abortion

The Transplantation of foetal tissues or organs requires the avail-ability of an aborted foetus (since spontaneously aborted ones may be infected or defective). This is complicated by religio-political anti-abortion movements, fuelled by medical–scientific research in artificial reproduction and foetal medicine. These promote a concept of the foetus 'as a second patient', independent of the woman in whose body it lives, and speak of foetuses as 'babies' or 'children'. The rights of women and their freedom of autonomous action have been perceived as threatened by granting primacy to the rights and interests of the foetus over their own. It has been argued that 'technology redefines the meaning of reproduction in society to the detriment of women' (Spallone, 1989, p. 4). This view is bolstered by the finding that 46 per cent of US heads of fellowship programmes in maternal–foetal medicine 'thought that women who refused medical advice and thereby endangered the life of the foetus should be detained' (Kolder et al., 1987, p. 1192). This is true even though a US Supreme Court ruling (Thornburgh, 1986) indicated that any state interest in the potential life of a foetus must be subordinated to the health and safety of the pregnant woman. The finding (Kolder et al., 1987) that the majority of women so 'detained' were non-white, foreign born and socio-economically marginal supports the view that the relative 'rights' of the foetus receive greatest attention when the mother's cultural and social identity place her at greatest risk for denial of her own rights.

In the non-industrialized world some belief systems, especially those supporting reincarnation, oppose abortion and, indeed, any manipulation of the reproductive system. The Koran is subject to interpretation, but has been regarded as permitting abortion well into the second trimester (Newman, 1991). Other societies, opposed to or with mixed feelings about abortion, may permit 'menstrual regulation', that is, inducing a menstrual period after a phase of amenorrhoea (Brody 1981a).

Clinical Usefulness

Additional animal research regarding such basic biological processes as cell survival and the immunology of implant/host relationships has been suggested before uncontrolled trials with foetal transplants multiply (Sladek and Shoulson, 1988). However, there seems little doubt that both basic research on foetal physiology and studies of foetal tissue transplantation have great potential value for treating diseases of foetus, neonate and adult (Hansen and Sladek, 1989). Foetal tissue grows rapidly, is adaptable, and, with appropriate preparation, evokes a minimum immune response from the host. It seems to have the greatest therapeutic potential for neuro–degenerative disorders such as Parkinsonism, although its value for this and other diseases is not yet unequivocally established. Among other possible applications is the treatment of diabetes and immuno-deficiency disorders. Foetal tissue has also been transplanted on a clinical research basis in radiation anaemia patients (Lehrman, 1988), and in mice for immune system research (McCune et al., 1988). Yet, despite the recommendation of its Human Foetal Tissue Transplantation Panel (1988) that research should continue, the United States government, on political grounds (to win the favour of the anti-abortion movement), has established a ban on federal funding for foetal research. Following US congressional and other initiatives the ban has been modified to allow research on spontaneously aborted foetuses and embryos and will probably be overturned in time.

The Embryo and Foetus as a Person

Foetal transplantation has become a politicized moral issue at the level of governments and intergovernmental bodies, largely because of the source of transplantable tissue in induced abortuses, and fear that its approval will increase the incidence of abortions. The problem with abortion exists in so far as the foetuses it kills are regarded as potential or actual human persons, with their right to life taking precedence over the rights of the woman pregnant with them.

The designation of embryonic and foetal entities as persons has varied historically, just as there have been historical changes in the status of adults (for example, in relation to slavery, doctrines of racial and ethnic superiority, the subordination of women, and the human rights accorded to prisoners and the mentally incompetent). Contemporary science has contributed to some uncertainty about the accepted designation of the unborn (pre-embryo, embryo, foetus) at various developmental stages. The aggregate of cells or the blastocyst ensuing from successful fertilization, itself a process continuing over many hours, was first termed a pre-embryo in 1985 in the UK; this designation categorizes the developing organism during the period when, according to the UK Warnock Commission (1984), it may be used for research. This is prior to the appearance of the neural streak and developmental individuality at 10–14 days after fertilization. This blastocyst or pre-embryo is the cellular aggregate, extinguished by natural causes in three out of four instances, which is prevented from uterine penetration by RU–486, the 'morning after' pill. Cryo-preserved, it may be stored externally for a so far undefined period, or thawed and implanted into an available uterus which may not be that of its genetic mother. Ectogenesis, growing external human embryos from pre-embryos maintained by life-support systems, is a speculative possibility. Grobstein (1988) believes that, taking all these factors into account, a

> suitably framed . . . consensus position assuring respect and dignity to the human quality of the unborn might easily be included in their status assignment (p. 17); . . . it would be a useful objective to develop consensual guidelines on such prospects before they become possible. The general presumption might be that interventions practiced on human beings at any stage are unwarranted unless specifically sanctioned for consensually derived purposes through a formal process of decision which is accessible to all interests (p. 19).

The fate of unimplanted pre-embryos obtained for *in vitro* fertilization has become a matter of legal as well as ethical debate. Their status as property or as persons is among the issues in question.

After uterine implantation the embryo with the basic structure of a single organism begins to form. It changes with great rapidity, and, while embryogenesis is not fully complete by the eighth week, its functional development by that time is usually such that it is typically regarded as a foetus. Even before the eighth week advancing technology, such as ultrasound and chorionic villus sampling, can identify the presence of vulnerabilities or severe defects which may lead to decisions about pregnancy termination, that is, ending embryonic or foetal life through abortion. Waller (1989) believes that rulings regarding the use of foetal transplants should be integrated into national laws regarding organ and tissue transplantation in general. The appropriate body for making such decisions, he believes, is not the judicial system, but the national legislature; a clear, legal determination of the legal status of a dead foetus and acceptable ways of disposing of it (if it is not to be used for medical purposes) should be achieved in all countries. In a vein reminiscent of other observers who note the intuitive human distaste for converting human tissues into 'objects', he recognizes the wishes of some parents for memorial services and other manifestations of the humanity of the foetal products of late abortion, believing that this should be considered in any definition of 'foetal status'.

Insulating Abortion Decisions from Foetal Tissue Use

The cautious attitude of Western medicine and legislative bodies with regard to actions which might encourage abortions is revealed in the attention paid to the topic by the Parliamentary Assembly of the Council of Europe, a number of national bodies in Europe and Australasia, some US university committees, and advisory groups to the US Department of Health and Human Services. A general consensus has been achieved to the effect that decisions to utilize foetal tissue should be totally separated from decisions to abort (that is, there must be no abortions designated for the purpose of providing foetal tissue), the personnel involved in the two procedures should be totally separate from each other, foetal tissue should not be commercialized, local ethics committees should monitor the obtaining and use of foetal tissue, and consent of the woman producing the tissue should be obtained, after the abortion, for its subsequent use. These are the conditions under which foetal tissue transactions have been conducted. The Council of Europe (1986) has also declared that 'even when dead the embryo or foetus retains its human character and . . . respect for human dignity requires that any commercial or industrial use must be prohibited' (p. ii).

However, objections are emerging to the idea that human rights are best protected by rigid insulation of foetal abortion from foetal use decisions and personnel. Grobstein (1988, p. 93) argues that it might be more fitting 'in terms of human respect and dignity to put human embryos to use in ways that are fully reflective of their value as members of the human community . . . abortion procedures should be modified to conserve rather than to destroy the integrity and life of the abortus'. Annas and Elias (1989) predict that if it is confirmed that foetal tissue can be therapeutic and 'the abortion can be performed in a way that enhances the potential usefulness of the foetal tissue without additional risk to the woman, there will also be tremendous pressure to adopt this technique' (p. 1081). It seems likely, although not publicly confirmed, that some knowledgeable couples (with the collaboration of their physicians) have already produced and aborted pregnancies to gain foetal tissue for therapeutic use by loved ones.

The Research Domains of Foetal Viability and Sentience

Once delivered, the foetus is designated as an infant. Prior to this point there is a tendency, reflected in the laws of many countries, to adopt a gradualist view of the foetus's developing personhood with rights as a potential person increasing in the last phase of intra-uterine development (Newman, 1991). Foetal 'viability', however, does not imply a capacity for survival without care from parents, surrogates or technological life-support systems. The concept of viability has become socially significant with respect to abortion. The US Supreme Court *Roe* v. *Wade* decision of 1973, legalizing abortion in the first two trimesters of pregnancy, noted that the State does not have a compelling interest in the life of the foetus until after the twenty-fourth week. Despite occasional claims to the contrary, and the 1989 decision of the US Supreme Court that states may require viability tests in 20-week-old foetuses, the point of extra-uterine foetal viability has not been pushed back before the twenty-third or twenty-fourth week. It apparently will not be moved to an earlier date unless new technology enables the foetal lungs (not sufficiently developed before this time to permit breathing) to obtain oxygen without irreparable tissue damage.

Research on foetal sentience acquires human rights significance as it provides information allowing the avoidance of imposed suffering on the foetus. Although a 20-week foetus behaves in a way suggesting minimal sentience, central nervous system electrical activity patterns suggest that 'an adequate neural substrate for experienced pain' does not exist until approximately 30 weeks, 'well into the period when prematurely born foetuses are viable with intensive life support' (Grobstein, 1988, p. 55).

Science, Autonomy and Beneficence Rights in Foetal Transactions

Beyond these concerns are many discussed above in relation to the transplantation of adult organs. Still other human rights concerns continue to emerge with regard to transplanting foetal tissue. The US National Organ Transplant Act (1988) addressed to adult organs was amended in the same year to include prohibitions on the sale of foetal tissue. It has also been proposed that the United States Uniform Anatomical Gift Act (1983), which provides that either parent may donate dead foetuses for medical use if the other parent agrees, be amended to prohibit gifts of foetal tissue by the woman producing it (Stanford, 1989). Other familiar problems with human rights significance are how to provide equitable access to these scarce tissues, as to any scarce resource; how to ensure the rights to adequate treatment of persons with diseases which might be improved by such tissues;

how to protect the rights of couples (or women) to produce foetal tissue to help loved ones; what is the social wisdom of devoting public funds to expensive esoteric treatments rather than to basic public health responsibilities; and how to avoid the possible exploitation of poor women everywhere, but particularly in the Third World, who might produce and sell foetuses for financial gain – their own, and, perhaps, that of others (Brody, 1989b).

5 The New Genetics: Manipulation, Screening, Prediction

The Power of Hereditarian Concepts

The Socio-political Context

The role of hereditarian concepts in modern science and society has been explored by Bowler (1989) who provides a social–historical context in which 'the new genetics' might be viewed. The contemporary era began with the independent rediscovery in 1900, by Carl Correns, Hugo De Vries and E. von Tschermak, of Gregor Mendel's laws, and the later work of T.H. Morgan and his school showing that chromosomal behaviour during *Drosophila* reproduction followed the Mendelian transmission of characters. It was now possible to 'exploit the concept of the gene as a discrete material unit on the chromosome, coding for a particular character that could be transmitted from parent to offspring, isolated from all external influence'; this allowed 'the "genetical theory of natural selection" to become the dominant paradigm in evolutionary biology' (Bowler, 1989, p. 4).

This paradigm was part of the body of natural science with its emphasis on a value-free truth. However, there has been a growing realization that, despite the undoubted sincerity and dedication of its practitioners, science does not constitute a disinterested, value-free search for the truth, but is influenced at every step by factors inherent in the socio-cultural-economic-historical context in which it exists. Such 'contextual variables' are increasingly identified by those who regard science as 'social knowledge' (Longino, 1990). The rediscovered Mendel's laws were used to support the argument, prominent at the turn of the century, that social reform was doomed to failure because of the hereditary predetermination of human capacities; the inevitable corollary was a focus on eugenics as the only effective method of protecting future generations: 'It is difficult to escape the feeling that the success of genetics came about at least in part because it could be presented as a plausible scientific foundation for these social attitudes' which, in the early 1900s, could be extended to include support of a capitalistic free-enterprise economy (Bowler, 1989, p. 10).

The embrace of eugenics and its later abandonment by the leaders of the industrialized democracies has been noted earlier. Many thousands of people defined as mentally retarded, significant proportions of whom appear to have been socio-economically deprived and members of minority groups, were sterilized in the USA in the period between 1920 and the early 1950s, mostly under state laws upheld by the US Supreme Court. The eugenics courts of Nazi Germany had earlier required the sterilization of an unspecified number of people, estimated by some as approaching one million, between 1933 and 1940. Beginning in 1988 the People's Republic of China, through various provincial laws, has required the sterilization of mentally retarded persons. For those who become pregnant abortions are compulsory. Some laws, for example that of Henan Province, mandate the sterilization of all married persons with 'serious hereditary diseases including mental disease, hereditary mental incapability, hereditary deformity and so on' (Kristof, 1991). In response to the Chinese move, UNFPA, the United Nations Fund for Population Activities, has offered to pay for a national study on the causes and prevention of mental retardation.

Genetic Variability, and Gene–Environment Interaction Determining Individual Behaviour and Social Organization

There is no longer serious scientific argument about the significant contribution of genetics to virtually every aspect of organismic function. This is widely accepted for most behavioural traits as well as intelligence measured by conventional tests. However, the proportion of variance for any particular feature which might be assigned to genes or environment remains uncertain. There is argument about data from 14 countries which suggest that 'in the current environments of the broad middle class in industrialized societies, two-thirds of the observed variance of IQ can be traced to genetic variation'; but this heritability estimate should not be extrapolated to the extremes of disadvantage found in these social contexts (Bouchard et al., 1990). It remains essential that enthusiasm for the new genetics does not obscure the crucial role of environment in determining the impact of genetically coded information on both the developing and mature individual. A succinct description of the current place of scientific knowledge in this respect states: 'Unlike simple Mendelian characteristics, genetic variance for behavioral dimensions and disorders rarely accounts for more than half of the phenotypic variance, and multiple genes with small effects appear to be involved rather than one or two major genes . . . the importance of non-genetic factors and multigenetic control of behavior require new strategies to detect DNA markers that account for small amounts of behavioral variation' (Plomin, 1990). Among the complex diseases with public health significance which appear to involve both environmental factors and multiple genes, at least as many as three to five acting together, are various forms of arthritis, cancer, hypertension, obesity, diabetes, multiple sclerosis, some forms of mental illness, and a range of autoimmune disorders. Long-term studies of psychological differences and similarities in twins reared apart suggest the general nature of the interaction of genetic and environmental determinants, although the specific linking mechanisms are unknown. When environmental variation is lower (that is, when social context is similar for everyone growing up within it and the cultural influence is relatively homogeneous) heritability is higher. Conversely, in a heterogeneous setting (where there is increased phenotypic variance), the heritability of specific behaviours, such as linguistic or religious, is low. The generalization encompassing these findings is:

> The institutions and practices of modern Western society do not greatly constrain the development of individual differences in psychological traits . . . the diverse cultural agents of our society, in particular most parents, are less effective in imprinting their distinctive stamp on the children developing within their spheres of influence . . . than has been supposed. . . . It is plausible . . . that a key mechanism by which the genes affect the mind is indirect, and that genetic differences have an important role in determining the effective psychological environment of the developing child (Bouchard et al., 1990, p. 227; Lumsden and Wilson, 1981).

These considerations are significant in estimating the consequences of deliberate genetic manipulation aimed at producing a desired human type with its corollary reduction in genetic heterogeneity. Genetic variability has been a fundamental influence upon the nature of human society and the intrinsic nature of human beings.

> A human species whose members did not vary genetically with respect to significant cognitive and motivational attributes, and who were uniformly average by current standards, would have created a very different society than the one we know. Modern society not only augments the influence of genotype on behavioral variability . . . but permits this variability to reciprocally contribute to the rapid pace of cultural change (Bouchard et al., 1990, p. 228).

Mapping and Manipulating the Genome

The Composition of the Genetic Regulators

Every cell of the normal human body, regardless of location or function, contains 23 pairs or a total of 46 chromosomes, one of each pair being transmitted by the male and one by the female parent. Each chromosome contains from 3000 to 4000 genes totalling altogether an estimated 100 000 genes made up of molecules of hereditary material (deoxyribonucleic acid, or DNA). The genes themselves are composed of 150 million chemical building blocks or base pairs. Of the approximately 30 000 base pairs per gene, approximately 10 per cent are effective protein-production regulators; they carry the encoded information, transmitted from parent to child across generations, which directs the production of crucial life-sustaining and life-shaping proteins. The rest contain filler DNA material constituting a matrix for the active elements. The DNA of the genes includes, at the molecular level, all the information necessary to lead to a complete organism, whether bacterium, plant, animal or human being. It is this fundamental information, the directions for characteristic patterns of living and growing, contained by the DNA which constitutes the 'genome'. Given this background it should be noted that research continues to discover new significance for non-genic elements of the chromosomes, and new influences, such as parental gender, upon the function of particular genes.

As has just been noted, half of each individual's hereditary material comes from each parent. Some genetic disorders stem from problems in the genes; others are associated with extra chromosomes or extra or missing bits of chromosomal material – a majority of naturally aborted or miscarried embryos and foetuses probably have serious chromosomal defects. Approximately 4000 such disorders have been identified as possibly resulting from defects in a single gene. The ability to predict the occurrence of such a disorder is increased with each new discovery about human genetic endowment.

Mapping the Genome

One of the most ambitious international scientific projects of the late twentieth century is the effort to map and sequence the human genome, which has been called the new anatomy (McKusick, 1989). Since the first genetic linkage map in 1913, continuing research has produced genome comparisons between organisms, functional groups of genes or dispersed gene families, and chromosome regions associated with pathologies. The primary goal of the current effort is to describe order and spatial relationships among such genetic landmarks as polymorphisms, genes and DNA sequences in order to produce a linkage map, a variety of physical maps, and the beginnings of a composite DNA sequence (Stephens et al., 1990). In short, the goal is knowledge of the information contained in the genome and the physical and functional relationships among its various regions.

James Watson who, along with Francis Crick, formulated the structure of DNA, has predicted (understanding the arbitrary nature of the date) that the human genome will be mapped and sequenced by 30 September 2005 (Powledge, 1989). By that time maps should be completed not only of a range of micro-organisms, yeasts, plants, and non-human primate and other creatures, but, perhaps, of the progenitors of modern man whose tissues are available for examination. This prediction understands that the expression of the genome is modulated by extra-genetic information, leading to not always predictable differentiating pathways. Genetic determination is continuously modified in a random way by environment, with exposure to significant elements often determined by seemingly random individual behaviour. Mutations in the sequence of the billions of purine and pyrimidine nucleotides (basic subunits of DNA) within the genome are continuously produced in a random manner so that each individual's genome is unique and in a process of continuous transformation. This spontaneous diversity, articulated by Charles Darwin ('life is endless polymorphism'), has been termed 'a basic human right which would be violated by artificial modifications of the genome' (Mayor, 1985, p. 17).

However, most mutations are functionally silent. Those which alter the ability of resulting proteins to carry out their specific functions become apparent in succeeding generations as the gametes (sperm and ova) are affected. Mutagenic conditions are stimulated by physico-chemical or biological agents which increase the transformation of chromosomal endowment. The intervention of human beings in the process of natural selection (of the random product of mutations) must appreciate 'the amount of freedom which may be risked to obtain a benefit' (Mayor, 1985, p. 17). At the same time it has been considered a 'government responsibility', at least in some quarters, to maintain 'ecological conditions free from mutagens' (Mayor, 1989, p. 22).

The Value of Genome Mapping

A detailed chart of the genes is essential to ultimate progress in understanding the biology of living organisms and, specifically, to the clinical biotechnology aimed at the prevention and cure of genetic disease. Despite the ultimate value of the genome-mapping project, however, it has evoked some opposition within the scientific community, in part because of its massive potential drain upon funds, time and personnel.

Speculation about the eventual significance of the new genetics at a global level is difficult. In the short run its public health impact will be minimal. For most of the world's populations the death rates of infants and children from infection, malnutrition and injury are so high that saving a few from genetic disease is numerically insignificant. Even in the industrialized democracies the number so afflicted is relatively small. For individual parents and children, however, the human value of prediction, prevention and, perhaps, cure is incalculable. Furthermore, as elements of scientific knowledge are increasingly mixed with culturally transmitted myths, and the media carry more and more accounts of research, public interest in heredity remains high. Along with a general interest in science it is especially prominent in literate industrial societies in which the values of autonomy and justice are sometimes perceived as conflicting with those associated with order and predictability.

Legitimation, Priority, Public Costs

Questions of legitimation, potential use in the service of prejudiced viewpoints, and cost-effectiveness have been raised with regard to contemporary gene research. The scientific community is not unanimous in favouring a massive investment of time, energy, talent and money in the genome-mapping effort, draining it from other research activities. Some point to the tedious, routine nature of much of the research; they suggest that it will wastefully generate unlimited quantities of information with no use or ultimate value – catalogues of genes, units, filler material – requiring additional specific research which might have been undertaken more efficiently and less expensively without the enormous genome project. Criticisms of this kind, including accusations of inappropriate publicity and claims, have become a matter of public and media concern (Angier, 1990). Other negative points, relative especially to the question of just distribution of scarce resources, have been made: the probable multigenic origin of many diseases diminishes the likelihood of clinically useful results from the project; the continuing investment of limited resources in high-technology bioscience is irrelevant to the health needs of a large proportion of the world's peoples; and, especially, the mapping project (with its commercial potential) is capable of being self-supporting and could proceed without public funding draining much-needed resources from other endeavours (Cooper, 1989). At least one view holds that the 'real crisis in biomedical research today lies in maintaining the infrastructure of a rich variety of laboratories in academic institutions and in the training of eclectic, creative new investigators. Imbuing the human genome project with unearned moral status will not help in this pursuit' (Cooper, 1989, p. 874). Despite these concerns, however, it seems that the genome-mapping project enjoys sufficient international support to continue.

Clinical Gene Therapy

Therapeutic Introduction of the Normal Gene

As noted above, many hereditary diseases appear to be caused by a mutation in a single gene. The bulk of those which permit foetal development to the point of producing a living infant are, except for the blood diseases, due to defective or absent enzymes (Nichols, 1988). Immune deficiency diseases and single-gene enzyme disorders thus appear to be good candidates for gene therapy.

Gene therapy refers to the insertion of genetic material into a cell to correct a defect. It is based on the assumption that genetic disease should be treated by altering the mutant gene itself rather than focusing on the effects of its products. The therapeutic effort is to replace or supplement the defective genetically based information with that present within normal, functional genes. Copies of a normal gene, which has been isolated and cloned, are inserted into the patient's cells located within an organ or tissue, perhaps from the bone marrow. The inserted genes are expected to produce proteins which can correct the enzyme or biochemical defect.

Somatic versus Germ Line Therapy

The procedure described above is known as 'somatic line' treatment because the new gene is inserted into ordinary organ or tissue cells in a postnatal individual. In contrast to germ line therapy it does not lead to heritable changes. The latter refers to insertion of the gene into germ cells, such as sperm or ova. Such germ cells, or those of an early embryo, treated to correct a genetic defect would affect all of the cells of the body. Gene therapy can also involve the modification of a gene already in place, or surgery in which a particular gene is excised and may be replaced by a normal counterpart.

The introduction and incorporation of the gene utilizes an externally originating vector or carrier. Retroviruses, or RNA tumor viruses, can act as carriers for transplantation, inserting the fresh gene into the invaded cells. Although RNA viral vectors can be infectious, a safe vector for transplanting exogenous genes into human cells has been obtained by deleting a fragment of viral RNA responsible for disrupting the host cell after infection. Another step is designing tissue or cell-specific vectors. The most widely used models of gene therapy for cancer, hormonal disorders, and those of bone marrow, liver, and the central nervous system, are based on altering mutant target genes by gene transfer with recombinant viruses 'in order to express new genetic information and to correct disease phenotypes – the conversion of the swords of pathology into the plowshares of therapy' (Friedmann, 1989, pp. 1275–81).

In the USA, where all proposals for trials in this field require approval from the National Institute of Health's DNA Advisory Committee, few contemporary discussions of somatic cell gene therapy still argue its ethical acceptability. Concerns continue, however, about germ line therapy. These relate mainly to the transmission of unpredictable genetic effects into future generations, and diminishing genetic diversity among human populations. It is even possible that genes causing known genetic diseases may have other undiscovered survival functions so that their elimination might prove ultimately harmful to the human population. Fears also continue about the consequences of the human species' attempts to control its own heredity. Thus the prospect remains that, once gene therapy is available, individuals may take advantage of the opportunity to select their own genes on the basis of personal prejudice, caprice or, in any event, scientifically uninformed short-term bases (Congress, 1984, pp. 27–32). More drastically, 'Once we decide to begin the process of human genetic engineering, there is really no logical place to stop' (Rifkin, 1983, p. 232). If it alters parental expectations, and is 'applied over time to progressively milder medical problems . . . parents may more and more expect "perfect" children' (Congress, 1984, p. 34). The Parliamentary Assembly of the Council of Europe, with the possibility of centralized government control in mind, suggested that 'the rights to life and human dignity . . . imply the right to inherit a genetic pattern which has not been artificially changed' (Parliamentary Assembly, 1983).

The Commercialization and Patentability of Genetically Engineered Products

Biotechnology

Controlled biological processes were employed for human use long before the formal advent of biotechnology. Many products depending on such processes are so familiar that they are accepted without thought: vaccines, beer, wine, cheese, bread, and more recently antibiotics. Modern biotechnology follows in the course already begun by those who attempted to control biology, but did not have the knowledge and skill to modify cells. It has been defined as 'the genetic manipulation of cells to enhance the production of substances beneficial to humankind' (Joseph, 1987, p. 3; National Institute of General Medical Sciences, 1986, pp. 14, 20). In agriculture, gene-splicing technology has been used to increase animal and plant resistance to disease, control pests, regulate growth, and improve the overall quality and quantity of food for human consumption. In medicine, gene technologies have created a large, and growing, number of health care products and procedures (see, for example, Guyer and Koshland, 1989). A commercial interest in modern biotechnology became apparent in the USA by 1976 with the establishment of the first new firm to apply recombinant DNA technology to medicine and other areas. The field was opened to general entrepreneurial activity in 1980 when the US Supreme Court determined that a petroleum-consuming bacterium was patentable. By mid-March 1987 the US Patent and Trademark Office reported that more than 6000 patent applications were pending for bio-technology-related products. Under a new policy adopted on 3 April 1987 the Office agreed on the patentability of all life forms except *Homo sapiens* (still protected by US constitutional safeguards against slavery). The new policy regarded an animal engineered through human intervention, that is by methods of gene-splicing, as having characteristics not attainable through historic breeding techniques.

This method was also clearly differentiated from that of inserting genes into newly fertilized embryonic cells before implantation into a uterus (a technique already experimentally employed with humans who would otherwise be born with a hereditary disease). The engineered creature was designated a 'human invention', and, therefore, patentable. In the language of the Patent Office this 'invented' life-form was definable as a 'manufacture or composition of matter'. The new policy was disturbing to many observers. As one noted, it transforms all living things on the planet into the exploitable raw materials of a 'biotechnology age'. The biotic community is no longer a common heritage, but 'the private reserve of major corporations' (Rifkin, 1987).

Potential problems lie in the differences between national legal frameworks inevitably reflecting the societies in which they arose. While the US Patent Office, for example, 'now considers non-naturally occurring non-human multicellular living organisms, including animals, to be patentable subject matter' (United States, 1987), European nations still struggle with this issue and in much of the world it has not yet been addressed. The European Patent Convention of 1973 specifically included micro-organisms and their productive processes within the realm of patent protection. The same convention, however, prohibited granting patents on plant and animal varieties. Its Clause 53(b) was invoked in the European Patent Office's provisional rejection of an application for patenting a mouse genetically altered through insertion of an artificial cancer gene (Dickson, 1989). The rejection quoted the clause stating that no patent can be granted on an invention 'whose exploitation would be contrary to *ordre publique* or morality'. In Germany a historically rooted fear of anything related to genetic 'engineering' or manipulation has led to public attacks on biotechnology laboratories and one of the world's most comprehensive and, possibly, restrictive laws intended to regulate the deliberate use of recombinant organisms (Kahn, 1992).

In partial consequence of progress towards European economic integration a series of regulations regarding genetically engineered products (placed, in contrast to the US Food and Drug Administration, in a special category) will deal with the approval process, guidelines for worker safety, contained use of genetically modified organisms (GMOs), the deliberate release of GMOs, and, most relevant to human rights, the socio-economic effects of biotechnology products. These will be regulations enforceable throughout the European Community (Balter, 1991). However, the European Commission has also proposed that an invention should not be considered unpatentable solely because it is composed of living matter (Dickson, 1989). Further, the European Community's Committee for Proprietary Medicinal Products has been able to give more rapid marketing permission to biotechnological firms than the US FDA. On the other hand, in 1992 the US FDA made a ruling that appears to exempt genetically engineered food products from special testing before they are released to the market. Some observers feel that this may endanger the food supply (Krimsky, 1992). It is pointed out that allergenic substances may be introduced into food, a foreign gene may not behave in the same way in a new host as in the original species, and the nutritional value of particular foods may be affected. As Krimsky (1992) points out, it is a mistake to initiate genetic engineering by exempting large classes of products from a case-by-case review under the same laws that protect consumers from synthetic food additives.

Conflicting Investigative Interests: Exclusivity and Sharing

Academic investigators, often working in publicly supported laboratories, may experience a conflict of interest when they engage in research for commercial, or even political, rewards (see Chapter 8). The conflict is between the desire to know and to help, and that for personal profit in terms of money, power and prestige. Preserving new genetic products for commercial gain may deprive individuals or populations of their benefits. Loyalty to shareholders is not compatible with loyalty to the welfare of needy persons. Monopolies and patent applications maintain consumer prices for medical products at high levels. 'There is anguished ethical study of the dangers to academic research of the new practicality of biological research' (Koshland, 1986, p. x). An illustration of this complex issue concerns the relative costs of streptokinase and TPA, both used for dissolving blood clots after heart attacks. The former, costing a fraction of what is charged for the latter, is preferred in most countries. The latter is preferred by most US doctors, justifying their decision on theoretical grounds, although many are changing because they do not believe that the possible advantage is worth the extreme difference in cost. The manufacturer of the more expensive drug has engaged in aggressive marketing, an alleged consequence of which was to make some cardiologists afraid not to use it for fear of malpractice suits (Pollack, 1991). The legal battles between two corporations which have cloned and expressed recombinant human erythropoietin, an expensive drug used as replacement therapy for persons undergoing haemodialysis, have raised another issue. While those who invest in the development, manufacture and distribution of this and similar products are entitled to 'fair and reasonable profit', the scientific advances that made them possible are based on many years of research in government-supported laboratories: 'the public also deserves that these drugs, the products of long-standing public investment, be made widely available at fair and reasonable prices' (Doolittle, 1991).

Another aspect of commercial research is its semi-secret nature. This leads to a restriction on the flow of information about molecular biology and other scientific fields with potential commercial application. The pursuit of basic knowledge is limited at the source by the often easier availability of support for short-term, commercially useful, than for long-term basic research. Similar considerations apply to university-based cost-effectiveness research funded by pharmaceutical companies. It has been noted that the main interest of these companies in providing such research funding is to promote sales, and that they fund projects with a high likelihood of producing favourable results. Since many such companies expect to review manuscripts of results prior to publication a number of guidelines to preserve investigative objectivity in this kind of study have been suggested (Hillman et al., 1991).

Research knowledge is also removed from the public domain on military security grounds. Access to data related to such areas as biological warfare, the medical care of casualties or other aspects of military conquest has routinely been kept secret. In contrast, international health agencies recognize that health (as well as welfare) problems in one part of the human family inevitably place the rest of the family at risk. If funding health-related biological research of international significance is not to impair basic health services in particular nations, it must eventually be organized on an international basis. The moral value of sharing versus exclusiveness is a human rights issue. Unlike some nationally or commercially based centres the international Human Genome Organization, HUGO, has stated that all of its data should be freely available to the world's scientists, and 'not used to secure narrow national interests'.

Predicting the Life Course: Genes, Environment, Disease

Popular Concern with Genetic Testing

For most people an interest in heredity is highly personal with reference to particular diseases identified in their own families. For some this extends to members of their ethnic, cultural or racial group. With increasing information about inherited disease vulnerability, and the possibility of avoiding it by testing or behavioural change, the literate citizens of the industrialized democracies have begun to demand more understandable information about the hereditary process.

Consent to Genetic Testing and Medical Responsibility for its Results

A Committee of Experts of the Council of Europe (Muller, 1990) notes that autonomy requires full information, and that to be fully informed in regard to genetic testing people must know the following:

> 1) the purpose of the test; 2) the risk of the test itself, if any; 3) the risk that the test results will be incorrect or that the test will produce a finding not searched for; 4) the implications of a positive result; 5) the nature of the condition/disease the test is intended to detect; 6) the options available to reduce the burden of the disease in the event of a confirmed positive test; 7) the alternatives if the individual decides not to have the test (p. 11).

The 'sources of misuse of genetic tests' are recognized as 'numerous': 'inadequate methodology, insufficient numbers of properly trained test providers, a lack of understanding of genetics and genetic testing by health care professionals or by the public', and the use, the interpretation and the follow-up of genetic tests, particularly for 'common diseases', are recognized as 'difficult' (p. 9). The committee strongly recommends that national laws permit long-term data storage in the interest of multigenerational health care and urges the development of genetic registers 'kept according to strict rules concerning data protection' (p. 17). Finally, it suggests considerations to be taken into account in testing for genes which predispose to common disorders later in life:

l) There must be an improvement of the quality of life through medical measures for the predisposed person if a predisposition is detected; 2) Any preventive measures which can be taken in persons having a given condition should not be heroic but generally acceptable; 3) The psychological burden caused by a positive test result must be alleviated by adequate support systems which have to be established; 4) There must be no social or financial pressure against someone with a positive test result; 5) Data protection rules should be strict and secured with laws (p. 29).

Privacy and Control of Individual Genetic Data

Prenatal and postnatal genetic screening can add to personal autonomy by obtaining information which can broaden the scope of individual reproductive choice and improve the possibilities of individual disease prevention, including that which may not emerge until middle or old age. The information could also be beneficial to relatives, especially offspring. The new ability to obtain data allowing the prediction of life courses, as well as monitoring to identify the possible genetic impact of occupational hazards, has been considered valuable by health experts.

However, the newly available information has raised questions about personal privacy, access to this kind of knowledge by others whose interest may not be beneficial to the subject, and the possibilities of restrictive or exclusionary action based upon it by public and private institutions such as insurance companies, employers, health care providers and governments. These concerns are inherent in the Council of Europe's Expert Committee recommendations (above) for data protection. It may be difficult to weigh the potential benefits versus the social harms of disclosure of genetic information. Requested access to information by those not genetically related to the subject, such as insurance companies and employers, with the capacity to reject insurance coverage or not to hire, raises issues of fairness or justice (Congress, 1984). New genetic screening technologies can give insurance companies even more data for stratifying the risk in the pool of potentially insurable people, for example in a particular workplace, and thus for excluding them from coverage. The likelihood is high that such genetic knowledge may be used inappropriately, resulting in an overestimation of individual risk. Many whose potential genetic disease will never emerge can be excluded. Perhaps in consequence of the growth of a legal structure aimed at protecting workers from discrimination there appears to have been 'little or no growth' in the use of genetic monitoring or screening technologies in the workplace between 1983 and 1990 (Congress, 1990).

Other commentators have discussed the question of who should be informed about the results of such testing, and when, if ever, incidental findings, such as paternity, should be disclosed. Among the controversial possibilities are screening workers for susceptibility to certain occupational diseases. According to one view, 'the tests are morally justified to the extent they enhance worker health in a manner consistent with established ethical principles' (Congress, 1988d). The problem seems to be the possibility that if tests are administered by management (rather than voluntarily taken by workers) their results will be used in ways which will enhance management's power rather than workers' health.

Genetic Counselling

This is an area in which human rights, personal psychosocial and scientific–clinical considerations overlap more obviously than in many aspects of medical practice. Many illnesses are due significantly to single chromosomal or gene effects, or stem from developmental or environmental factors (such as diet, smoking, alcohol ingestion, viral infections, chemical exposures, solar ray exposures) interacting with genetically induced vulnerability. However, as Eric Lander has stated, 'The frontier is diseases of more complex inheritance' (Marx, 1990, p. 1540). As noted above, susceptibility to many of the diseases with major public health significance appears to be multigenic. In these instances the genes may contribute only 10–20 per cent of an individual's susceptibility to illness, rather than 100 per cent as in the case of single-gene disorders. None the less, genetic information could provide the possibility of early warnings of such illness with the opportunity for intervention.

Prenatal screening and prediction has developed as part of the effort to ensure the birth of healthy offspring. In this setting genetic counselling has usually been requested by couples prior to conceiving, most often on the basis of their family histories, or having already had a diseased or defective infant. It was not until 1976 in the USA, however, that the National Genetic Diseases Act made counselling generally available through federal funding. Now prospective parents can learn about the nature of particular disorders and the likelihood of their occurrence. Crucial to the counselling process, as it takes all available information into account, is a non-directive stance increasing the potential parents' ability to make the choices which fit their own needs, desires and backgrounds – but with full understanding of the possible outcomes.

Routine Prenatal and Neonatal Screening and Testing for Genetic and Congenital Disease or Defect

Prenatal and newborn screening of all mothers and infants on a routine basis vary from country to country. A central human rights issue is the potential parents' freedom to choose, within the context of counselling and discussion with trained individuals, what they consider the most desirable response to knowledge that they are carriers of genetic disease, or that they are pregnant with a damaged or potentially damaged or diseased embryo or foetus. The response could include pregnancy termination (abortion), preparation to care for a defective child or to consider institutionalizing it, or even foetal therapy. Neither public education nor personal preparation for an emotionally disturbing outcome in this area can be taken for granted. It falls within the purview of the right to knowledge essential for the preservation of life and health.

There is no substantial database about the actual post-diagnosis behaviour of pregnant women in response to their knowledge of a damaged or potentially damaged or diseased embryo or foetus. One US study of 395 parents of children diagnosed as having cystic fibrosis elicited a 68 per cent response. A majority supported legal abortion in the first trimester for all of 23 sample situations depicting status as a carrier of a serious illness, or actual embryonic–foetal damage or disease. In respect of a guess at one's personal behaviour, 58 per cent said that they would abort for severe mental retardation, 40 and 41 per cent for genetic disease leading to death before the age of 5 or a child bedridden for life, and lesser degrees for less severe conditions. Twenty per cent said that they would abort with prior knowledge that their child would have cystic fibrosis (Wertz et al., 1991).

All 50 of the US states routinely screen all newborns for the genetic diseases of phenylketonuria and hypothyroidism, which occur with low frequency (approximately 1 in 12 000 children has phenylketonuria and 1 in 4000 has hypothyroidism). This permits treatment before the full-blown disease develops and before growth and development are impaired. Some states screen for other rare inherited disorders as well. The screening is so generally accepted as a hospital routine that parental objection is rare. However, mandatory or even elective predictive screening can be problematic because of the fallibility of available methods.

Of the large number of gene-induced disorders some 250 diseases and birth defects can be diagnosed prenatally (Nightingale and

Goodman, 1990). The available prenatal tests are not usually used for routine screening, but on an individual basis, often requested by people who consider themselves at risk. Even before a pregnancy occurs it is possible to detect whether either prospective parent carries genes for certain disorders. However, without a family history there is no reason for a person to regard himself or herself at risk, and general population screening for this purpose is not yet feasible. Prenatal testing, depending upon the procedure and the disorder for which it searches, has varying degrees of certainty. A negative finding will be reassuring. A positive finding could permit intra-uterine treatment if such is available; more often it helps parents anticipate the birth and treatment of an affected child, or it may be a reason to consider pregnancy interruption. Details of the available tests which can 'assist in one of the most formidable of life's choices' are now accessible to the educated, non-professional public (Nightingale and Goodman, 1990, p. 43). But in every instance personal counselling is essential.

The AFP (alpha-fetoprotein) determination to detect neural tube defects, leading to such disorders as anencephaly, spina bifida and meningomyelocele, is routinely offered to patients by many US obstetricians. In some parts of the world, such as Cuba, it is used as a screen and positive findings are, reportedly, more often than not followed by abortion.

For some parents in a private practice setting, a positive test, also indicative of about 20 per cent of cases of Down's syndrome, may also be taken as an indication to terminate the pregnancy. For others, it is the cue to arrange for necessary surgical care immediately after birth (Nightingale and Goodman, 1990). However, all positive tests do not necessarily mean pathology, and negative tests are not invariable assurances of normality. If there is reason to suspect difficulty additional studies, as with the ultrasonogram to visualize the embryo or foetus, should be undertaken (see Chapter 3).

Each of the other commonly used tests has its own scientific or clinical, personal or psychosocial and human rights advantages and drawbacks. Amniotic fluid testing does not usually produce useful data until the pregnancy has entered its second trimester, when interrupting a pregnancy can be more traumatic than in earlier periods of development. Or, if laboratory error requires another sample, by that time the foetus may be old enough to survive in an advanced neonatal intensive care unit, severely curtailing the parents' options (Nightingale and Goodman, 1990, p. 35).

Cells from the chorionic villi, containing the same genetic information as the foetus, can be obtained as early as nine weeks into pregnancy and analysis, indicating a number of disorders, is rapid. Genetic disorders can also be diagnosed by direct 'gene probe' techniques with foetal tissue, and by an indirect method, the RFLP test, which has been used to track the epidemiology of Huntington's disease. Other techniques are being developed. Again, however, on a global basis, these options are available only to a tiny minority of the world's parents.

In the USA, despite the increasing frequency of pregnancy monitoring in vulnerable women, it is estimated that well over 100 000 infants are born yearly with genetic disease. The most common are Down's syndrome, cystic fibrosis, neural tube defects, sickle-cell disease and Tay–Sachs disease. The last two characteristically appear in families of particular racial–ethnic descent which may have minority status, depending upon national or social context – sickle-cell disease in persons of African, and Tay–Sachs in those of Eastern European Jewish background. In the case of Tay–Sachs the US Eastern European Jewish community has become a strongly involved constituency for prevention, and through a system of confidential testing has been able to avoid a significant number of marriages between carriers (Merz, 1987).

The diagnosis of sickle-cell disease, in particular, became traumatic for African–Americans, since no treatment was available and the label became stigmatizing. The injustices stemming from thoughtless legislation by some state governments in this instance have been reviewed by Nightingale and Goodman (1990, pp. 64–5). Programmes mandated the sickle-cell trait screening of specific, arbitrarily chosen groups (typically those with little social power) rather than encouraging voluntary participation. Many laws did not provide confidentiality, public education about the disease, or other safeguards. Discrimination against trait carriers came to include higher life insurance premiums, and recommendations that certain jobs be closed to them. Since carriers were predominantly (though not exclusively) African–American, the racist implications of these restrictions created concern. Since that time it has become possible to justify screening. Antibiotic therapy to infants with sickle-cell disease reduces the likelihood of infection with early death, and new possibilities of definitive treatment are changing the social significance of the diagnosis.

Should Development of a Genetic Test be Followed by Routine Screening? The Case of Cystic Fibrosis

The genetic disorder receiving greatest US attention in the 1980s and early 1990s is cystic fibrosis; it is the most common lethal genetic disease, affecting, according to various estimates, 1 in 1800 to 2500 newborns. It can be identified in 85 per cent of newborns by measuring the pancreatic enzyme, trypsin, in the blood. While the remainder can be identified by testing sodium chloride in sweat, this cannot be done until the infant is two months old and may already show signs of disease. This has added urgency to the search for the abnormal gene, even though the long-term value of early diagnosis and treatment is not yet established. However, as guidelines to incorporate screening for the abnormal gene into routine medical practice were being organized at the US National Institutes of Health (NIH), evidence became available that the cystic fibrosis mutations are much more complex than had been anticipated (Roberts, 1990). A major basis for testing was to have been the finding (by Lap-Chee Tsui and by Francis Collins) of a simple mutation responsible for most cases of the disease in about 75 per cent of those carrying the abnormal gene. The 'entrepreneurial interest . . . in what could become a billion-dollar industry' (Wilfond and Frost, 1990, p. 2777) is illustrated by the speed with which a number of biotechnology companies offered a DNA test to detect this particular mutation. However, a considerable number of other, albeit rare, mutations have since been identified, and it is suspected that a significant proportion may remain unaccounted for even after continuing and extensive research. This complicates the question of widespread genetic screening in general since the same problem, of differing mutations in different unrelated persons, is true for other disorders linked to the x-chromosome, such as haemophilia and Duchenne muscular dystrophy. With a 75 per cent accurate test, the disease could be precluded or its severity reduced in 56 per cent of those affected. As reported by Roberts (1990), however, some investigators fear that screening with an imperfect test would do more harm than good, particularly for couples receiving inconclusive reports, some of whom might decide to abort healthy foetuses. Other investigators, including members of the NIH panel, agree that testing should be available, but on a specific rather than a routine basis. It should be voluntary, with protected confidentiality and informed consent, and should be accompanied by appropriate education and counselling. Emphasis should be on high-risk individuals and families rather than on mass screening. Wilfond and Fost (1990) conclude:

> Regardless of improvements in the detection rate, implementation of population screening should be delayed until pilot studies that demonstrate its safety and effectiveness are completed . . . pre-conception testing should be offered to adult relatives of cystic fibrosis patients . . . following institutional review board approval . . . to ensure that strict standards of informed consent, education, quality control of the testing procedure, and counseling are followed (p. 2777).

Genetic Screening and Counselling with Regard to Mental Illness

Uncertainty is particularly high in counselling people with family histories of mental illness as to whether or not they should reproduce, since their potential child-rearing behaviour, as well as their genetic loading, must be taken into account. In the absence of valid and reliable data for use by trained counsellors, the enthusiasm of psychiatric investigators for a genetic aetiology of mental illness, and the ready incorporation into popular wisdom of a hereditary basis for 'insanity', make it especially important that predictions on the basis of biological markers take the influence of the social–interpersonal context into account. Investigators with a strong commitment to the biomedical model sometimes ignore the fact that phenotypic expressions of genic tendencies require significant inter-action between the predisposition and particular environmental elements, and may even require specific diseases as co-factors.

While a large scientific literature supports the probability of some genetic predisposition to schizophrenia, there is also evidence that the appearance of clinically diagnosable schizophrenia can be made more likely by neurological defects (such as may be incurred during difficult births, or in consequence of infantile or maternal viral or other disease), or environmental stresses; similarly it may be less likely because of interpersonal, protective factors (Watt et al., 1984). Available data suggest that 'rarely . . . does genetic influence account for more than half of the variance of behavioral characteristics . . . non-genetic sources of variance must be given serious consideration' (Plomin, 1989, p. 645). The genetic source of variance appears to be multiple: 'results . . . suggest heterogeneity in the genetic factors predisposing to schizophrenia' (Kidd, 1989, p. 645). Cerebral ana-tomical abnormalities in the schizophrenic member of monozygotic twin pairs discordant for schizophrenia were attributed to non-genetic factors (Suddath et al., 1990). These findings from magnetic resonance imaging were present in 12 of 15 twin sets, including the only two with a family history of schizophrenia. Data of this kind support two overlapping ideas which have been in the research literature for approximately 75 years. One is that 'schizophrenia' comprises a group of disorders and may represent a final common pathway reachable through more than one route. The other is that brain structure and function are implicated in its development. It appears, nevertheless, that neither brain damage, even early in development, nor a family history, nor a particular developmental experience are necessary, unique or sufficient causes of this compli-cated disorder.

The hereditary predisposition to variants of manic-depressive disease has seemed more likely on the basis of family pedigrees than that for schizophrenia. However, the data do not yet permit absolute certainty. Reports, for example, by Janice Egeland and her group that manic-depressive disease in a particular family in an inbred community was caused by a single gene on chromosome 11 (although approximately 40 per cent of those with the genetic finding did not develop the disorder) have not been replicated. Among the research problems identified by Kelsoe and colleagues were consistency and clear definition of the clinical diagnostic criteria used for case identification and the need to follow the reservoir of potential patients for a sufficiently long time to identify additional cases of disease as they appear in individuals not meeting the criteria at the time of the study (Barinaga, 1989). Such findings lend credence to those of Kendler et al. (1987) who appear to have demonstrated through methods of multivariate genetic analysis that genes act largely in a non-specific way to influence the overall level of psychiatric symptoms. In predisposed persons environmental stress seems to have a more specific impact on associated anxiety symptoms than on those of depression itself. Linkages between manic-depressive illness and gene markers on a number of chromosomes may point to different hereditary forms of manic depression (Baron, 1989). All these findings indicate the difficulties in making unequivocal predictions about the emergence of disease, even in the presence of a positive family history, and the possible cost in stigmatization, mental pain and unsupported decisions when counsellors fail to take all variables into account.

Genetic Prediction of Degenerative Brain Disease

In this instance, as in others, advances in genetics may lead to improved diagnostic capabilities more often than effective therapy. The ability to diagnose, and thus for the afflicted individual to predict personal death or disability, often adds to the burden of pain while contributing little or nothing to the ability to cope with it. In some cases, therefore, vulnerable people may not wish to take advantage of predictive technology. For example, predictions of the clinical appearance of untreatable, hereditary and always deteriorative and fatal Huntington's disease can influence a personal decision not to take the risk of producing a child who might be doomed to the same fate. However, persons with a family history of the disease, who have already decided not to have children, may not wish to know whether they are themselves at risk for this fate. Another kind of ethical problem has arisen because of obstacles encountered by the French Institut National d'Etudes Démographiques in its plan to notify potential carriers of a hereditary form of juvenile glaucoma (approximately 30 000 families were at risk for the disorder) that can lead to blindness in order that they could receive early treatment aimed at preventing blindness (Dorozynski, 1991). In this instance, although the INED investigators felt that notification with its promise of prevention was urgent, and that nationwide screening as a possible substitute was not feasible, they were blocked by the French privacy law, controlled by the Commission Nationale d'Informatique et des Libertés (CNIL). CNIL has ruled that INED can only notify physicians to be alert to the possibility of juvenile glaucoma among their patients, and its hereditary nature, but cannot give them the identities of vulnerable or affected families or individuals. According to the law, 'even in the domain of medical research such information can, in certain cases, cause prejudice to a patient because it informs him he is affected by a severe disease'. Proposals to change it have been rejected because, in the words of CNIL president at the time (1989) Jacques Fauvet, 'they did not provide for a satisfactory equilibrium between the interests of public health, the respect of fundamental liberties, and the rights of men, notably the right to respect privacy' (Dorozynski, 1991, p. 370). An emphasis on patient autonomy, equitable access to treatment, action based on emotional bonds between family members and health providers, and an informed public, would clearly argue in favour of notification and treatment of vulnerable persons, and against an abstract, and possibly distorted, view of 'fundamental liberties' which deprives families and their members of informed consent.

Research on Alzheimer's disease, called presenile dementia in an earlier era, suggests that its neuropathology is the basis for much, although not all, of the clinical pictures once designated as senile dementia. It has been reported that, at least in some familial lines, it is caused by a defective gene located on chromosome 21, the same which has been identified as causing Down's syndrome (St George-Hyslop et al., 1987). A marker has also been discovered on chromosome 21 for the gene that produces amyloid, a protein found in the neural tangles and clumps characteristic of the brains of several species of aged animals as well as in human Alzheimer's patients. These findings will ultimately make it possible to clearly distinguish familial Alzheimer's disease from other forms (Barnes, 1987). However, while it may have eventual familial usefulness, it so far promises no immediate relief for individual sufferers since the two forms of the disease are clinically similar and there is no available treatment for either. Further, there is a possibility of overevaluating the hereditary aspects of the disease with the needless imposition of anxiety, decisions not to reproduce, and other consequences as individual information is disseminated into various computerized data banks (as for insurance, employment, or social security).

Finally, the emergence of clinical disease may require exceptional longevity in many persons. Thus, if they live into their 90s, half the immediate family members of any Alzheimer's patient may develop the disorder; with this longevity close relatives appear to have four to five times the risk of developing the disease as the general population (Mohs et al., 1987). The most general human rights question raised by this research domain concerns how society should deal with the kind of predictive information which it supplies.

It is especially important when evaluating the genetic loading for any disease with a hereditary component to remember, as noted above, that genes do not act in isolation. Thus, a viral infestation in a mutant gene, or cumulative environmental stress over a lifetime, may be necessary to bring out the genetic effect. Knowledge of the possibility of future occurrence alone cannot be used for intelligent medical counselling, because mere identification of a predisposition does not permit prediction as to the timing of a disease's occurrence, or whether or not it will, indeed, occur.

Predicting Socially Condemned or Deprecated Behaviours

A major area of uncertainty in the definition of behaviour patterns as disease involves those which are socially condemned or defined as deviant. Genetic, as well as early behavioural, screens to predict the later possibility of psychosocially deviant behaviour have raised fears about violating the civil rights of those about whom the predictions are made. If childhood predictions for poor learning ability, later anti-social, asocial or aggressive acts, or a sexual orientation not fitting the approved norm, become known to teachers and parents, this may result in expectations of socially unacceptable behaviour. The ensuing attitudes of these and other adult reward-givers and punishers can facilitate the appearance of the unwanted behaviour; knowledge of the screening result, valid or not, creates a 'self-fulfilling prophecy'. The availability of such information may also lead to invasions of privacy as it is included in the records of insurance companies, third-party health service payers, potential employers, potential marriage partners, and others, including government agencies. In these instances predictions could be used by third parties to grant or deny access to opportunity, as in education or employment, which may be considered essential to the full development of innate potential and, hence, a human right.

Socio-medical Corollaries and Consequences of Predictions

The most pervasive issues regarding prediction relate to health care. In most of the world basic health care is simply unavailable. In the USA, and less obviously in countries with national health systems, there are significant inequities in its availability (see Chapter 8). These inequities are determined mainly by the social or economic status of those in need which, when low, often overlaps with ethnic minority status. It makes little sense from the pubic health standpoint to emphasize prenatal testing for genetic disease in a setting in which significant numbers of pregnant women receive inadequate general prenatal care, or none at all.

Prenatal testing, whether for congenital defects which may be of genetic origin, or for other foetal abnormalities, raises basic questions of cost, equitable distribution and access. There are also frequently overlooked problems of reliability and validity. For example, a variety of studies in Europe and Canada have suggested that chorionic villus testing, adopted with enthusiasm by many physicians and their patients, may be less accurate than amniocentesis and more often yields ambiguous results requiring subsequent amniocenteses (Rosenthal, 1991).

As noted in Chapter 4, 'government's obligation to ensure the provision of medical services is not unlimited' (Blumstein, 1989, p. 9). Care involving the unborn, infants and children, however, has particular symbolic significance in terms of a government's benevolent, paternalistic image. To the degree that some ethnic populations utilize resources not needed by or unavailable to others, particular problems of justice, that is to say, equitable access, may arise. The high prevalence of cystic fibrosis in a reservoir including 'essentially the entire population of Caucasian ancestry' could lead to the largest demand for genetic screening and counselling ever experienced; by the same token, 'members of non-Caucasian races also get CF, but at much lower rates, raising very difficult issues in this regard' (Nightingale and Goodman, 1990, p. 72). Screening for the most serious and prevalent genetic disorders for which technology is available (cystic fibrosis, sickle-cell disease, haemophilia, Duchenne's muscular dystrophy) would require more than four million tests yearly, with follow-up for at least 46 000 women – those who have tested positive and seek care in the first two months of their first pregnancy (Holtzman, 1988). No industrial nation has the capacity to manage this kind of demand, and none is making the effort to train genetic counsellors who could handle it.

In most industrialized countries administrative factors associated with how medical practice is organized are as important determinants of whether a screening test is used as are its medical indications. In the USA the possibility of malpractice suits has led to the development of screens aimed at excluding potential litigants. The varying personal circumstances of those who are screened contribute to variation in the rights-related consequences of predictions from case to case. For example, if the prediction is prenatal, as in the case of neural tube defect through alpha-fetoprotein determinations, which also detect between one-quarter and one-third of foetuses with Down's syndrome, there has been argument between the scientific and legal advisers of obstetricians over the best course to take (Elias and Annas, 1987b). Parents may wish to take the chance of having a healthy infant, but the hazards of congenital defect have usually been sufficient to make them consider terminating the pregnancy. (Professional pressure in this respect is not acceptable in the USA, where non-directive genetic counselling has been agreed upon by the American Society for Human Genetics.) Most recently the sono-graphic diagnosis of neural tube and ventral wall defects has become so accurate as to question the wisdom of routine amniocentesis for women with elevated alpha-fetoprotein levels and a structurally normal foetus as determined by ultrasonography. The risk level of having an affected foetus under these circumstances is stated to be less than the reported risk of abortion due to amniocentesis (Nadel et al., 1990). Regardless of specific indications for the use of these predictive techniques, there is general agreement that they should be preceded and followed by counselling, covering both their aims and consequences (Elias and Annas, 1987a).

If a prediction of defect or disease is postnatal the person is, as suggested above, at risk of stigmatization and impaired ability to become employed, married or otherwise involved in rewarding pursuits. As already noted it is possible to predict, although without absolute accuracy, the possibility of other conditions for which no treatment or prevention is possible. Multi-battery screening, inclu-ding the detection of 'pre-symptomatic disease' has already led to predictions being used for economic reasons by gatekeepers of the health care system. Nelkin and Tancredi (1989) emphasize the human rights hazards to vulnerable socio-economically dis-advantaged persons identified by the screens. Hospital administ-rators try to separate out patients whose future illnesses can be expected to require expensive care, for which they may be unable to pay, from those who can be expected to have few illnesses, respond quickly to treatment, and, therefore, be profitable. In the USA reports are multiplying about insurance discrimination against persons with genetically based disorders, or even those vulnerable to them by virtue of family history, of the sort usually encountered by chronic-ally disabled or diseased individuals. This has extended to health maintenance organizations' refusal to pay for amniocentesis in women with family histories of genetic disease unless assured that positive findings would be followed by abortion, or for tests confirming neural tube defects on the grounds that a 'pre-existing condition' was present (Blakeslee, 1990). Some scientists have recommended that genetic testing for insurance and employment should be halted until these human rights issues are clarified.

Other Human Rights Hazards of Genetic Technology

The new possibilities of controlling life have raised widespread concern about changes in the human view of human nature, and in the ultimate nature or essence of being 'human'. In 1983 a resolution signed by 56 US religious leaders, sent to Congress and introduced into the Congressional Record, urged that 'efforts to engineer specific genetic traits into the germ line of the human species' should not be undertaken. This touches on a concern for the sanctity of human life addressed by many thinkers, including the President's Commission (1982).

A committee of the European Parliament has proposed that European efforts to map and sequence the human genome should include substantial support for studies of the social and ethical implications of such research (Dickson, 1989). The international Human Genome Organization (HUGO) has its own ethics committee. Workers based in various national centres all recognize that social and ethical problems will arise in consequence of the effort, and all have their own ethics advisory bodies. In the USA the editor of the journal of the American Association for the Advancement of Science recognized the potential human rights significance of genome mapping when he wrote:

> A genome sequence should not be a precondition of employment, and legislation might be needed if that problem were to arise. However, less accurate data of the same type would be available today from family histories, and that does not seem to be part of current employment forms. If more accurate information provides temptation for abuse, action will be needed (Koshland, 1989, p. 189).

It may be more accurate to say that, if there is a temptation for it, that abuse will occur, sooner or later. Protective or preventive interventions are essential to prepare for these and cope with them as they occur.

The possible production of aberrant life forms, such as interspecies hybrids including 'humanoids', and changes in the essential character of human beings through genetic manipulation have been a greater concern in Europe than in North America. The prospect of cloning human beings, a topic of great popular interest, has been so universally rejected as to preclude extensive scientific discussion. The year 1975, however, saw creation of a French national 'Commission d'Ethique' which paid attention to this issue; in 1982 the

'Comité de Bioéthique Médicale' of the French National Institute of Health and Medical Research was requested to advise on genetic manipulation research. In 1982 the Parliamentary Assembly of the Council of Europe, responding to warnings of potential danger from the application of genetic engineering techniques to human beings, adopted a system of reciprocal information-sharing on this score and in 1984 recommended to its 21 Member States that similar information-sharing be initiated about all projects involving the use of recombinant DNA. By now interest was widespread. In 1984 and 1985 multidisciplinary conferences in several countries considered the new reproductive technologies, genetic engineering and other developments in applied science with a focus on the protection of individual integrity. Mayor has emphasized the possibility that genetic research might fundamentally alter the human genome, interpreting the Spanish Constitution's declaration, 'All have a right to live' as guaranteeing each person's right to his or her individual genome. He considered that

> the greatest danger to human biology and personal rights lies in the manipulation of human genes before and after fertilization . . . by different methods of artificial procreation, the manipulation of fertilized ova, modifications introduced into somatic cells with thera-peutic objectives, and alterations of gametes (Mayor, 1985, pp. 5, 6).

A number of other potential human rights threats from gene research have been noted, although not thoroughly studied. Among them are the possible development of a parental obligation to remedy the genetic problems of foetuses *in utero* various eugenic possibilities in pursuit of a culturally or otherwise prescribed 'perfect child'.

It has also been asserted that promotion of the genome mapping programme has proceeded with insufficient discussion either by professionals or the public: a 'real danger' may be 'the possible emergence of an establishment program to invade the rights and privacy of individuals, whether in the area of sexual preference, or right to abortion, or drug addiction, under cover of beneficent eugenic intervention' (Luria, 1989, p. 873). Similarly, critics have attacked the implication that 'human beings reduce to their genomes' and wonder about the possibility that genetic engineering may be used to create human beings with characteristics considered desirable by those with social power: 'How would the cost of dehumanization inherent in fabrication of people compare with the benefits of eradicating certain diseases?' (Berkowitz, 1989, p. 874). In contrast, 'there is the immorality of omission – the failure to apply a great new technology to aid the poor, the infirm, and the under-privileged' (Koshland, 1989).

Other Social Issues Arising from Genetic Research

Human Rights Concerns in Forensic Medicine

Gene technologies bear on human rights issues in forensic cases such as the identification of lineage in paternity suits and identification of suspected criminals. Understanding their role and relevance in such cases requires discussion of the admissibility of scientifically obtained evidence (the result of a potentially fallible technology) into the legal process with its inevitable consequences for the civil rights of the persons involved. A review by Stenson (1989) compares the Frye standard (*Frye* v. *United States*, 293 F 1013, 1014 [D.C. Cir. 1923]) of evidence with the relevancy standard in this respect. Frye states:

> Just when a scientific principle or discovery crosses the line between the experimental and demonstrable stages is difficult to define. Somewhere in this twilight zone the evidential force of the principle must be recognized, and while courts will go a long way in admitting expert testimony deduced from a well-recognized scientific principle or discovery, the thing from which the deduction is made must be sufficiently established to have gained general acceptance in the particular field in which it belongs.

The issues in summary form are: 1) What constitutes 'general acceptance'? 2) Which scientific community will accept the technique? 3) What methods will the court use to decide whether the technique has gained general acceptance?

The alternative relevancy standard, associated with Charles T. McCormick, states that courts should admit relevant conclusions supported by a qualified expert witness unless their admission will prejudice or mislead the jury or consume undue time. An obvious problem concerns the jury's ability to understand and properly evaluate novel scientific evidence such as DNA typing. Another problem is that the relevancy approach does not involve verifying the reliability of the scientific procedure prior to admission. Users assume that the adversarial process of the courtroom will allow the opposing side to criticize scientific evidence.

DNA 'fingerprinting', which reveals an individual's unique alleles in several DNA regions, and the genetic analysis of blood and other tissue samples have been major tools. In view of the extreme unlikelihood of two people (excluding identical twins) having the same DNA type, 'virtual certainty' has been the typical maxim communicated in the literature to describe confidence in accuracy of identifying the person in question. Tommie Lee Andrews in 1987 was the first person in the USA to be convicted on the basis of DNA printing, and her case was the first appellate decision on the admissibility of DNA prints (Rymer, 1989). However, the Andrews court rejected the requirement that scientific evidence be 'generally accepted' (the Frye test) and substituted the relevancy standard – ruling, in effect, that novel scientific evidence could be admitted by the same standard as used for other expert testimony. The human rights concern here related to a potential 'information gap' between the introduction of a new technique and its subsequent independent validation: at the time of the trial the reliability of the DNA test developed by Lifecodes, the company doing the typing, had yet to be verified by the scientific community (Bechtold, 1989).

Since that time two rebuffs of Lifecodes' fingerprinting evidence have changed the legal picture. On 14 August 1989 a judge refused to allow DNA evidence in court after the data and Lifecodes' evidence had been discredited at a pre-trial hearing. Forensic experts for both the defence and the prosecution testified that the laboratory procedures used to match bloodstains found on the defendant's wristwatch with blood samples from the victim were so flawed as to render the resulting evidence 'unreliable'. However, the judge did rule that other DNA typing could be admitted if processed under recognized guidelines. This case set the precedent for the reopening of 60 convictions in 27 US states which used DNA-related analyses (Anderson, 1989).

In the other case the failure of Lifecodes' DNA semen typing results, received on 18 August 1988, to confirm an obvious suspect identified by every other possible means, and its subsequent indication on the basis of blood studies that another suspect was the culprit, led to an examination of whether the DNA data could, indeed, be admitted in court. By December 1989 repeated examinations revealed a series of irregularities in handling the data, evidence of problems of measurement and in accounting for expectable data variations, as well as apparent mislabelling and failures to carry out independent checks. These had resulted in the failure to identify the apparent criminal and the misidentification of another suspect (Norman, 1989). The evidence that DNA 'fingerprinting' is subject to both human and technical error, and does not, in fact, result in 'virtual certainty' of identification has led to the appointment of a committee of the US National Academy of Sciences to draw up guidelines for the procedure.

Most commentators on DNA technologies in forensic settings have noted similar human rights issues. Basic is the lack of scientific standards for technological data to be admitted to the courtroom (Hoeffel, 1990). The US Supreme Court has classified taking blood samples as a search and seizure under the fourth amendment so that police can take samples only after obtaining a warrant based on showing probable cause. However, DNA testing seems most useful when the police lack probable cause (Tande, 1989). Tande (1989) suggests that law enforcement authorities should automatically destroy all tests and related records of non-matching suspects after their completion. Concern has been expressed about the lack of accreditation of forensic laboratories, the importance of guaranteed access by indigent defendants to free testing by a neutral laboratory, and the opportunity for opposing sides to retest their own samples (Pearsall, 1989). Forced or even voluntary submission to testing could constitute a threat to privacy if the information were placed in an available computer database. Thus a 'genetic fishing expedition' could involve a search for all people in a certain area with a similar genetic anomaly. Calls for massive voluntary DNA testing to solve a crime could make a suspect of everyone who refuses (Moss, 1988).

More recent techniques have involved the use of maternally inherited mitochondrial DNA. These have been used in establishing the parentage of children suspected of being the offspring of kidnapped or murdered victims of the Argentinian military during the approximately seven years beginning in 1976. Some of these children were adopted by couples unaware of their circumstances; others were reportedly kept by guards at secret detention centres where victims were held. Among the issues raised is whether 'one who was involved in the military repression should be allowed to benefit from it by keeping a child obtained under such conditions', and the possibility that 'it would be severely damaging to find out in adulthood that an adoptive parent was connected to the torture and death of one's biologic parents' (Raymond, 1989, p. 1393). In these instances psychotherapists are also involved, in the interests of the child. This work carried out by geneticist Mary-Claire King has been reported by her in several lectures and publications since 1984 (Raymond, 1989).

The US National Academy of Sciences report was issued in April 1992 (Roberts, 1992). Recognizing the scientific and technical problems involved it called for quality assurance with mandatory accreditation and proficiency testing to be overseen by scientists, not practitioners, and agreed with the need to establish population frequencies for each allele as a baseline for estimating the likelihood of a match. Among a series of other recommendations it called for the establishment of a National Committee on Forensic DNA Typing with the primary task of evaluating new approaches, and dealing with a variety of statistical, ethical and technical questions. From the human rights standpoint it is noteworthy that the committee favoured overall responsibility for the effort by the US health rather than the justice establishment, and recommended against a comprehensive national DNA profile data bank as premature and interfering with the privacy of genetic data.

The Dangers of Uncontrolled Genetically Altered Organisms

Much concern has centred on the possibility of releasing new strains of genetically altered organisms into the environment. The 1973 Gordon Scientific Conference on Nucleic Acids led a group from the US National Academy of Sciences to recommend in 1974 the cessation of some experiments pending the development of methods to prevent possible dissemination of artificially created recombining molecules. Recommendations also included the establishment of an advisory committee to assess the dangers inherent in genetic alterations, and to develop safety and ethical guidelines for future research (Ribes, 1978). In 1975 the US Asilomar Conference authorized resumption of experiments, while laying down stringent safety requirements both for the laboratories in which such investigations would be carried out, and for the biological systems studied. Although in 1981 the Social and Economic Committee of the European Community had decided that the risks of recombining DNA were less than previously feared, it none the less established rules for special protective measures and microbiological safety. In 1988 the UK Department of Trade and Industry, responsible for fostering biotechnological development, began a formal programme of Planned Release of Selected and Modified Organisms. Preliminary data on one type of seed suggest that the ensuing plants do not overwhelm their competitors in the wild or pass on their foreign genes to other species (Cherfas, 1991). However, the possible escape into the environment and proliferation of genetically produced new life-forms, mainly bacterial, continues to receive public attention. A Committee of the Ecological Society of America (reported by Roberts, 1989) concluded that most genetically engineered organisms will pose minimal ecological risk when released to the environment. However, important exceptions, while very rare, could occur. Organisms with 'novel combinations of traits are more likely [than others] to play novel ecological roles' (Ecological Society of America, 1989, cited by Simon, 1991). It is possible that 'too little attention is given to the dangers of an accidental rapid dissemination of bacteria carrying hybrid molecules which could affect man by bringing about aberrant genetic information or an infection resistant to antibiotics; or which could devastate flora and fauna, and even cause irreversible imbalance in the biosphere' (Ribes, 1978). Hypothetically, a newly acquired property could give the host organism a selective advantage over unaltered members of its species. Even if an organism's fitness or survival capacity is reduced by adding a gene or genes, natural selection over hundreds of thousands of generations will tend to increase fitness; if the organism passes on the new gene to other organisms, that trait can persist even after the modified organism itself has died out. Thus, regulatory oversight is recommended with a case-by-case review of environmental releases.

6 Biomedical Science and the Rights of Persons Defined as Mentally Ill

Medical Paternalism and Mentally Ill Persons

Benevolent Paternalism: the Parent–Child Model

The traditional attitude of clinicians to help-seeking sufferers is one of benevolent paternalism. In this respect it is modelled after that between parent and child. The parent feels justified in prescribing actions which limit the child's freedoms because the child, unlike the parent, is regarded as lacking in capacities for reasoned judgement and intelligent choice (Tormey and Brody, 1978). This attitude is not confined to scientifically trained Western physicians with their biomedical technology; the traditional folk healer or shaman, and the contemporary practitioner of 'alternative healing', as well as the psychiatrist or non-physician mental health professional, all presume that their judgement is superior to that of the help-seeker because of their specialized training, experience and command of esoteric knowledge and methods, however unvalidated. This presumption is heightened in dealing with persons defined as mentally ill. The diagnosis of mental illness suggests that a person has impaired autonomy, diminished capacities for reasoned judgement, and is not fully responsible for his or her acts and opinions.

When such a person enters into a systematic relationship with a mental health clinician or institution (in other words, becomes a 'patient'), the assumption of interpersonal impairment is further strengthened; she or he is seen as having abandoned some decision-making prerogatives to the clinician. This issue also emerges in relation to persons who are not defined as mentally ill, but as handicapped for a variety of reasons – severe developmental disability with mental retardation, traumatic brain damage impairing judgement and problem-solving ability, or degenerative brain disease with dementia. One pilot programme empowered volunteer committees, including physicians, to make decisions about medical care for incompetent mentally disabled persons without family or guardian. While unanimity about its value was not achieved, both

157

advocates for the mentally disabled and health care providers have preferred this approach to the judicial process (Sundram, 1988).

Compulsory Mental Hospitalization and Treatment

Compulsory or 'involuntary' treatment is by its nature administered to the patient in the role of an object rather than a collaborating subject (as in the case of psychotherapy). Aside from sequestration in a seclusion room, or forcibly administered baths or packs, available psychiatric technologies with intended therapeutic significance are limited. Their therapeutic goals also tend to be limited: tranquillization or sedation, the alleviation of depression, and interruption of psychotic behaviour ('antipsychotic' agents). They include psychosurgery (various forms of lobotomy), electroshock (electroconvulsive, ECT) therapy, and the psychopharmacological agents which are widely employed not only by psychiatrists but by non-psychiatrically trained physicians. Even these latter, despite an accelerating volume of research, are used largely on empirical grounds; the ability to predict the nature, timing and duration of outcome is variable and as often due to the clinical skills of a psychiatrist familiar with the history and reactivity of a particular patient, as to generally applicable knowledge of the agent itself. While knowledge about the role of such neurochemicals as serotonin and dopamine is significant there are still no definitive theories of action, and much of any clinician's thinking about what is happening in a particular case is unsubstantiable speculation. As Silove (1990) has pointed out, the much-vaunted 'biological' psychiatry would more accurately be termed 'biologism', and much of what is considered 'scientific' in the field would be considered by some as 'scientistic'. Biological research certainly holds great promise for understanding brain function in relation to behaviour. Practically, however, biological determinism in psychiatry is premature; it involves expensive neuro-imaging and other diagnostic approaches, but deprives patients of adequate care since it offers little of therapeutic significance aside from the pharmacological treatments (Brody, 1990d).

The more complex the ramifications of a technology the more difficult it is to acquaint a patient, relative or guardian with its meaning. This is especially true if the clinician recommending the treatment has no definitive understanding of its mode of functioning or its outcome. Yet all such procedures, under laws in most of the industrialized democracies, may be applied to patients without their consent if the situation is definable as an 'emergency' – a definition which often involves a judgement that 'the public health' is threatened (emergencies usually imply temporary forcible restraint). This is generally also true if the patient is defined as mentally 'incompetent'.

Clearly, all these definitions are subject to interpretation by professionals and government officials. But physicians are traditionally unquestioned by those in acute need of care, afraid of death and disability. Under these circumstances they and their anxious families are more likely to accept their recommendations and to become dependent rather than critical. Relatives in particular, burdened by the care of mentally ill family members, may be easily persuaded, especially under frightening and exhausting circumstances, that involuntary treatment is necessary.

Psychiatrists, too, are subject to persuasion and coercion, and in any event are creatures of their cultures. Totalitarian governments, through their controlled hospital systems and ability to label social protests as 'sick', can persuade psychiatrists who are state employees that compulsory hospitalization and treatment are indicated, and might even be humane alternatives to imprisonment. These include Member States of the UN which have been accused of applying the available psychiatric technologies to political dissidents under the pretence of treating them for mental illness.

Patient Advocacy and the Voluntary Mental Health and Consumer Movement

Challenges to Coercion

Medical status, in so far as physicians have wielded status as well as healing power, has been intermittently challenged by civil rights activists most of whom were patient advocates. This has been especially true for psychiatrists who can commit persons to involuntary confinement on the basis of their own systems of classification (that is to say, diagnoses). Challenges to physician power and patient restraint have been especially prominent during social crises with heightened emphasis on the values of individual freedom and self-determination. It was in the climate of the French Revolution, in 1793, that Philippe Pinel made his dramatic effort to free the mentally ill from their chains at Bicêtre. He wanted to do away with the public perception of psychotic persons as 'wild beasts', to stimulate a recognition of their humanity and, thus, their right to be dealt with as human beings.

In Florence, Italy, almost simultaneously, a new law was passed requiring a mental examination to be performed on people after their hospital commitment on grounds of insanity. The 1793 rules of the newest mental hospital there, prepared under the direction of Vincenzo Chiarugi (1759–1820), stated: 'It is a supreme moral duty and medical obligation to respect the insane individual as a person.'

The problem of disease state versus learned incapacity or simple deficiency emerged at almost the same historical moment in what was called the 'moral treatment' of insanity. In 1796 the Quakers in England, under the leadership of William Tuke, established an asylum, the Retreat, for the care of members of their group who were considered to be insane. Its 'moral' treatment was marked by an absence of coercion and a deliberate decision to use not fear but the disturbed psychotic patients' own desire for self-esteem as motivation to develop their capacity for self-restraint and to interact usefully with others. Tuke, however, in keeping with the philosophy of benevolent paternalism, none the less regarded the patients as essentially childlike, requiring humane treatment within a framework of re-education for living.

The French law of 1893 governing the medico-legal status of the mentally ill remains in force as a direct consequence of Pinel's work. It 'took the greatest care to underline the fundamental difference existing between the restriction of freedom imposed on mentally ill patients and the restriction of freedom imposed on criminals by courts of justice' (Pichot, 1967). Yet, despite the care taken to guarantee the liberty of those designated as patients, criticism began almost immediately to focus on the risk of arbitrary confinement. People were afraid that a mentally normal person might be committed to an institution for ulterior reasons. This bears on contemporary patients' rights movements as they reflect the distrust, co-existing both with respect and fear of the unknown, which is accorded to physicians. The ambivalence is compounded for psychiatrists, stigmatized with their patients as peculiar, along with the popular difficulty in understanding that a particular pattern of behaviour need not simply represent personal idiosyncrasy, badness or a response to stress, but can reflect a disease process.

Patients' Rights and the Voluntary Mental Health and Consumer Movements

The world's first voluntary mental health association was established in Finland in 1897 and continues to be a major force in the Finnish public health and patients' rights field. Although other beginnings were made in the UK and elsewhere, the next major impetus for patients' rights was the US publication in 1909 of *A Mind that Found Itself*. Its author, Clifford Beers, a sufferer from what was diagnosed as manic-depressive psychosis, devoted his life to the improvement of mental hospitals with special reference to preserving patients' rights; his efforts were instrumental in establishing the forerunner of the US National Mental Health Association in that same year, 1909. Beers's achievements also signalled the beginning of a fight against stigmatizing the mentally ill, and paved the way for others who had learned about such illness from their own experience to enter the ranks of leaders in the voluntary and consumer movement. An International Committee for Mental Hygiene, formed in 1919 with primary support from the USA and Canada, initiated the first international gathering devoted to the ideal of mental health. Professional groups, mainly psychiatrists and psychologists but also many others, joined the work and became prime movers in this First International Congress of Mental Hygiene which attracted 4000 people to Washington DC in 1930. From that conference an effective International Committee was founded on 6 May 1930 with representative groups and individuals from 29 countries. It sponsored, along with French organizations, a Second International Congress in Paris in 1937, but then the Second World War intervened. In 1946 an international Preparatory Commission was formed at the suggestion of still infant UNESCO and the newly formed Interim Commission for the World Health Organization. They suggested 'that a body representing voluntary services in the mental health field was needed to co-operate with the UN agencies that would be thoroughly interprofessional and completely international'. The new organization, the World Federation for Mental Health, was formally founded on 21 August 1948 during the Third International Congress of Mental Hygiene in London, with 22 member organizations from 22 countries. In 1992 WFMH had over 200 member organizations, about half representing national or international groups and half representing local or state groups, as well as 2400 individual members. The total reflected a presence in 194 countries.

Patients' Rights in the Context of Civil Rights

In the USA rising public sensitivity to patients' rights accompanied the social upheavals associated with the unpopular Vietnam war. One psychiatric consequence of the social protest movement, in which many offspring of upper-class, educated families participated, was a shift from considering social protesters as psychopathic or psychologically deviant to accepting their behaviour as a legitimate attempt at coping, changing a situation which they found morally and psychologically wrong. Also at this time, previously deprived, discriminated against or ignored groups who had served in the armed forces began to insist on their own civil and political rights. These included African–American and Native Americans (Indians, Eskimos, Aleuts), to a lesser degree those of Oriental descent, and more recent immigrant ethnic minority groups, particularly those termed 'Hispanic'. This period also saw the rise of the physically disabled as a political power able to insist on special facilities for wheelchair users. In Europe, particularly France with its large population of Algerian and sub-Saharan African *émigrés*, and the UK with its West Indian and Asian migrant populations, similar phenomena emerged.

In this context health consumerism became a major movement, not only in the USA but in industrialized Europe and New Zealand (in which the health rights of the Maori were becoming a political issue). In Australia the health and mental health rights of the Aborigines are gradually being politicized and recognized as relevant to psychiatry. Just as doctors were increasing their power with the new technologies, large segments of the educated public became no longer willing to accept their orders passively. Mutual participation of professional and patient began to threaten professional dominance as the social ideal in medicine (Benson, 1984). Mental patients and their families became a self-aware, right-seeking minority, comparable in some ways to other previously ignored groups emerging as socially and politically active collectivities. They accused psychiatrists of depriving non-conforming individuals of their freedom and, indeed, of fostering a type of oppression. In the industrialized democracies where such movements were free to arise psychiatry was accused of doing this, in part through diagnostic labelling which deprives persons of responsibility for their acts by defining them as irrational or symptomatic, and in part through compulsory hospitalization and treatment.

Much of what came to be called the 'anti-psychiatry movement' was fuelled by informal organizations of former mental hospital patients. In some areas, however, the voluntary mental health movement itself became caught up in an adversarial relationship with organized psychiatry. MIND, the Mental Health Association of England and Wales, for example, lost many of its prominent psychiatric members, especially in 1980, as it mounted a media campaign against psychiatry focused on an academic leader whom it accused of depriving an anorexic patient of her rights by administering intravenous nourishment to her against her will. The psychiatrist in question (personal communication) noted that the patient was semi-comatose and in imminent danger of death, and that while he would have no objection to her transfer to another hospital he felt that so long as she was entrusted to his unit he could not allow her to die. The issue finally subsided as a media concern, the Executive Director of MIND left his post, and the organization's usual relationship with the profession resumed.

The Political Abuse of Psychiatry

During the decades of the 1960s and 1970s the world also became aware of the use of psychiatric hospitalization by totalitarian leaders, particularly in the USSR, as a means of discrediting the political opinions of 'dissidents' who did not agree with state-approved policies. In 1971 the World Federation for Mental Health was the first international non-governmental organization to issue a resolution condemning the Soviet abuse of psychiatry, and it repeated its resolutions during its annual congresses for several years thereafter.

The most widely used 'diagnosis', justifying involuntary confinement in a mental hospital, was that of 'sluggish schizophrenia', coined by Andrei Schnevnesky, the USSR's chief psychiatrist and leader of the 'Moscow School' of psychiatry. The pathognomic feature of 'sluggish schizophrenia' was 'anti-state' behaviour including 'delusions of reformism'. Once hospitalized a variety of mind-altering and painful 'treatments' were administered to the incarcerated victims. *The Right to be Different: Deviance and Enforced Therapy* (Kittrie, 1971) was an outstanding example of scholarly reflection on this era.

The present author was labelled by the Soviet psychiatric system as a proponent of 'bourgeois individualism' when, in response to an official invitation during a 1972 consultation in Leningrad, he urged abandonment of 'anti-state' behaviour as a basis for psychiatric diagnosing, and advocated individual psychotherapeutic approaches with persons diagnosed as schizophrenic.

The Rights of People Confined in Mental Hospitals: Towards International Recognition

Despite efforts to bring this situation before the UN, and despite the guarantees contained in its 1948 Universal Declaration of Human Rights and subsequent elaborations, it was difficult for the inter-governmental system, sensitive to the national sovereignty of its Member States, to arrive at guarantees for the protection of persons detained on grounds of mental illness. In 1980 the UN Working Group of the Sub-commission on Discrimination and Protection of Minorities, on behalf of the Commission on Human Rights, its parent UN agency, the Economic and Social Council (ECOSOC), and the General Assembly, began work on such a document. Its unofficial 1983 report with an appended list of 'principles' reflected mainly the views of its author, the rapporteur of the Working Group (Daes, 1986). The anti-psychiatric tone of the report provoked protests by such professional groups as the World Psychiatric Association and the American Psychiatric Association, but their efforts to rectify it through governmental channels were ineffective. By August 1987, however, following changes in the political orientation of involved governments, particularly that of the USSR, and increased pressure for action by NGOs, particularly WFMH, the process of developing a declaration began to accelerate. WHO, influenced by NGO activity in Geneva, contracted with WFMH to produce a draft version of a new document. This was elaborated by the working group in 1988 and used as the basis for another version which was circulated by the full commission after its 1989 meeting.

The responses to this version permitted yet another revised draft which was debated in 1989 by a newly formed Joint International NGO Working Group on Mental Health, formed under the leadership of WFMH, and hosted by WHO, Geneva. Six NGOs, representing psychology, the law, multidisciplinary health groups and psychiatry participated. Except for the World Psychiatric Association, which differed on some points touching on their professional prerogatives as medical practitioners, it came to significant agreement on a common position. Following this yet another working group was authorized by the commission and ECOSOC, reconvening in January 1990 to produce a revision to be submitted, yet again, to the commission. The report of this group was eventually issued by the Economic and Social Council on 5 February 1991 (UN Commission on Human Rights, 1991) and passed without a vote by the UN General Assembly on 17 November 1991.

This document, entitled *Human Rights and Scientific and Technological Developments* (Doc. E/CN.4/1991/39, 5 February 1991), reiterates in many of its sections and in many ways the principle of treating mentally ill persons with respect for their dignity as human beings, and the importance of protecting their freedoms, rights and autonomy. Treatment is to be carried out in 'least restrictive' settings, using the least restrictive and intrusive appropriate methods. The principle of consent to treatment is also hedged with as many protective clauses as possible, although it remains vulnerable. Thus, consent is not required if the patient is held involuntarily, has an approved 'personal representative' who may speak for him or her, and if a legally qualified mental health practitioner believes that an emergency exists. Psychosurgery, however, and 'other intrusive and irreversible treatments for mental illness shall never be carried out on a patient who is an involuntary patient in a mental health facility' (p. 12).

Meanwhile, individual nations and regions have been clarifying their own guidelines. Thus, a series of revisions, aimed mainly at preserving patients' rights, were being accomplished in the British Mental Health Act first enacted in 1959 (Gostin, 1986). The Mental Health Acts Commission, composed of volunteer advocates, including some professionals, was empowered to hear complaints. Its definitive manual (Mental Health Act Commission, 1985) stimulated a 1986 meeting by the Royal College of Psychiatrists; a discussion contained in that meeting's proceedings (Murphy, E., 1988) indicates the nature of the continuing conflict with advocacy groups as it is experienced by UK psychiatrists. The main problem is the Mental Health Act Commission's 'essentially legalistic approach' (p. 63) which attempts to balance two opposing rules of British common law. One is that any form of care applied without the patient's consent is defined as 'battery'; the other is that the care giver 'is under a duty to use reasonable care and skill' which in the case of a physician means accordance with practice 'rightly accepted as proper by a responsible body of skilled and experienced doctors' (p. 63). This latter means that 'a patient can bring an action alleging negligence if he can prove he has suffered damage resulting from the doctor's failure to give adequate care' (p. 66). This legal approach 'ignores the spirit of intention of the action and . . . the manner in which it is carried out' (p. 66) which, in accordance with formal and informal codes of practice, involves 'the style of behaviour and emotional tone in our dealings with patients' (p. 67). The commission, as other similar bodies, must inevitably act at times in a paternalistic manner, making decisions against the will of particular patients in whose interest they presumably act. An unpublished example was the desire of a convicted rapist, diagnosed as suffering from an impulse disorder, for oestrogen treatment to reduce his sexual-aggressive drive. Although his psychiatrist supported his application for the treatment it was denied by the commission.

At the regional level the Council of Europe has been especially concerned with these matters, issuing a general set of recommendations (No. R 83 2) regarding 'the legal protection of persons suffering from mental disorder placed as involuntary patients' after the 22 February 1983 meeting of its Committee of Ministers. This required NGO action and in 1984 the newly formed European Council of the World Federation for Mental Health, meeting in Copenhagen with representatives of health ministries of a number of European governments, called upon the United Nations 'to establish a body with continuing responsibility to consider the rights of those called "mentally ill" and to work for adequate safeguards which do not of themselves give rise to discrimination'. It requested the co-operation in this endeavour of 'all relevant bodies, including non-governmental agencies with special experience and knowledge of the subject'. Although the request reached the appropriate UN agenda, there was no response to the idea of a permanent monitoring body. In 1989, anticipating the eventual formulation of a human rights guarantee for mentally ill persons by the UN, WFMH issued its

Declaration of Human Rights and Mental Health as a guide to the intergovernmental system, individual governments and institutions and other NGOs (Appendix 3).

Psychiatrically Applicable Biomedical Technologies

Psychosurgery

Procedures applied with therapeutic intent by physicians to psychiatric patients, consenting and non-consenting (and typically with an insufficient scientific basis for predicting the desired outcome) have included those which disrupt the integrity of the brain. Prior to the contemporary neuro-science research era most central nervous system investigation involved ablation of discrete portions of the brain, or their electrical stimulation. During this period, beginning after the First World War and continuing through the Second, some crudely defined brain treatments were applied to psychiatric patients in an atmosphere which was not sensitive to human rights. A prominent example was prefrontal lobotomy initiated on humans by the Portuguese neurosurgeon, Egas Moniz, in 1936 (Moniz, 1937). Moniz's first attempt involved a partial isolation of the frontal poles in chronic schizophrenic patients. His inspiration came from reports of frontal pole inactivation used for the treatment of 'experimental neuroses' in two chimpanzees by Carlyle Jacobsen in John Fulton's laboratory at Yale (Jacobsen, C., 1936). By the time Walter Freeman and James Watts published the first major book on the subject (Freeman and Watts, 1942) several thousand patients had been lobotomized with a variety of methods, all of which involved interruption of the thalamo-frontal projection tracts and some of the neuronal paths from the frontal poles to other parts of the brain. Striking from the human rights viewpoint was the fact that these procedures were carried out in an almost complete absence of animal research after the initial chimpanzee studies. It was not until the early 1950s that the kind of animal research which should have preceded the human applications began to emerge (Brody and Rosvold, 1952).

The broad and enthusiastic application of the various lobotomies (now known as leucotomies, especially in the UK) to human beings placed those subjected to it in the position of experimental objects. However, this was not a concern to long-hospitalized patients, many already recipients of prolonged courses of electroconvulsive therapy; they were accustomed in that era to passively conforming to medical orders. Nor was it a concern for their families, often desperate for some change in an incurable condition, sometimes made worse by prolonged hospitalization; or to doctors habituated to act as benevolent paternalistic figures and, in any event, regarding the presence of a possibly effective treatment as a moral imperative to use it.

The procedure was also applied, however, to non-psychotic patients by clinicians whose research aims appeared to be at least as important as their therapeutic intentions. (Most research was carried out by investigators who did not participate in the joint psychiatric–surgical decision to do the operation.) An illustrative example is published work from a leading London medical institution entitled, *Personality and the Frontal Lobes: An Investigation of the Psychological Effects of Different Types of Leucotomy* (Petrie, 1952). The psychologist–investigator noted: 'Investigators in the past who have worked with psychotics undergoing leucotomy have been confronted with the difficulties arising from having too many unknown variables. The patients used for the investigations to be reported in this book were probably as near the normal as any likely to be operated upon. They were in the main neurotics, and the operation was carried out to relieve them of their neurosis. Their personalities were so well preserved that they could co-operate through the many hours of testing necessitated by this investigation' (p. 3).

During the 1940s and 1950s, until the introduction of antipsychotic drugs, lobotomy was widely used in the treatment of hospitalized chronic schizophrenics, and to a lesser degree for crippling obsessive–compulsive states and the pain of advanced, disseminated metastatic carcinoma. Other variants of brain surgery were used, largely in a semi-experimental way, for intractable, impulsive aggressive outbursts. This usage, along with the behavioural sequelae of the operation in many patients, inaccurately described as 'vegetables', stimulated charges that it was carried out largely as a method of controlling unruly hospital inmates – a charge which appeared to have merit in some instances. Lobotomy, in this last view, was regarded in the same category as seclusion, physical and chemical restraint. There is some reason to believe, however, that the behaviour of lobotomized patients characterized as 'vegetables' was less a function of the brain lesion itself than of the interpersonal neglect after surgery preceded by years of hospitalization for treatment-resistant schizophrenia. At least one study (Brody, 1958) demonstrated that chronic patients who had undergone a modified lobotomy (undercutting areas 11 and 13) produced dreams, free associations and psychodynamically relevant interview material when seen for an hour daily in psychoanalytically oriented interviews.

Public concern about direct invasion of the brain stimulated proposals in the US House of Representatives (1973a) and the Senate (1973b) to suspend federal support of research projects involving psychosurgery and to prohibit its practice in federally connected health facilities. A major concern of the US professional community was with the implications of governmental assumption of clinical decision-making power (Brody, 1973b). Rather than allowing government to assume responsibility for particular medical procedures it seemed more desirable that commissions or task forces, including a range of scientists and clinicians, as well as representatives of the lay community, should be appointed to study the matter. The various proposals to limit the procedure in the USA did not pass, however, in part because the advent of easily available and progressively more effective pharmacological agents made the application of brain surgery to psychiatric patients less urgent. It also diminished the research enthusiasm of some clinical investigators. The US National Commission on the Protection of Human Subjects of Biochemical and Behavioral Research (1979), charged by the US Congress with considering this topic, noted positive evidence that the more refined, less broadly destructive procedure of cingulotomy may be useful for patients with intractable pain, severe excessive compulsive states and severe emotionally agitated depressions (Klerman, 1989, p. 1741). However, charges about its destructive effects led in some countries to all psychosurgery being outlawed as a violation of patients' personalities and human rights. In the USSR, for example, the procedure was banned in the early 1950s, although after 1973 N.P. Bekhtereva in Leningrad used stimulation and auto-stimulation with implanted electrodes in the treatment of mental disturbances associated with temporal lobe epilepsy; in Japan, under pressure from a movement of 'militant psychiatrists and medical students', no lobotomy was performed in 1975 (Pichot, 1983).

Contemporary psychosurgery survives in the USA and the UK in refined form, mainly the highly controlled destruction of thalamic nuclei and other neural way-stations, and is rarely used except in cases of severe social crippling where there is reason to believe that some functional recovery is possible. It is occasionally considered, along with the use of psychoactive drugs, as treatment for intractable pain in patients with terminal metastatic carcinoma. An estimated 400–600 patients per year undergo psychosurgical procedures in the USA (Klerman, 1989).

Electroconvulsive Therapy (ECT)

The other widely used form of directly intrusive brain-focused treatment is electroshock or electroconvulsive therapy (ECT). It was preceded by a variety of chemical agents applied on a trial-and-error or clinical-intuitive basis, primarily by European academic psychiatric leaders. Insulin was used in psychiatry almost immediately after its discovery in 1922 because of its sedative and appetite-stimulating effect. Manfred Sakel of Vienna, who also used it for withdrawal from morphine addiction, first realized that its behavioural effects were most marked when doses sufficient to induce coma were administered. His first report on its favourable effect on schizophrenia was presented in 1933 (Sakel, 1938). Meanwhile, Lazlo von Meduna of Budapest and colleagues were experimenting with chemical substances such as camphor and Metrazol to lower the seizure threshold, thus inducing generalized seizures (Pichot, 1983). Despite dramatically positive results with some patients suffering from what was then diagnosed as schizophrenia (in an era when disorders currently called depressive were often so diagnosed), and with some who apparently had psychotic depressive disorders, technical difficulties with these chemical agents led to the introduction of electrical methods by Hugo Cerletti and Lucio Bini in Italy. In April 1938 Cerletti, Professor of Neuropathology and Psychiatry at the University of Rome, applied the method to a schizophrenic patient who was hallucinating and incoherent and had responded temporarily to Metrazol the year before. After eleven treatments a 'spectacular remission' occurred (Pichot, 1983, p. 125).

Although Sakel, who emigrated to the USA in 1936, remained in New York until his death in 1957 his insulin coma technique, requiring close, intensive nursing supervision, was gradually abandoned as the much more easily and inexpensively applied ECT became widely used, especially in the 1940s. During the 1950s and 1960s ECT was 'perhaps overprescribed' (Welch, 1989). Excessive use reflected both ignorance (in other words, lack of sufficient rigorously controlled and analysed data) and therapeutic enthusiasm in the absence of any other so quickly and easily administered treatment. The manufacture and sale of ECT equipment for use in private offices as well as hospitals became a burgeoning industry in that era, one which continues.

ECT was also used as a means of reducing the frequency and intensity of impulsive aggressive behaviour. However, alternate modes of non-destructive therapies were also receiving major attention in this pre-psychopharmacological era. Efforts begun earlier in Germany and Austria to work psychotherapeutically with schizophrenic patients, with elaborations flourishing in the USA after the Second World War, began to spread to leading medical schools (Brody and Redlich, 1952). However, the requirement of intense, prolonged personal involvement with very sick patients discouraged most psychiatrists after drugs became available – and, indeed, the use of psychotherapy with such patients in lieu of available pharmacological agents came to be regarded by some as a questionable practice. With the passage of time, however, as it became evident that the available drugs are not universally effective and that for many their therapeutic benefit is transient, there has been renewed interest in psychological approaches to treatment. But interest has shifted from the former psychodynamic emphasis to a 'psychosocial' one involving training in interpersonal and social skills, as well as work within a relationship with a therapist.

The use of ECT also declined as antipsychotic drugs became available. After several years, however, when ECT was often regarded as undesirable, it resumed its place in the accepted psychiatric armamentarium with more specific indications and more refined means of administration. Undesirable side-effects have been diminished through the use of anticonvulsant and anxiety-reducing medications and procedures. It is recognized as especially effective for severe life-threatening agitated psychotic depressions, often in the post-middle-age period, when drugs are ineffective. According to an American Psychiatric Association report (1978) it is the only effective treatment for many drug-resistant or drug-intolerant depressed patients. Most informed patients, especially when the family is included in discussions about therapy, consent willingly to ECT as a relief from the almost intolerable anguish of otherwise treatment-resistant severe depression. However, special efforts are often necessary to safeguard the rights of those whose ability to comprehend may be impaired by illness. Thus, videotape presentations of ECT have been used to help demystify it (Remick and Maurice, 1978). There is also general agreement within the profession that when patients are 'too inert to carry out meaningful consent or oppose treatment because of negativistic or paranoid ideation that is part of their depressed illness . . . it is incumbent upon the physician, and in the patient's best interest, to seek substituted judgement regarding treatment' (Welch, 1989, p. 1807). Such judgement usually comes from relatives advised by physicians. Beyond this there has been a trend, despite treatment delays, to require court review of contested individual cases prior to involuntary treatment (Winslade et al., 1984). For a time an absolute legal prohibition was imposed on administering ECT within the town limits of Berkeley, California. This was regarded by many as an unconstitutional denial of access to appropriate treatment and made it necessary for families to move patients to other jurisdictions where ECT could be legally administered. None the less, occasional efforts in this direction continue, and some organizations of former patients (frequently called 'users' or 'consumers') oppose ECT as a brain- and personality-destructive process.

Psychopharmacology

The aspect of advancing biomedical science most relevant to the rights and vulnerabilities of mentally ill persons is the rapidly growing field of psychopharmacology. The advent of psychotropic or neuroleptic drugs has been credited in many quarters with creating a revolution in psychiatric care, helping to empty the mental hospitals and restoring large numbers of persons, who would otherwise have remained hospitalized, to community life. (Earlier, the advent of therapeutic community concepts, psychosocial treatment and the application of psychoanalytic principles to hospitalized patients were also credited with revolutionary consequences.) The possibly undesirable social consequences for family life and patient protection of an early return to the community of still vulnerable persons continue to be debated. For many, fragile mental stability continues to be dependent upon regular medication which they may forget or resist. Beyond these therapeutic concerns are the legal ones related to forcible medication, or to the impact of medication upon the mental status of someone on trial for a crime who pursues the insanity defence. These pose difficult problems, but while they are relevant to human rights issues they fall more in the field of legal than health concerns (Gutheil and Appelbaum, 1983).

Another rights-relevant issue is the fact that, while some of these drugs can produce rapid and dramatic alleviation of the most disturbing psychotic symptoms, as well as of less disturbing, non-psychotic distress, particularly depression and anxiety, they can produce undesirable side-effects over the long term. Different classes of drugs have different effects. Some benzodiazepines, for example, have been shown in non-psychotic patients to produce dependency of a degree which makes it difficult to discontinue their use. The production of new drugs and their approval and release to the market have been so rapid that it is difficult for many practitioners to remain knowledgeable about their potential side-effects. Thus, physicians are dependent for necessary information upon the drug companies which produce the agents in question and are inevitably motivated by profit considerations. Patients, as well as their physicians, may find themselves taken aback by unexpected consequences – as when a medication taken to relieve depression produces serious anxiety.

Physicians' responses to these consequences also reveal the value connotations of particular symptoms. Depression, for example, is often taken more seriously by the medical community than anxiety, although anxiety can be at least as crippling. Similarly, the value of controlling seizures may be overestimated in comparison with the cognitive hazards of seizure-controlling drugs. While most physicians, for example, have suspected that the long-term administration of phenobarbitone (phenobarbital) to infants and children with febrile seizures could have adverse effects upon intellectual development, they regarded the seizures as the greater of the two evils. One consequence was a delay of many years before systematic research demonstrated not only that the drug does, indeed, have a negative effect on development, as indicated by lowered IQ, but that its effectiveness in lowering seizure frequency is less than originally thought. It was concluded that 'phenobarbital depresses cognitive performance in children treated for febrile seizures and that this disadvantage, which may outlast the administration of the drug by several months, is not offset by the benefit of seizure prevention' (Farwell et al., 1990, p. 364).

Some patients, although relieved of psychotic feelings by major tranquillizers and other antipsychotic drugs, complain of a sense of being placed in a chemical strait-jacket. Others have side-effects which are less disturbing, but still enough to make non-compliance with a treatment regimen a major clinical problem. It has been demonstrated that even psychotic persons can benefit from careful education regarding the purposes, benefits and risks of antipsychotic medication (Benson, 1984, p. 651). Frightening and unexpected drug effects often lead to the abandonment of antipsychotic medication (Van Putten et al., 1984). Non-compliance in the administration of oral neuroleptics measured by tests of venous serum was reported in 24–63 per cent of outpatients (Carman et al., 1984). It is likely that the full extent of the potential harmful or unpleasant effects of long-term medication with neuroleptics is not yet known. An example of a potentially lethal condition, still not highly prevalent, but reported with increasing frequency (perhaps because of the increased education of clinicians), is NMS, the neuroleptic malignant syndrome. This has been reported as a potential response to all commonly used neuroleptics as well as to discontinuation of dopaminergic agents and at least one antidepressant, amoxapine (Taylor and Schwartz, 1988), and with the concomitant use of neuroleptics and lithium (Susman and Addonizio, 1988).

Scientific Knowledge as the Necessary Basis for Estimating Human Rights Violations: the Example of Tardive Dyskinesia

A large literature exists on the most prominent side-effect of prolonged neuroleptic medication, namely tardive dyskinesia. This is one of four extrapyramidal syndromes; the other three, occurring with much less frequency, are pseudoparkinsonism (sometimes described as a hypokinetic syndrome), acute dystonic reactions found most often in young males, and akathisia (Sachdev and Lonergan, 1991). The actual prevalence of these syndromes in the population at large is unknown since clinicians appear to be quick to diagnose movement disorders as hysterical. The establishment of research-oriented clinics for such disorders is of relatively recent occurrence. It is especially important to note the possibility that dyskinesia can occur spontaneously, that is without drug administration, and that the incidence of its spontaneous occurrence and its prevalence in non-neuroleptically treated psychotic patients remain uncertain.

Tardive dyskinesia, which has proved irreversible in many cases, began to be reported worldwide in the early 1960s. Despite the lack of definitive knowledge court judgements have been rendered in the US against physicians, hospitals and pharmaceutical manufacturers in favour of patients suffering from this disorder; plaintiffs have sued because of alleged failure to obtain their (or their client's) informed consent to administration of the drugs, as well as for negligence or malpractice. A wide range of specific accusations includes: failure to inform the family; failure to justify neuroleptic treatment; failure to monitor the effects of continued neuroleptic administration; the simultaneous administration of many drugs ('polypharmacy'); failure to stop neuroleptic administration upon the onset of tardive dyskinesia; the use of neuroleptics for behavioural control in the interest of hospital management; and failure of manufacturers to include sufficient warnings on the product or its packaging.

Here, as in most instances in which human rights are the focus of concern regarding biomedical technology, advancing knowledge about the drugs and their presumed side-effects makes the determination of medical negligence problematic. Thus, there is increasing evidence that a certain number of schizophrenic patients develop dyskinesia in the absence of drug administration. Emil Kraepelin made a long-forgotten observation in this respect. He wrote in 1902 of the appearance of 'peculiar choreiform movements of the mouth' as well as other signs of dyskinesia in a significant number of patients diagnosed, in the terminology of the era, as having dementia praecox. Contemporary research indicates that, while such evidence of dyskinesia is found in children, the likelihood of it developing without, but especially with, neuroleptic administration increases with age. Again, this suggests the possibility of aetiological factors other than, or acting in combination with, neuroleptic drugs.

Another type of rights question is raised by psychiatry's increasingly biological and pharmacological orientation. Stone (1984) noted that 'when courts enforce a psychotic person's right to refuse . . . treatment prescribed by a competent biological psychiatrist, the question [arises as to] whether the alternative effective treatment is possible' (p. 1385). He wonders if it is ethical 'for a psychiatrist to continue to assume professional responsibility for a patient whose treatment, limited by legal constraints, does not meet minimal standards of care' (p. 1386). In terms of the UNESCO–ISSC (1985) conclusion that access to appropriate care should be considered a right, it is possible to conclude that a psychiatrist in this position is violating that right. On the other hand, it is immediately evident that the opinions of the 'biological psychiatrist', however 'competent', might, in the light of rapidly changing clinical scientific knowledge, be considered arguable by a number of equally competent peers. That is, the definition of 'minimal standards of care' remains scientifically uncertain. The converse question has also been raised as to whether a patient treated with drugs by a 'biological psychiatrist' is being deprived of more effective psychotherapeutic treatment. The evidence is mounting that for many patients psychotherapy alone or a combination of psychological and drug treatments are more effective than drugs alone. It has been reported, for example, that cognitive therapy without drugs (and their possibly adverse effects) has been effective in patients diagnosed as having panic disorder; patients with a personality disorder or depression were also effectively treated but required a longer duration of treatment to become symptom-free (Sokol et al., 1989). Cognitive–behavioural treatment without drugs produced major improvement not only in panic symptoms, but in associated phobic avoidance and generalized anxiety (Shear et al., 1991). This has been replicated with psychopharmacologically oriented clinicians trained by a behavioural psychologist (Welkowitz et al., 1991). There is also new evidence that an interpersonally oriented psychotherapy is more effective in the treatment of non-psychotic depressions that either drugs or a combination of drugs and psychotherapy (Wexler and Cicchetti, 1992).

Apparently Competing Rights: Freedom versus Care

While 'access to appropriate therapy' may be considered a human right, the definition of what is 'appropriate' is still determined by physicians or members of other professions. Clearly, the definition of needed treatment can reflect the professionals' own needs for money, power, or clinical excitement – and, if they are state employees, their allegiance to the perceived desires of the government which gives them security and status. At the same time, this seems preferable to having clinical decisions explicitly made and options restricted by clinically untrained persons such as lawyers, legislators and judges.

The dramatic advances of psychopharmacology, combined with the consumer health movement, have intensified interest in a universal human challenge: how to foster individual dignity and freedom, and the patient's right to autonomy while, at the same time, preserving the social fabric. Within it lies a specific challenge to psychiatry, the other mental health professions, mental health advocates and governments: how to balance the civil rights of persons labelled mentally ill against the clinically required limitations on their freedom (Brody, 1985, 1988b). Stated simply, are there occasions when preserving an abstract right to autonomous self-determination is destructive to the patient, and in some instances to the family and society? In this respect it is essential to remember that civil rights have been construed, in local and national as well as international settings, to include access not only to appropriate therapy, but to the protection essential to survival when one's capacities are impaired. Abandoning resistant patients to death, or increased physical morbidity by suicide, chronic exposure, exhaustion or victimization by others, cannot be viewed as protecting their rights. Limiting a mentally ill person's access to scarce technical resources by easy agreement with his or her resistance to their prescription may delay regaining lost powers of self-determination. Even within the hospital failure to medicate may increase the likelihood of mental deterioration, the use of seclusion and delayed release.

On the other hand, available data do not support the universal desirability of rapid medication and, as noted above, they make it clear that the benefits of neuroleptic drugs must be balanced against the costs of such side-effects as tardive dyskinesia. A determination of the potential effectiveness of pharmacological agents versus a variety of psychotherapies, or a combination, requires careful diagnostic appraisal. The scarcest diagnostic and treatment resource for mentally ill or emotionally disturbed patients is the time of well-trained, empathic evaluators and psychotherapists, or even of untrained but humane and empathic hospital staff. Time, always in short supply, has become even scarcer since psychopharmacological advances have made psychotherapy less attractive to physicians. In the absence of psychotherapeutic time and interest drugs may be administered as substitutes for human contact.

Part of the problem of reconciling autonomy with beneficent paternalism, that is, making decisions for the patient according to what the decision-maker regards as the patient's best interests, lies in the characteristic uncertainty of medical practice. It is often necessary to make rapid judgements in crisis situations on the basis of limited information. Thus, court decisions in a number of US states noting the risks (such as tardive dyskinesia) of neuroleptic drug treatment require the patient's informed consent to medication, but exempt the informed consent requirement in 'emergency circumstances' (as in a case of threatened suicide) – a feature allowing very broad interpretation. Beyond emergency decisions, while the issue of informed consent remains unarguable in the abstract, it is highly problematic in actual practice. With non-psychiatric patients the paralysing effects of 'full disclosure' of all possible pathogenic or undesirable consequences of taking a medicinal drug are well known. Many, perhaps the majority, of patients suffering from pain, anxiety and threatened death or disability wish only to place themselves in the hands of a competent, caring physician who will make these decisions for them. Psychiatric patients, whose cognitive capacity is impaired by anxiety or psychosis, will find it difficult to understand the situation sufficiently to give a consent that is truly 'informed'; or they may be so mistrustful of physicians and medicines that they are unable to arrive at any decision.

A Right to Just Treatment in the Context of Unequal Resources and Opportunities

Justice, reflected in equitable access to treatment and equitable freedom from restraints, is widely regarded as a civil or human right. Even in the absence of mental illness the likelihood of just dealing is diminished when suffering requires dependent interaction with another (Veatch, 1981), in this case a doctor possessing significantly greater means than the patient. Here the means refer less to money than to knowledge and social power. Under these circumstances an equitable distribution of self-esteem (Rawls, 1971), and the development of a sense of community between help-seeker and help-giver, may be almost impossible.

The situation is complicated by patients' differing life circumstances and the contexts in which the clinical encounter takes place. It is self-evident that treatment varies with the social and cultural context in which a patient lives, including its available resources, as well as the patient's socio-economic, ethnic and other statuses carrying differential power and prestige. It was suggested in Chapter 2 that in an era dominated by biological in contrast to psychosocial theories of mental illness minority-group persons denigrated by members of the majority may be dealt with less optimistically, and be deprived of some opportunities because of predicted inability to benefit from them. As Gould has noted, 'Theories of biological determinism gain attention in conservative [political] climates' (*New York Times* book review, 20 August 1984, p. 7). And the prediction itself may be based on misperceptions, because psychiatric deficit is sometimes difficult to separate from the combination of social deficit and cultural distance from majority norms.

In multi-ethnic societies a patient's ethnic and social class status may be significant predictors not only of the availability of the most effective treatment, but whether or not the doctor discloses the possible side-effects of particular technical approaches. This concern is increasing with the increasing migratory flows throughout the world. It has been widely reported, by WHO as well as by individual investigators, that immigrants, including guest workers, from the less developed world to the European industrialized democracies do not effectively utilize available health resources (Colledge et al., 1986). Relations between physicians and help-seekers migrant from countries only recently emerged from colonial rule can be made difficult by the latter's defensive behaviour in the face of perceived authority. Avoiding or refusing the use of medical technologies, including psychopharmacological agents, can be a way of maintaining cultural boundaries and personal identity in an alien setting. In the less developed world itself, technical medical treatment offered by foreign physicians, in contrast to that available from native healers, can be resisted, as incompatible with the tradition of operating within familial limits, values and loyalties (Brody, 1981b).

Within the USA the greater probability of psychiatric hospitalization (often on an involuntary basis) for African–Americans and Native Americans, in contrast to outpatient or general hospital treatment for whites (Snowden and Cheung, 1990) suggests that the first two groups receive less psychotherapy and more drug or physical treatments than the last. This finding is compatible with that reported two generations earlier (Hollingshead and Redlich, 1958) that patients of the lowest socio-economic status, usually diagnosed as schizophrenic, in contrast to those more socially advantaged, tended to accumulate in public mental hospitals and to receive only custodial care or ECT. Private US psychiatrists tend to give more information about drug side-effects to their voluntary patients than hospital staff doctors to their committed patients. Patients of high socio-economic status receive more voluntary explanations about illness and treatment, regardless of diagnosis, than patients of lower socio-economic status (Benson, 1984). These differences between public and private are even greater in the developing world where the socio-economic and cultural gulf and the differences in social power between physicians and patients impede mutually trusting communication (Brody 1973a, 1981a). In large public mental hospitals doctors have little relationship with and little or no individual knowledge of the many patients about whom they make important decisions. In the industrialized democracies, exemplified by the USA with its vast medical training and research establishment, the problem is intensified by the large numbers of immigrant physicians from other countries. Under these circumstances the treating clinician has only limited mastery of the patient's language and culture. The cultural–linguistic gap added to the socio-economic and power differences between doctor and patient, one of whom as a mentally ill and severely distressed person is already in some measure a cultural alien, can paralyse effective communication. This reduces the patient's sense of security, increases the likelihood that treatment methods will be confined to impersonally administered drugs or other physical methods, and makes a mockery of full disclosure and informed consent.

The relatively anonymous patient within a large public mental hospital, regardless of humane physical care, is at a further disadvantage. As he or she must conform to the ordinary logistical requirements of the institution, administered by a staff smaller than the total number of patients, deviations from ordinary rules (which in therapeutic terms might be regarded as healthy efforts at individuation) are regarded as infractions requiring discipline or as symptoms requiring medication. In this context the culturally different, foreign-born, or rural, uneducated, low-status patient, and others without special claims to individual attention, are at a clear disadvantage.

The low staff-to-patient ratio in large public mental hospitals throughout the world poses another problem, most marked in relation to the drug therapy which is, typically, the central mode of treatment. The clinician initiating the pharmacological intervention is often not the one who observes the outcome. This is frequent when the patient must make repeated transitions between inpatient and outpatient care and back again. Since the clinical course of psychiatric illness is influenced by context, including both social support and the negative impact of demands and fears from family and acquaintances, the possibility of tense emergency situations involving disturbed members of the community is high. The clinician is often under pressure from community and family to compulsorily administer sedative drugs, the outcome of which will have to be judged by someone else, and it becomes almost impossible for doctor and patient to develop mutual trust.

The Right to Respect and Justice, Embodying Full Disclosure and Informed Consent, Regarding Mental Hospitalization and Drug Treatment

In English law a 'fundamental principle, plain and incontestable, is that every person's body is inviolate' (Sullivan, 1988, p. 1). The US legal doctrine of informed consent enunciated by Supreme Court Justice Benjamin Cardosa in 1914 states that 'every human being of adult years and sound mind has a right to determine what shall be done with his own body'. But since psychiatric patients are not considered to have sound minds this basis for the doctrine is difficult to apply. Similarly the 'free and rational' or 'self-legislating will' postulated by Kant (1785) as prerequisite to common membership in a moral community does not encompass mentally impaired or defective individuals. Since membership in this moral community brought with it rights to justice, individual autonomy and equality of respect it appears that Kant would not grant such rights to these impaired individuals. However, they constitute, significantly, the community to which medical practitioners are dedicated, and are among the reasons for the durability of benevolent paternalism as a basic philosophy of medical care. There exists on *a priori* grounds no reason to deny psychologically inadequate persons the basic respect accorded to other human beings. One is forced to conclude, therefore, that (considering the difficulty in deciding upon the rationality of all persons under all circumstances) such rationality should not be the sole, certainly not the unique, basis for respecting an individual's human status.

Various attempts have been made to solve this issue. One basis of respect for mentally impaired, psychologically immature or other persons, which could include everyone else, is Bernard Williams's concept of a common humanity with moral worth independent of 'natural capacities, unequally and fortuitously distributed' (Williams, 1971). This concept could be a basis for the right-making principle of justice as the affirmation that all 'people have a claim on having the total net welfare in their lives equal in so far as is possible to the welfare in the lives of others' (Veatch, 1981, p. 268). Psychiatry is not alone among medical specialities in confronting the challenge of deciding whether its patients are competent to refuse treatment. It shares this with all of medicine, most obviously with neurology, geriatrics and pediatrics, as well as, at times, internal medicine and surgery. In 17 per cent of a series of US general hospital admissions, for example, the physicians' primary response to refusal of drugs by patients whom they regarded as psychiatrically or neurologically incompetent was to force treatment over their continuing specific objection (Appelbaum and Roth, 1983).

Diagnosed patients for whom involuntary, compulsory hospitalization and treatment is considered necessary constitute a relatively small group of the total population definable as psychotic, incompetent or in need of care. US studies in a number of different localities suggest that the great majority of involuntary patients are admitted on the basis of physicians' subjective impressions of their potential for violent behaviour; this impression is often, it appears, a function of the emergency context in which psychiatric consultation was requested. In terms of diagnostic nomenclature such patients tend to be manic, overactive, grandiose and alternately euphoric, irritable or hostile; those who are depressed, burdened with delusions and hallucinations stimulating desires to kill or mutilate themselves; or those who suffer from paranoid delusions and hallucinations and are acutely fearful, angry and suspicious. Typically such behaviour diminishes after hospitalization and is not associated with exceptionally high use of restraint or seclusion. The legal psychiatric problem usually begins after they have become part of a therapeutically calming milieu, or treated sufficiently with drugs to relieve their acute symptomatology. At that point, with their faculties returned to a level permitting greater reflection and self-awareness, they may begin to protest their incarceration. Patients in these circumstances in the USA have initiated a number of lawsuits. Those concerning the right to treatment, that is, the right to be released from custodial care when no active treatment is available, are reported in a large literature. They have been generally effective and have resulted in marked improvement in the environments of many large public hospitals.

Another issue concerns the presumed right of patients to treatment in community settings. A claim in the early 1970s against the state of Massachusetts (Okin, 1984), for example, asserted that patients living in state hospitals, or at risk of being so hospitalized, have a right to treatment in community settings. A 1978 decree following that suit resulted over a period of five years in a tenfold increase in state expenditures for community mental health services, a 49 per cent decline in the state hospital census, and a 15 per cent drop in state hospital admission rates in the involved region of the state. The author commented that such a 'least-restrictive alternative suit', unless it indicates the ultimate aim of 'providing a system of services that would make institutionalization unnecessary for most patients . . . provokes the fears of the community at large [and] tends to increase the destructive polarization that often exists between clinicians and lawyers' (p. 788). They may improve mental health care if they have 'a concern for the patients' need for treatment and not simply their rights to liberty' (p. 789).

The Right to Autonomy in Relation to Determinations of Competence

The view that a patient's right to autonomy is violated by compulsory hospitalization or treatment presupposes that his or her autonomy is not already impaired by illness. Autonomy in this usage does not refer simply to the capacity for free voluntary action in pursuit of conscious goals, as such freedom is retained in most mental illness. It refers rather to 'effective deliberation' (Miller, 1981), making reflective choices on the basis of clear awareness of alternative courses of action and their consequences, which is not always possible for mentally ill persons. To this may be added (Dworkin, 1976; Miller, 1981) the element of authenticity, acting in a manner 'consistent with the person's attitudes, values, dispositions and life plans' (Miller, 1981, p. 24). Again, while such consistency may extend to periods of mental illness it is not always present. The appropriateness of paternalistic medical intervention, presumably impairing autonomy, thus requires careful determination on a case-by-case basis. It may conceivably be regarded as helpful when it compels treatment aimed at transforming an impaired person into one capable of exercising independent, authentic, rational choice. In this sense a clinician may act within a close therapeutic relationship to restore a patient's authenticity, independence and rationality even while failing to respect his refusal of treatment (Cassell, 1978). At the same time, as noted above, the clinician, urged on by the community, is less likely to look for lucidity behind the apparently disturbed behaviour of a non-hospitalized patient, more likely to find it threatening, and more likely to impose hospitalization or treatment without informed consent when the patient is of lower socio-economic class or different ethnic status. In some US states, for example Massachusetts in terms of a 1981 decision of its Supreme Judicial Court (Arkin, 1984), an incompetent person may have the right to refuse medical treatment if it is exercised for him or her by another. The right is hedged by the requirement that, in the absence of an emergency, because of the intrusiveness of treatment, the possibility of adverse side-effects, prior judicial involvement, and the likelihood of conflicting interest (in psychiatrists as well as family members) that other person must be a duly constituted judge. Some patients' rights and self-help groups, particularly in the UK and Northern Europe, have proposed that members of the patient's friendship network and advocacy groups be involved in such proceedings. They have expressed particular concern about families who may be more interested in keeping a patient securely confined than in his or her freedom or autonomy. In contrast, the author's inspection of several Soviet facilities in 1990 revealed, even in the most enlightened, and despite the advent of *glasnost*, an almost total lack of comprehension of the self-help and volunteer concepts, and insistence that if professional control were to be loosened it should only be to give families a greater voice in the handling of their sick relatives.

A number of proposals have attempted to separate the restraint aspects from the therapeutic aspects of involuntary hospitalization. A suggested *parens patriae* commitment requires that 'the patient suffers from a severe mental disorder, lacks capacity to make a reasoned decision concerning treatment, is treatable and is likely to harm himself or others' (Stromberg and Stone, 1983). This is contrasted with police power commitment which permits evaluation while not allowing long-term custodial involvement in the mental health system unless treatment is available. However, a variety of patient advocate groups recommend that psychiatric commitment for purposes of public protection, especially 'preventive detention', be totally eliminated. This position is supported by a significant literature affirming the inability of psychiatrists to make predictions about the future dangerousness of mentally ill persons who have not previously engaged in violent action.

The situation is complicated, as already suggested, because estimates of competence are often ambiguous in the clinical situation. A position paper of the American Psychiatric Association (Bonnie, 1982) stated that 'patients have a right to participate in the decision-making process in the most meaningful manner consistent with their clinical conditions'. But the criteria for judging that clinical condition are not listed. Further, although the right to refuse treatment was regarded as derived from the constitutional right of freedom from unwarranted intrusion into one's person, the principle of patient self-determination was not considered to be a legally enforceable right. Psychiatrists are left with the question as to whether and when intrusion into another's person, however sanctioned by law and culture, is ethically justified. Further, they must decide if such intrusion is warranted on clinical grounds as beneficent, that is, promoting the patient's well-being. And if they conclude that it is indeed beneficent, is it possible that they are embracing a paternal-istic, beneficence-based theory with no genuine commitment to autonomy (Macklin, 1983)?

Competence is not an all-or-none condition, but a continuum, just as treatment is not an event, but a process. Diagnosed illness cannot be equated with incompetence, just as it does not always require invasive treatment or restricted liberty. Decisions about 'competence' should recognize that, as a concept, it is a social artefact responsive to particular social needs. Its definition has fluctuated throughout history and with values and available technologies, both for measuring and for modifying it. It has also varied with the performance demands of society upon individuals. These are different, for example, in agrarian from those in industrial societies.

In addition, competence is increasingly considered to be related to context; the presumption of incompetence no longer follows commit-ment based on behaviour in a specific situation, but depends upon capacity to make decisions about specific problems in a range of situations (Bonnie, 1982). A sliding scale of competence has been proposed requiring an increasingly stringent standard as the consequences of the patient's decisions embody more risk (Drane, 1984). At the incompetent end of the scale are those delusional, depressed and confused persons who wish only to die or those panicky, paranoid ones overwhelmed with fears of attack or persecution who see hospitals as gaols and torture chambers, and proffered treatments as poisonous or death-dealing. Here any decision other than to be treated is regarded as irrational, that is, incompetent. In these situations the physician's power to prescribe compulsory hospitalization and treatment is routinely accepted. This degree of incompetence is often encountered in the kind of emergency circumstances under which US courts exempt the informed consent requirement. An emergency can allow the state to override a person's rights in order to assure the protection of others or of himself or herself (Arkin, 1984). However, in Massachusetts, as enunciated in 1983 by its high court, forcible medication, even under these circumstances, is regarded as restraint rather than treatment.

Towards New Relationships between Help-seekers and Helpers

Some of the differential means, that is, some of the inequities, between patient and clinician are being balanced out by the growing power of self-help and advocacy groups in the USA, Europe and Oceania. In Japan mental health law reform, beginning in 1989, is contributing to a decline both in the almost absolute power of private hospital superintendents and in that of families over their sick members. In the Western industrialized democracies in particular there is a growing availability of settings in which social support is combined with opportunities for self-determination, and in which the facility-users themselves have a voice in governance. The success of life in such settings may require sensitive employment of anti-psychotic drugs (often feared or disliked by the patient) as well as counselling and social support; hence a mutually trusting relationship between patient, community (both within and outside the facility) and clinician is essential. All this represents a move away from the tradition in which the professional holds complete authority while the patient is essentially disenfranchized. At the same time, if the professional is to function optimally, Veatch's reminder (1981) is crucial: if a lay person is given complete authority for specifying the framework of the relationship the professional loses all sense of being an autonomous agent with the right to make moral and other value choices.

The solution requires that the clinician always be regarded as the patient's advocate, even with a clearly specified obligation to society. The patient–physician relationship has always been regarded as a fiduciary one: the physician is held to a higher standard of performance than in ordinary contracts, with an obligation to protect the broad interests of the person who has entrusted himself or herself for care. This fiduciary and advocacy role is equally applicable to non-physician clinicians. It will become increasingly important as more patients are able to live in autonomy-enhancing settings with their own non-professional support groups. It should be preserved even if the psychotic person has a legal guardian or a family member who insists on acting in his place. Guardians and family members may have their own private aims which do not coincide with the best interests of the patient, who may be perceived as a burden and an embarrassment.

It is recognized that the effort to reconcile the principles of justice, autonomy and beneficence with treatments (sometimes resisted by the patient) aimed at restoring the welfare of persons defined as mentally ill or legally incompetent is an ideal. It is possible that a relationship between such persons, their communities and their professional helpers may never completely fit the ideal. However, it seems that the solution does not lie in relegating the issue to lawyers and the courts. As the Royal College of Psychiatrists' discussion indicated, 'good practice will not be established by balancing legal niceties, but by consensus within the professions and the general public about what ought to be expected of professional carers in relation to incapable patients' (Murphy, 1988). An open society requires negotiation, taking into account the rights of both helper and help-seeker in the context of community values about how people should be treated (Tormey and Brody, 1978). This is difficult when only one party, the helper, belongs to an elite with social power, and when diagnosis and treatment are determined significally by socio-economic status and context. It is made even more difficult by the social and ethnic diversity within the world's communities, a diversity progressively increased by accelerating flows of inter-national and rural–urban refugees and other migrants. Under these circumstances the tendency of clinicians to depend upon pharma-cological therapy instead of personal communication is increased. However, even the intergovernmental health arm, WHO, appears to be moving towards a more flexible, less legalistic stance with regard to psychiatric patients' rights, one emphasizing relationship and collaborative engagement in therapeutic efforts rather than the administration by a professional of a treatment to the patient as object. One WHO working group report (1987) describes 'the medical relationship' as 'an unusual mixture of a relationship between intimates . . . usually governed extra-legally' and a relationship 'between strangers . . . often governed by law'. This unusual mixture requires a special 'need for honesty and integrity' (p. 14).

All emotionally distressed and mentally ill persons, however disturbed, and even when defined as severely psychotic, should be given the opportunity to relate to another empathic, compassionate human being. Improved communication between helpers and help-seekers would do much to resolve some of the individual dilemmas of compulsory treatment and reduce the tendency to rely upon courts for solutions (Macklin, 1983). Along with the increased availability of user-controlled living facilities it would reduce the preoccupation of professional ethicists, lawyers and legalistically inclined citizens commissions with compulsory hospitalization and treatment. The increased participation of local support groups will help redress the inequity in social power which impairs communication between helper and help-seeker and precludes genuinely informed consent. The education of clinicians not to depend totally upon methods of physical or pharmacological treatment when human personalities are involved will foster recognition of the essential humanity of their patients. The dialogue between clinician and patient, as that between power-holder and help-seeker, is fuelled, as in Hegel's discourse between master and slave, by the mutual requirement of each to be recognized by the other as human. It is evident that the claims of mentally ill persons to respect and just treatment cannot be based upon a fluctuating standard of rationality, which may be bound by time or context, but must rest upon the qualities which they share in common with the rest of the human family.

7 Sustaining or Ending the Life of Dying or Comatose Patients

Introduction

Human Control of the Moment of Death

All societies and cultures recognize the transience of human life and the inevitability of death. However, they differ in their views of the meaning of death for individual and community life, and in their tolerated or preferred attempts at life prolongation for terminally ill persons, especially if they have lost their ability to maintain meaningful contact with families, friends and caretakers. The frantic efforts of modern medicine to defer death for even a brief period can be understood in part as reflecting the cultures in which the new technologies have arisen. They attach high value to individualism, self-reliance and dominance over other people as well as nature (see Chapter 1). While fear of death is ubiquitous among humankind it is plausible to suggest that such fear in individualistic cultures may be heightened by the approved early separation of adolescents and young adults from their parents, the pressure for independent living (autonomy) and, at the end of the life span, the continued attempts at independence by aging persons who, if they have the financial resources, may move themselves into retirement homes for their last years of life. Under these circumstances recourse to any means of extending personal control over one's own destiny, including the use of biomedical technology, seems a natural part of individual coping and defensive repertories. The most important research-based attitudinal contrast between individualistic cultures and those of the rest of the world is a factor called 'family integrity' which includes the items, 'Aging parents should live at home with their children' and 'Children should live at home with their parents until they get married' (Triandis et al., 1986). In general, the individualistic cultures here studied were exemplified by the USA, Canada, Australia, New Zealand and Europe, and the more collectivist cultures by East Asia. It is evident that, in the individualistic cultures, staving off or actively seeking death are the private (autonomous) concerns of the persons involved, perhaps collaboratively with their mates or other family members; their main allies or adversaries in the effort are their society's designated professional life-sustainers, the physicians. In the industrialized democracies, notably in the USA, physicians are sometimes forced into denying individual and family wishes with regard to life maintenance by prosecuting attorneys and courts. Under these circumstances the wishes and biases of the professionals may take precedence over those of the death- or life-seekers and families.

In the collectivist cultures, in contrast, death (including its timing) appears to be more acceptable as an inevitable element of life. It would be neither culturally nor personally acceptable to struggle for a brief moment of survival, often in highly constrained and painful circumstances, involving the massive expenditure of financial and human resources. If there are questions to be answered and decisions to be made, the family rather than the health professional (or the law or the courts) would be crucial. The individual is not regarded as a discrete unit, but rather as part of an interdependent web of mind and body, ancestors and the living, person and family. The immense investment of the industrialized democracies in artificial life extension represents a major change from the traditional world-views of pain, sickness and death as natural and unavoidable reflections of humankind's place in the universe. But while these have characterized preliterate and pre-industrial communities, they continue to be present, with modifications, in every society. Thus, in late twentieth-century rural Sweden an elderly person feeling the approach of life's end may still decide to 'go upstairs' and turn his or her face 'to the wall'.

For most of the world's peoples, of course, technological life-sustenance, whether for seriously defective neonates or for terminally ill adults with no hope of definitive recovery, is not part of consciousness or expectation. However, expensive technologies, sometimes in their own countries, but more often via travel to other parts of the world, are available to the affluent or politically powerful elites of less developed or authoritarian states. This is true both for those in which the privileged classes have accumulated great wealth by exploiting natural resources purchased by the industrialized nations, and for former colonies in which the values of the colonizers continue to motivate the elite. Artificial life extension is also possible for the less privileged citizens of the industrialized democracies; for them, however, while the opportunity for such life support exists, it is severely constrained by the excess of demand over supply and, in the absence of state subsidies, their inability to buy it (see Chapter 8).

At the same time, experience with the new death-deferring technologies is creating a new set of attitudes in the industrialized democracies which, paradoxically, may lead to a reduction in the values of individualism, independence and autonomy. The possibility of perceiving dying or defective individuals as collections of body parts to be used to repair others who are still viable or are economically able to purchase them have been discussed earlier (see Chapter 4). But, in addition, industrialized cultures may be returning to some perceptions of human life characteristic of the less developed world. A difference lies in the increasing power of society's designate (rather than the family), that is to say, the medical profession. Modern societies are coming to realize that 'human finitude is a reality, that physicians cannot cure all patients, that many patients are "saved" but remain with severe disabilities, and that we possess only finite resources', the allocation of which is significantly in the hands of physicians (Sprung, 1990, p. 2211).

The Impact of Biomedical Technology on Two Populations

In the industrial democracies and among the elite of the less industrialized world, biomedical technology has resulted in the existence of whole new populations of human beings. Few would have survived in earlier periods. The financial and emotional expense of maintaining them has sometimes been viewed as conflicting with the needs and rights of their families and society as a whole. Those evoking most intense debate about their possible rights are at the two extremes of the life cycle.

One population is at the beginning of postnatal life. The rescue of the most premature and low-for-gestational-age, as well as defective, neonates who require heroic, expensive and continuing treatment for survival of unpredictable duration with varying degrees of intactness have been widely debated. They owe their existence to the technologically based and still evolving field of neonatology. Here, as in other advancing biomedical fields, the research interests of physicians and their desire to use the most advanced available technologies may conflict with compassionate care. However, aggressively treating neonatologists are reinforced by popular movements devoted to sustaining all human life, including that of the unborn. For pro-life activists, and for many physicians, as well as some ethicists and theologians, the fact that survival technology is available constitutes a moral imperative to use it.

The other population is at the end of the total life cycle. Considerations similar to those involved in caring for defective infants with minimal expected life spans have been voiced in regard to sustaining the lives of terminally ill adults, including those who are competent and wish to die, or who are comatose, seriously brain-damaged or demented. In contrast to the neonates these have been self-aware, self-determining persons who have achieved identities in which there usually remains a community investment. For them the use of advanced directives regarding the withholding of life-sustaining technology, prepared when they were competent, is becoming more prevalent.

What Technologies are Considered Life-sustaining?

Life-sustaining technologies are 'drugs, medical devices, or pro-cedures that can keep individuals alive who would otherwise die within a foreseeable, but usually uncertain time period' (Congress, 1987, p. 8). They are not all 'high technology'. Cardiopulmonary resuscitation (CPR), for example, an interruption of 'the "normal" dying process' (Sprung, 1990, p. 2211), may be carried out by means ranging from vigorous external cardiac massage and mouth-to-mouth ventilation, to electrical defibrillators and temporary pace-makers. Other categories of life-sustaining technology include those which support or replace the functioning of a vital organ such as mechanical ventilation, or renal dialysis; nutritional support and hydration by parenteral means; and antibiotics. Except for the last, none can cure the underlying condition which makes their use necessary. Thus, many patients who survive an acute episode of illness because of life-sustaining technology may require it for the rest of their lives. If they become chronically dependent on such technology, this inevitably means dependence upon a range of other supportive persons, services and facilities.

The Human Consequences of Life-sustaining Technologies

On a global basis the disparities between human groups in access to technologies are clearly unjust. Awareness of denied access with its implicit denial of personal worth is a painful consequence. However, the most widely publicized human rights problem in this respect is not that of equal access. It is rather the imposition of, often temporary and unrewarding, survival upon patients and families who may not wish to have it. This is in significant part a consequence of the shift from home to hospital as a place to die. 'While hospitals were once feared as "places to die" because so little could be done to avert death, some people now fear [them] as places to die because so much can be done' (Congress, 1987, p. 17). Becoming a hospital patient means becoming subject to the legal as well as moral and clinical concerns of hospital managers and professional staff. Technological methods of diagnosis, treatment and life support are now available to physicians, sometimes backed up by lawyers and judges, who often feel that it is morally wrong not to use them, reinforcing their 'bias to treat'. The presence of technology rather than patients' needs becomes paramount. 'When resources are available, patients with life-threatening conditions are more likely than not to receive aggressive treatment' (Congress, 1987, pp. 27–8).

The fears of patients and their families that technological survival may be imposed upon them are well known to clinicians responsible for maintaining delirious, stuporous or comatose older persons after cerebral haemorrhage or metabolic failure, or younger ones unlikely to regain consciousness after serious brain injury. Concern is highest among educated middle-class adults in individualistic cultures attaching high value to personal autonomy. For them, loss of independence and the need to be cared for by children or other family members is not as acceptable as it is in more traditional and collectivist cultures. Informed, reflective, elderly persons in particular in these societies have become so concerned with the possibility of becoming imprisoned in a hospital bed that apprehensive discussions of how to cope with that possibility have become commonplace. The new technologies have already condemned enough people to a limbo between life and death to make anguished discussion about rights to live or die and the quality of life familiar. Proposed solutions range from escape through suicide or avoiding medical institutions in cases of life-threatening illness, to the construction of living wills asserting a desire to be allowed to die in case of persisting coma or loss of mental, communicative or motor functions. These patients, including those in persistent vegetative states, whose lives 'may be filled with suffering, but [are] sometimes . . . devoid of anything – of pleasure, sensation, or comprehension', have been called 'prisoners of technology' (Angell, 1990a, p. 1226).

Some of the new clinical options also raise questions about beliefs in the benevolence and omnipotence of nature or an all-powerful deity once felt to be stable and timeless. They are complicated by anxiety about assigning new death-dealing duties to a privileged class of health care providers whose past activities were traditionally constrained by a commitment to sustaining life. At a more concrete level a right to die, or not to be sustained by artificial means, may conflict with local moral interpretations, and with legal structures protecting the *status quo*. In this sense comatose or terminally ill demented patients whose families request their removal from life-support systems, and especially those who are rational (and not diagnosably depressed) but find their lives intolerable, impose a burden of decision-making on hospital staffs. In the most widely publicized instances relatives and patients have been painfully cast as adversaries to hospital staffs concerned with legal prosecution if they do not rigidly guard the lives of those whom society has assigned to their care.

The Role and Responsibilities of Physicians

While health economists have addressed these issues in terms of costs, and lawyers, jurists and legislators have considered their impact on society, at the individual human level they cannot be separated from clinical considerations, in other words, those controlled by physicians. Both 'prisoners' and beneficiaries of technology are 'patients' engaged in highly individual relationships with medical institutions and practitioners. Technological advances in medicine are always mediated for the individual patient through interaction with a physician who cannot ethically consider these issues without 'specific and informed attention to the psychological well-being of all concerned' (Brody, 1989b, p. 293). The application of life-sustaining technologies to individuals for whom death or personality dissolution is imminent makes it clear that the 'ethical' or 'human rights' issues involved in these clinical situations cannot logically be considered apart from those involved in giving humane, psychologically and culturally sensitive medical care to both patients and their families.

Care-givers themselves are being recognized as a third constituency (in addition to the society and patients and their families) with needs, demands and possible rights of its own. It has been suggested that as 'society upholds the rights of patients to forgo treatment, it should . . . avoid encroaching . . . on the moral sentiments of individual health care professionals'. Patients should be able to seek care from facilities and professionals who will affirm their own preferences without negating their 'preeminent right to decline any life-prolonging treatment' (Miles et al., 1989, pp. 49–50).

Continuing controversy about the allocation of scarce resources, and the existence of 'prisoners of technology', confirms that the assessment of hazards, and of burdens versus benefits, the adequacy of informed consent, and preservation of individual autonomy have lagged behind the technical progress of biomedicine. Hazard assessment requires attention to the value of treatment versus non-treatment, and of one kind of treatment versus another. It also requires attention to the appropriateness of aggressive versus supportive treatment in a particular situation. Some people 'may be willing to give up a small chance for survival in order to avoid the pain and indignity of death following aggressive medical care' (Murphy and Matchar, 1990, p. 2103).

An extensive literature suggesting physician discomfort with dying patients has resulted in new attention to these issues in medical school curricula. However, this tends to be overshadowed by the increasing emphasis on high-technology medicine which focuses the attention of student doctors on procedures and machines rather than the persons they are intended to help. This is strikingly evident in the neonatal intensive care nursery. Its patient population is totally dependent for its survival on life-sustaining devices, beginning with the bassinet. Work with fragile low-birthweight, sick and defective newborns who die easily (and who if 'salvaged' may survive only for short and pain-filled lives) can threaten the intern's self-esteem. It evokes anxiety, shame and guilt, intensified by the criticisms of supervising physicians, as well as doubts about the ultimate meaning of their work. At the same time the clinical demands upon the intern are so unceasing that personal discomfort must be ignored in order to permit continued functioning. The adaptive and defensive processes triggered by the anxiety, shame and guilt engendered by the work may be reflected in cynicism, denial and avoidance of contact with patients and families. It can impair the young physician's ability to deliver empathic clinical care (Brody and Klein, 1980).

How Life-sustaining Technologies are Used

Institutional Protocols: Public and Private Concerns

Health care institutions are expected to simultaneously serve the public interest and protect that of individual patients. This entails apparently conflicting goals, for example, respecting a patient's right to refuse treatment while, at the same time, trying to provide a high standard of health care to the community. A medical judgement that resuscitation efforts would be futile must be balanced against a legal or hospital requirement to resuscitate, or the need to respect a family's wish that resuscitation should be attempted. In order to satisfy sometimes incompatible interests most institutions depend in some measure on protocols or standard operating procedures. Protocols are one of several complementary mechanisms for clinical decision-making. They are usually formulated by committees from institutional staffs, but may represent compromises between medical, ethical and political judgements as the committees include advisers representing the community at large, religion, ethics, and the law. Such protocols are unevenly developed in countries which use them. This is true in the USA despite their advocacy by the President's Commission for the Study of Ethical Problems in Medicine and Biomedical and Behavioral Research (1983), public and private agencies, professional associations, and educational and advocacy groups, such as the American Association of Retired Persons. At the same time, concern with their development as a way of ensuring the consistent, ethical and humane use of life-sustaining technology has continued to follow increased public concern with patients' rights. Simultaneously, the concept of medical paternalism has been subjected to increasing scrutiny with regard to the welfare of incompetent patients.

Futility Judgements and Physicians' Decisions Not to Treat

The introduction in the late 1950s of effective technologies for cardiopulmonary resuscitation (CPR) brought an almost immediate need for a 'standing order', since imminent death from cardiac arrest does not permit time for deliberation. Soon, however, it was recognized that it could often be determined in advance that the attempt would be futile. Futility judgements tend to be made with success rates between zero and 14 per cent; more valid clinical predictions may become possible with the use of new predictive scoring systems (Murphy and Matchar, 1990). In their absence futility judgements continue to be based, as in the past, on informed guesses that the patient cannot be saved by CPR and would, indeed, be subjected to needless pain. The first hospital 'do not resuscitate' (DNR) policies were developed in the 1960s. In the 1990s CPR for cardiopulmonary arrest is usually required by institutional policy unless a DNR order with patient or family permission has been written. However, one ethics institute, while agreeing that a health care professional has no obligation to provide a treatment regarded as clearly futile, added an element of ambiguity. It stated that 'the health care professional's value judgment that, although a treatment will produce physiological benefit, the benefit is not sufficient to warrant the treatment, should *not* be used as a basis for determining a treatment to be futile' (Hastings Center, 1987). There is widespread agreement among physicians that treatment or no-treatment decisions should always be made on a case-by-case rather than a categorical basis. None the less, the importance of guides for clinical decisions 'responsive simultaneously to the needs of patients and the obligations of health care institutions and professionals' has been a major concern of the OTA (Congress, 1988b, p. 1).

Assertive hospital policies against using life-sustaining technologies clinically predicted to be futile (Massachusetts General Hospital, 1976; Rabkin et al., 1976) came at the same time as a 1976 judicial decision opening up the question of preserving 'life' at any cost. This decision permitted the removal, upon her parents' request, of a persistently comatose young woman, Karen Ann Quinlan, from a ventilator to which she had been attached for several years (see below). However, the concept of a DNR order was thrown into question by the President's Commission (1983, pp. 240–41) finding, on grounds of preserving the patient's autonomy, that it is 'necessary for the patient or surrogate to have given valid consent to any plan of treatment, whether involving omissions or actions'. This position has been increasingly challenged. A review of the problem (Tomlinson and Brody, 1990, p. 1276) notes arguments 'that judgments of futility should have the authority to limit the patient's or surrogate's autonomous choice of treatment' for adults, low birthweight neonates, and severely burned patients. It makes the point that 'certain sorts of value judgments must be made unilaterally by physicians as part of reasonable medical practice. Moreover, the mixed messages inherent in requesting patient consent to withhold futile therapy serve to undermine rather than to enhance autonomous choice' (p. 1276).

The American Medical Association (Council on Ethical and Judicial Affairs, AMA, 1991) notes the two exceptions to presumed consent to administer CPR. First is the patient's advance directive (a written statement of preference) for withholding CPR, or a decision made by the family or other surrogate. Second is the treating physician's judgement that CPR would be futile. The futility judgement is made in the context of the prevalence and established effectiveness of the procedure. CPR is attempted before approximately one-third of the two million annual patient deaths in US hospitals; approximately one-third of these survive the resuscitation effort, and of these survivors approximately one-third remain alive until discharge from the hospital (Schiedermayer, 1988). The life of those who die before hospital discharge is typically confined to an intensive care unit, subject not only to constant technological monitoring, but to invasive therapies (Congress, 1987). On the other hand, those who survive past the time of discharge usually do so without severe persisting impairment (Council on Ethical and Judicial Affairs, AMA, 1991).

Conflict has arisen most typically when family members want CPR performed despite a medical judgement that it would be futile. However, even if in a particular instance CPR is not clearly futile and requires discussion, an argument has been made against always requiring family agreement to the treatment (or no-treatment) plan (Hackler and Hiller, 1990, p. 1282). It recommends that hospital policies should allow physicians to write a do-not-resuscitate (DNR) order over family objections when

> 1) the patient lacks decision-making capacity; 2) the burdens of treatment clearly outweigh the benefits; 3) the surrogate does not give an appropriate reason in terms of patient values, preferences, or best interests; and 4) the physician has made serious efforts to communicate with the family and to mediate the disagreement. Most drastically, when resuscitation would clearly provide no medical benefit to the patient, policy should not require that it be discussed with either the patient or the family (Hackler and Hiller, 1990, p. 1281).

Other observers also believe that 'care-givers should have no obligation to discuss this useless therapy' (Murphy, D., 1988). Less drastically, the physician should be able to place at least some limitations on patients' demands for treatment, understanding that 'the moral basis of the physician–patient relationship is the obligation of the physician to attempt to do the patient some good' (Tomlinson and Brody, 1990).

The limitation of families' and other surrogates' wishes for continuing treatment continues to be opposed by many on the grounds that it violates the patient's rights to dignity and respect. Most students of the problem urge that patients or surrogates be informed of the futility judgement even if consent is not required. This does not negate the necessary and routine judgements made by physicians between good and evil, couched in terms of whether or not a particular treatment may do more harm than good. It fits the argument that the legitimacy of treatment goals must be determined in part by whether they are empirically possible as well as ethically justified (Steffen, 1991). An extension of this view might be that the pursuit of therapeutic aims, especially those imposing great discomfort on patient and family, is not ethical if there is little or no possibility that the aims can be achieved. This authority to make such judgements is based on societal concern with physicians' professional rather than their personal or individual integrity:

> the protection of this integrity is necessary for creating and sustaining a profession . . . [which must] make some judgments about the means to be employed in achieving the social goods for the sake of which medicine is instituted. . . . Social judgments about the range of rational conceptions of the good set the boundaries within which individual, instrumental rationality can competently operate (Tomlinson and Brody, 1990, p. 1279).

This is the background for an argument that failure to make futility judgements can undermine autonomous choices by patients and surrogates. It does not regard limitless options for patients as a safeguard against professional arbitrariness, but instead urges social dialogue to ensure that the value judgements of physicians have an adequate social warrant. In this context the use of the consent process as an organizing theme should be replaced by discussion aimed at enhancing the patient's and public's understanding of the limits of medical intervention (Tomlinson and Brody, 1990, p. 1280).

There appears to be general agreement that, under the circumstances of shared decision-making necessitated by multiple care-givers and family members, physicians should ensure that relatives and staff as well as competent patients are as well informed as possible. This is despite the fact that even well-informed people, especially dependent patients and their families, may be moved by anxiety, denial or hope to make decisions that are not fully rational. Discussing the futility of therapy may be useful in dealing with the family's denial of the patient's impending death, and thus helping them prepare for it. Discussion rather than unilateral DNR decision-making is essential to maintain the trusting relationship between physician, patient and family (Doukas, 1991). In this situation the clinician may find it useful to review hospital protocols with staff, family and patient and indicate their relevance to the particular problem being faced. Even those family members who regard the DNR order as in the patient's best interests will probably accede to the request of one member who insists that the resuscitation efforts continue. 'In the painful and confusing last hours of life . . . demanding that family members agree to the specific moment of cardiopulmonary death is occasionally cruel, leaving them with the belief that they may have made the wrong decision when there was actually no decision to be made' (Paradis, 1991, p. 354).

Objectives of Decision-making Protocols

Clearly articulated protocols or standard operating procedures for employing life-sustaining technology constitute one approach to creating order from sometimes chaotic clinical situations. They offer protection from poorly considered decisions, provide guidance about ethical and legal dilemmas which may bring liability judgements against the institution and its staff, and can be tailored to fit the needs of individual institutions. But almost paradoxically a major purpose of such protocols is to encourage clinical decision-making which is 'appropriate' and 'individualized' (Congress, 1988b, p. 6). Among the corollary objectives are decreasing staff uncertainties; reducing conflict between professionals, patients and families; improving the ability to audit and establish accountability; and increasing the empathy towards dying patients by 'creating processes that articulate positive health care goals other than sustaining life when this is no longer possible or wanted' (Congress, 1988b, pp. 7–8). The cultural diversity of health care workers as well as patients is recognized by including among the objectives of protocols, 'protecting the civil liberties of individual staff, so as not to compel them to perform duties to which they have a moral objection' (Congress, 1988b, p. 9).

Protocols may be expanded to include factors bearing on decisions about technologies defined as life-preserving which may more accurately be described as life-sustaining. Outcomes research suggests, for example, the possibly inappropriate use of a number of procedures with chronically ill elderly people. These include mechanical ventilation for patients with haematologic malignancies, prolonged intensive care for patients with multiple organ system failure, hepatorenal syndrome, and severe closed head injury. At the other end of the life span is CPR for premature infants (Murphy and Matchar, 1990, p. 2105).

The Right to Die: Patients in Persistent Vegetative States

It is estimated that, up to 1990, there were approximately 10 000 Americans in persistent vegetative (comatose) states, with no possibility of recovery, whose bodies were being maintained through life-sustaining technologies. Many of these are cared for in special institutions. It seems likely that this number will increase. At the same time, public awareness of these unfortunates, and the emotional and financial costs of sustaining their vegetative functions, is also increasing and may lead to changes in accepted practice.

Public and Scientific–Clinical Opinion

Contemporary life in the industrialized democracies is characterized by the wide dissemination of medical scientific information which in an earlier period would not have been available to the public, or would have been deemed too esoteric for general interest. The advent of life-sustaining technologies, in particular, has brought the popular and scientific–clinical subcultures closer together as knowledge of the difficult decisions which they pose to specialists has become almost immediately available to the wider public. Much interest has been focused on who makes decisions in the best interests of patients with absent or severely impaired cognitive functions and no power of self-determination. Physicians still continue to apply inappropriately and persistently the full contemporary medical armamentarium to such patients who will never regain their capacities, not only because they are totally and permanently unconscious, but because of severe mental retardation, brain damage, or dementia; all are 'non-autonomous' even though not declared legally incompetent (Weir and Gostin, 1990, p. 1846). Most physicians tend to overestimate the possibility of adverse legal action if they were to abandon repetitive attempts to preserve the body's vital functions, overlooking the fact that the right to refuse medical treatment has been granted to non-autonomous patients by almost all US state courts.

The Cases of Karen Quinlan and Mary O'Connor

As noted above, it was only in 1976 that a US state court decision, that of the New Jersey Supreme Court in the case of Karen Quinlan, 'established the tentative and limited authority of a loving family to stop high-technology respiratory support for a woman who was, with great certainty, irreversibly comatose' (Veatch, 1989, p. ix). Removal of life support was based on the patient's constitutional right of privacy which, due to her incapacity, could only be exercised by her parents. Since then many study commissions have recommended that the patient, or the patient's representative, should have the right to refuse or to halt life-sustaining treatment including medication and artificially administered food and water (Hastings Center, 1987). It was specifically noted that artificial feeding should be considered medical care, just as the use of a respirator is regarded as medical care. Although a national consensus for this view seems to be developing in the USA, and courts have, in many cases, held that individual patients have a right to refuse treatment over the objections of a hospital or nursing home, conflicts persist. Annas (1987), suggesting the primary responsibility of individual physicians who work intimately with patients and their families, considers that health care facilities have no institutional responsibility for the morality of medical decisions made within them.

'The medical, ethical and legal consensus that families could make decisions based on the best interests of incompetent patients' was rejected by a New York Appeals Court ruling in October 1988 in the case of Mary O'Connor, a widow with multi-infarct dementia (Lo et al., 1990, p. 1228). When her two daughters objected to the use of a feeding tube to keep her alive, believing on the basis of her own previous unambiguously expressed wishes while working in an emergency room and with cancer-stricken relatives that she would not want any form of life support, the hospital asked for court authorization for such feeding. Although the trial and appellate courts denied permission to emplace the tube (the patient was fed intravenously during the proceedings) the appeals court ruled that life-sustaining treatment be continued in the absence of unequivocal evidence that the patient would have chosen to refuse it. The patient had not specifically mentioned tube feeding in her earlier statement that she 'would not want to go on living . . . if she could not take care of herself and make her own decisions', and the court rejected decisions about treatment that were based on assessments of 'the best interests of an incompetent patient' (Lo et al., 1990, p. 1228). Mary O'Connor died in August 1989 with the feeding tube in place.

The Case of Nancy Cruzan

The first 'right to die' case to reach US Supreme Court was that of Nancy Cruzan, a 32-year-old woman in a persistent vegetative state for seven years since an automobile accident in 1983. Tube-fed through a gastrostomy, she continued, even with an atrophied cerebral cortex, to be sustained by the state of Missouri at an annual cost of $130 000 (Angell, 1990a; Lo et al., 1990). After four years of this, in 1987, her parents requested that the feeding tube be removed so that she could die. The hospital's insistence on a court order to permit the parents' request was granted. However, in 1988, the Missouri Supreme Court reversed the lower court decision on the basis of an unqualified state interest in the preservation of life and lack of 'clear and convincing evidence' that the patient herself had rejected life-sustaining treatment. 'It held that Cruzan's right to refuse treatment was personal to her and no one could exercise it on her behalf' (Annas, 1990, p. 670). The patient had, in fact, once expressed a wish not to live as a 'vegetable' (Lo et al., 1990, p. 1229), but the state's presumed 'unqualified . . . interest in . . . life' was given precedence over whether she herself would have wanted the feeding tube removed, the quality of her life, and her parents' request. Her mother, unconvinced that 'the state has evidenced an unqualified interest in preserving life' pointed out that children in Missouri were unable to obtain possibly life-saving bone marrow transplants for want of the $130 000 that the state spent on Nancy yearly. 'Missouri also has a death penalty – hardly consonant with an unqualified interest in preserving life' (Angell, 1990a, p. 1227). Lo et al. (1990, pp. 1230–31) reviewed the following human rights positions (and the literature supporting them) which were not taken into account by the Missouri court: society has an interest in promoting the best interests of incompetent patients; decisions about life-sustaining treatment should respect the patient's views on quality of life; and the court should take the adoption of procedural safeguards into account when it is concerned about the 'slippery slope' possibility, that is, that unscrupulous families might wish to discontinue treatment inappropriately.

In 1990 the US Supreme Court in a five to four decision upheld the Missouri opinion. It concluded that the US Constitution did not prohibit 'a state from requiring clear and convincing evidence of a person's expressed decision when competent to have hydration and nutrition withdrawn in such a way as to cause death' (Annas, 1990, p. 670). The major dissenting opinion in the words of its author, Justice Brennan, noted that the liberty interest of competent adults in refusing treatment is 'fundamental'; 'the State has no legitimate general interest in someone's life, completely abstracted from the interest of the person living that life, that could outweigh the person's choice to avoid medical treatment'. Justice Brennan added that the decision not to terminate life support 'perpetuates a patient's degraded existence . . . his family's suffering is protracted; the memory he leaves behind becomes more and more distorted', and the procedure 'transforms [incompetent] human beings into passive subjects of medical technology' (Annas, 1990, p. 671).

The importance accorded to the Cruzan decision, and its potential for misinforming the medical profession, are reflected in a published statement by a group of 35 bioethicists, including physicians (Annas et al., 1990). It emphasized that the court had affirmed the right of competent patients to refuse life-sustaining treatment and it urged physicians to follow their usual ethical and clinical guidelines, and to discuss life-sustaining treatments with their patients. The Cruzan court decision did not, in fact, rule specifically on the right of competent people to refuse treatment. However, it did not preclude a future determination that the Constitution could require states to implement the decisions of a duly appointed surrogate. 'If the state of Missouri can inflict its will on Cruzan and her family, none of us are safe from states that wish to control our health care decisions and our deaths' (Annas, 1990, p. 672). Despite uncertainty, it is important to execute detailed 'living wills' and durable powers of attorney documenting a person's wish not to have life-sustaining treatment continued under certain conditions. Although living-will statutes have been enacted in more than 40 US states most do not make provision for surrogate designation or penalties if health care providers do not do so (Annas, 1991). Fewer than 10 per cent of Americans have either such advance directives or organ donor cards.

Advance Directives for or against CPR or Life-sustaining Care

The concept of a document, often called a 'living will', or embodying a still intact person's wishes for continuation or cessation of life-sustaining treatment in the event of incompetence, is widely accepted in the industrialized democracies of North America, Europe and Oceania. In these regions, although specific legislation varies, such efforts to extend one's autonomy beyond the time of personal competence are culturally and socially congruent. Elsewhere, the question is usually irrelevant, as the technology to defer death is not available, or such decisions are in the hands of the family. Most states of the less developed world have not articulated an interest in preserving the life of vegetative or severely incompetent terminally ill persons.

In the USA the actual effectiveness of these advance directives is uncertain. One prospective study in a single hospital and nursing home suggests that, while they constitute a significant improvement, their effectiveness is limited both by failure to pay attention to them and by placing priority on decisions other than those aimed at preserving the patient's autonomy (Danis et al., 1991). Among the reasons for the staff's ignorance of the patient's advance directive were high staff turnover and a failure to transfer the document from unit to unit. Perhaps the most remediable area with regard to this, with worldwide applicability, is the education of physicians. While limited available data suggest that most patients in the industrialized democracies might wish to have a say about their future with reference to either CPR or life-sustaining technology, only a small minority have been given the opportunity to discuss the issue with their physicians (Council on Ethical and Judicial Affairs, AMA, 1991). Even those who have produced advance directives may not wish them to be strictly followed. One hundred and fifty mentally competent dialysis patients in a US hospital were asked if they wanted their treatment continued or stopped if they developed advanced Alzheimer's disease, and how much leeway (flexibility) they would give their physician or a surrogate to override the directive. They varied greatly in their responses and in which factors they wanted taken into account in making the decision (Sehgal et al., 1992).

Surrogate Choice

The tendency in appointing surrogates or substitute decision-makers for incompetent patients has been to appoint a member of the patient's family as one most familiar with the patient's previously expressed values, beliefs and wishes. In some instances, however, depending upon the discretion of the courts, this individual has been a long-term friend, a homosexual partner, or a fellow resident in a nursing home. Through the surrogate the non-autonomous patient is considered able to exercise the right to choose or refuse life-sustaining treatments (Weir and Gostin, 1990). However, substitute decision-making for incompetent patients raises the troubling question, in the absence of prior direct discussion while the person was competent, of whether or not the surrogate's decisions will, in fact, fit those which the patient might have made, or of whether or not the surrogate's decisions are necessarily in the patient's best interests. It is, of course, impossible to know, even with a prior advance directive, if the substitute or surrogate's views correspond with those which the patient, hypothetically, might have had under the circumstances. In this context the physician's own opinions and attitudes, not necessarily based on technical considerations, may play a major role. A physician who believes on moral or clinical–scientific grounds that something is in the patient's best interests is not likely to attach high value to a surrogate's differing recommendation or attempt to demonstrate its similarity to the formerly competent patient's own views.

Recognizing these issues, it has been suggested that 'real patient interests can better be served by a broad public dialogue around judgments of medical reasonableness and medical futility, rather than concern for the form but not the substance of patient autonomy' (Tomlinson and Brody, 1990, p. 1276).

Parents sometimes make decisions contrary to the best interests of their child, and this has been proposed as the basis for allowing physicians to refuse requested treatments that they considered 'burdensome and without benefit' (Paris et al., 1990, p. 1012; Leikin, 1987). An illustrative case (Paris et al., 1990) in this instance was of a 23-month-old girl, neurologically depressed with no responsiveness except to pain, who with a history of repeated medical and surgical interventions required mechanical ventilation and cardiovascular support. She had had four cardiopulmonary arrests, but her mother had continued to 'demand that everything possible be done to ensure the child's survival' (p. 1013). A meeting of all responsible hospital service chiefs agreed that further intervention would only subject the child to additional pain without affecting the underlying condition or ultimate outcome, but the mother rejected that opinion and took the case to court which appointed a guardian *ad litem* for the child. A paediatric neurologist from another institution expressed willingness to accommodate the parental wishes and the child was transferred to her care. Two years later the child remained 'blind, deaf . . . quadriplegic . . . fed through the gastrostomy' and averaging 'a seizure a day. . . . Her mental status [was] that of a three-month-old infant' (Paris et al., 1990, p. 1013). This case was used to illustrate the point that 'responsibility should not be shifted onto the shoulders of the patient (in this instance the mother) in a misguided attempt to respect autonomy. The patient or family can of course accept or reject the physician's recommendation. They are not free, however, to design their own treatment; nor is the physician bound to provide it' (Paris et al., 1990, p. 1013) This fits the report of the US President's Commission (1983) which states: 'The care available from health care professionals is generally limited to what is consistent with role-related professional standards and conscientiously held beliefs.'

Euthanasia and the Right to Die

Patients Who Want to Die

The foregoing has focused mainly on withholding or terminating life support for sick, defective low birthweight infants and comatose adults or those for whom CPR is judged futile. Another population consists of conscious individuals, still self-reflective and as rational as one can be under their circumstances. Some, having accepted surgery or other drastic treatments in the hope of attaining a few more months or years of life, choose to have DNR, do-not-resuscitate, orders written for them. Their desires in this respect, however, are not always clear, and involved surgeons and anaes-thetists, despite the possible hazards of CPR, often prefer not to have such an order if they are to agree to operate, and to have a pre-existing DNR order temporarily lifted for the surgical and post-operative period.

Other patients are less equivocal. They are not trying new treat-ments, but are usually maintained on life-sustaining technology, and because of pain, immobility, and loss of active engagement with life (and, presumably, in the absence of endogenous depression) find their lives intolerable and wish for oblivion. Perhaps the largest group of such persons wishing for medically assisted death, some-times called 'active' euthanasia, is that of elderly adults suffering from incurable, painful disease who have lost their powers of self-determination, sometimes even of communication, or those not yet totally incapacitated who dread the inevitable progression of dis-ability. Most arguments in favour of medically assisted or active euthanasia refer to the patient's right to autonomy or self-determin-ation. Most clinicians who argue against it refer not only to the traditional focus on the sanctity of human life, but on its conflict with the physician's traditional life-preserving role and the possibility that once it is permitted it may constitute the thin end of the wedge for other, less beneficent, life-terminating possibilities at the hands of the State or the professions.

Active practitioners, however, especially those dealing with painful chronic diseases such as cancer in its various forms, under-stand quite clearly that many palliative treatments intended to relieve pain and suffering will, when taken to their logical, and sometimes inevitable, extreme, result in the patient's death, for example through depressed respiration after gradual increases in morphine dosage. The Council on Ethical and Judicial Affairs of the American Medical Association (1992) notes that public opinion polls have indicated that more than two-thirds of respondents believed that patients dying of incurable disease should be able to end their lives if they wish to do so. While recognizing that in 'certain carefully defined circumstances, it would be humane to recognize that death is certain and suffering is great' the Council is unequivocally opposed to physicians performing euthanasia or participating in assisted suicide: while 'support, comfort, respect for patient autonomy, good communication and adequate pain control may decrease dramatic-ally the demand' for these acts, 'the societal risks of involving physicians in medical interventions to cause patients' deaths is too great in this culture to condone euthanasia or physician-assisted suicide at this time' (p. 2233).

When Elizabeth Bouvia, a 28-year-old woman, quadriplegic with severe cerebral palsy and severe arthritic pain, maintained through mechanical ventilation, tried to end her life by refusing to eat, a nasogastric tube was inserted into her by hospital staff, against her will. After many appeals in April 1986 a California court ordered physicians to remove the tube, holding that her refusal of treatment was not suicide and that removing the tube would not make the hospital party to suicide (Sprung, 1990). One judicial opinion recognized a right to die with assistance, noting that the patient 'apparently has made a conscious and informed choice that she prefers death to continued existence in her helpless and, to her, intolerable condition. . . . This state and the medical profession instead of frustrating her desire should be attempting to relieve her suffering by . . . assisting her to die with ease and dignity. . . . The right to die is an integral part of our right to control of our destinies so long as the rights of others are not affected' (Sprung, 1990, p. 2213). Comparable was a 1980 case in which the Florida Supreme Court ruled that a patient with amyotrophic lateral sclerosis who requested the removal of his respirator and understood that death would ensue without it should have his request granted (Sprung, 1990, p. 2213).

There were no deliberate life-terminating acts by a physician in these instances. It is likely, however, that such assisted deaths do occur in the USA as elsewhere in the world without regulation or public acknowledgement. The American Hospital Association has estimated that many of the 6000 daily deaths in the USA 'are in some way planned by patients, families and physicians' (Cassel and Meier, 1990, p. 751). One of the first physicians to write about engaging in such an act was Max Schur who, following years of discussion with Sigmund Freud whom he had treated for recurrent carcinoma of the soft palate, administered a lethal injection of morphine because of intractable pain when Freud was 81 years old. In contemporary times such acts have become taboo, placing physicians who acknowledge them at risk of losing their licences and even of prosecution for murder. The new medical powers to sustain life beyond comfortable limits, however, and increasingly widespread information about medical research, have begun to change public opinion. Aided by the advancing health consumer movement, patients and families, again mainly in the industrialized democracies, have begun to expect their physicians to collaborate with them in supporting a 'right to die'. Consequently, a few of these physicians are revealing their efforts to respond to their patients' needs. One such, notice of which brought shocked letters, was the (unsubstantiated) case of a 20-year-old woman with terminal ovarian cancer, revealed by an anonymous correspondent to the *Journal of the American Medical Association* (Anonymous, 1989). This correspondent claimed to have given the patient a lethal injection of morphine on their first encounter. Another was the reasoned discussion of a physician who, after consultations with the family and referring the patient (suffering from acute leukaemia) for psychological consultation, prescribed barbiturates with which she committed suicide (Quill, 1991). In this instance the author deplored the secrecy which has surrounded such acts, believing that they should be open to public and professional discussion. These discussions are occurring in an atmosphere of increasing frankness, stimulated in part by the work of the US Hemlock Society which has published a text on how to kill one's self, understood as 'self-deliverance', and assisted suicide for the dying (Humphrey, 1991).

The headlined act in June 1990 of Dr Jack Kevorkian and his makeshift 'suicide machine' with which Mrs Janet Adkins, a member of the Hemlock Society, took her life fearing deterioration from Alzheimer's disease evoked great public and professional concern. This reflected the physician's atypical background, the currently excellent health and functioning of Mrs Adkins, the brief period that they had known each other, and 'the lack of any procedures to ensure the accuracy of her diagnosis and evaluate her capacity to make this decision' (Cassel and Meier, 1990, p. 750). However, at a civil hearing about the use of the device to help terminally ill people commit suicide, attempts to find relief through its use were recounted by a wheelchair-bound woman with multiple sclerosis, and the relatives of a man who was dying from AIDS. They regarded Kevorkian, who had declined his services, as a 'trailblazer' (Wilkerson, 1991b). The co-ordinator of the Hemlock Society in the state of Oregon noted that the patient, Mrs Adkins, had had 'a longstanding, voluntary, well-considered philosophy of life that included her wanting the option of a physician's aid in dying in case of terminal illness or a disease such as Alzheimer's' (Coppens, 1991, p. 1435). She did not begin to work with Dr Kevorkian until after the failure of an experimental treatment for Alzheimer's disease, and did so with the support of her minister, family and others. Her aim was 'to die before her mind escaped her and made her, in her eyes, a non-person' (p. 1435).

A differing view focuses on the dependence of the death-seeking patient upon the physician. It asserts that most people who wish to end their lives because of pain and suffering can obtain instructions for suicide from the Hemlock Society (if not elsewhere) and do not require active physician assistance. Accordingly, 'dependence on another moral agent (the physician) diminishes the capable patient's own moral integrity while unnecessarily compromising the physician's' (Spielberg, 1991). This formulation seems to negate the reality of the helper's specialized knowledge and social power sought after by the help-seeker in this unique circumstance. Obviously there are hazards in the unexamined and unregulated practice of suicide with the assistance of physicians who have not been intimately involved with the sick person and family over time. But a case can be made for physician-assisted suicide as the ultimate act of compassion by a caring, reflecting, socially sanctioned helper. Cassel and Meier (1991) present a view more congruent with an interhuman formulation of patients' rights when they state that 'patients should not believe they have to sever their relationship with their physician in order to have comfort in dying' (p. 1436). But they favour strict criteria and guidelines, as well as improved physician education in this area. Kevorkian himself has become an advocate for laws explicitly permitting assisted suicide under certain conditions with special clinics for those meeting the legal criteria (Wilkerson, 1991a). Benrubi (1992) makes the point that many painful deaths are a direct consequence of advances in medicine that make it possible to survive for a valuable period of time, but make it likely that death, when the disease (e.g., a carcinoma) ultimately overwhelms the treated body, will be much more protracted and uncomfortable than it might have been prior to the advent of the new technologies. In such a situation, which will often last for only a brief period if allowed to run its course, 'compassion, intuition, and common sense cry out for active inter-vention to stop the suffering for all' (p. 198). The proposed solution is to develop stringent, procedural safeguards involving at least three physicians: the patient's actual care-giver, an anaesthesiologist with special qualifications in pain management, and a psychiatrist to make sure that a treatable pathologic depression is not involved.

The advent of shock–trauma units with supporting helicopter services bringing badly injured patients who might otherwise have died quickly to treatment within minutes has added yet another group to this population. They are typically young adults, many of whom suffer brain damage or permanent paralysis from high spinal cord injuries. Some, just as others with congenital defects, or cerebral haemorrhages suffered early in life, have indicated that they find living under such circumstances intolerable. Some relatives of seriously impaired older people, particularly those whose minds and sense of self have vanished (as in the case of Alzheimer's disease or multi-infarct dementia), as well as the parents of young adults in persistent vegetative states, and of grossly impaired children, may also find their own situations intolerable.

Euthanasia as Defined and Practised

Euthanasia, sometimes qualified as 'active', has been defined as 'the deliberate action by a physician to terminate the life of a patient'; this may be differentiated from 'assisted suicide' in which 'the doctor prescribes but does not administer a lethal dose of medication; and "mercy killing" performed by a patient's family or friends' (Singer and Siegler, 1990, p. 1881). While still technically illegal, it is currently part of operating Dutch public policy, and between 5000 and 10 000 patients in the Netherlands are estimated to receive euthanasia by barbiturate and curare administration each year. National guidelines for physicians (deWachter, 1989; Rigter et al., 1988) require that there be no doubt about the patient's wish for death; severe suffering without hope of relief; lack of other treatment options; and free and informed decision by the patient. The practice is illegal if these guidelines are not met. However, while consultations are required, the exclusion of severe clinical depression is not clearly defined. On the one hand it has been suggested that euthanasia could be part of a physician's responsibility towards hopelessly ill patients (Wanzer et al., 1989). On the other, while many proponents of euthanasia fear the 'prospect of dying shackled to a modern-day Procrustean bed, surrounded by the latest forms of high technology', the ability of competent patients to 'exercise their right to choose or refuse life-sustaining treatment' has been taken to mean that 'they do not require the option of euthanasia' (Singer and Siegler, 1990, p. 1882). Similarly, a strong case can be made for improving the care of dying patients, especially with the appropriate use of analgesics. A central issue is involuntary euthanasia, active as contrasted to passive (via the withholding of treatment). Suggesting a likelihood of increased pressure to legalize euthanasia associated with spiralling health care costs, Singer and Siegler (1990) believe that it would endanger many vulnerable patients who could be killed without their consent, or persuaded to consent, and that it threatens the moral integrity of the medical profession. If euthanasia is legalized they recommend that physicians refuse to participate. Analogies to Nazi excesses, beginning with murders of mentally defective and chronically psychotic individuals, have been drawn. Published responses to their statement suggest an almost even split among physicians. Most agree that, while physicians should not be required to participate in carrying out euthanasia considered as a patient's right, the issues of right and wrong are not clearly defined and the abuse of the privilege by a few does not justify its denial to the many (Spital and Spital, 1991).

Indications of a possible shift in the climate of American public opinion include polls showing a majority in favour of active euthanasia under specified circumstances. Polls published by the national Hemlock Society, a pro-euthanasia organization (Roper, 1988), and in 1990 by the *New York Times*–CBS, reported that a majority of those responding believed that doctors should be allowed to assist a severely ill person to commit suicide. In November 1988 an attempt was made to place a law permitting euthanasia for terminally ill patients on the California ballot, and in Washington State there has been a move to broaden the definition of terminal illness and permit aid to competent patients wishing to die.

The dialogue now in progress and sporadic attempts at legislation indicate the need for more public as well as professional education in this area. Cassel and Meier (1990, p. 751) suggest that 'a more open process might allow a higher level of public and professional accountability, resulting in the effective limitation of assisted suicide to clearly appropriate cases and enhancing public respect for physicians'. They believe that 'the debate over assisted suicide and euthanasia should shift to an examination of the needs and values of patients in a context that recognizes the limits of modern medicine and the inevitability of death'.

Courts versus Physicians as Arbiters of Life-sustaining Technologies

A growing body of opinion among US physicians feels that courts should not be routinely involved in decisions regarding withholding or withdrawing life-sustaining technologies. Tomlinson and Brody (1990), above, have made a strong case for the physician's role as society's socially and culturally designated decision-maker in this arena. An opinion of the New Jersey court ruling on the case of Karen Quinlan stated: 'The morality and conscience of our society places this responsibility in the hands of the physician. What justification is there to remove it from the control of the medical profession and place it in the hands of the courts?' (Sprung, 1990, p. 2212).

Lo et al. (1990) believe that 'the legal process, by its very nature, may rely on inaccurate clinical data [and that] requiring advance directives to meet the legal standard of "clear and convincing" . . . promotes the . . . imposition of treatments that are neither beneficial nor wanted' (p. 1229). They believe that courts should be involved 'only when the surrogates are not acting in good faith or when the decisions of the surrogates cannot be considered by a reasonable person to be consistent with the patient's wishes or best interests' (p. 1231). Angell (1990a, p. 1227) suggests that court procedures are ill equipped for decision-making about life-sustaining technologies, and judges 'can certainly make no claim to any special understanding of the patient. The role of the courts might better be limited to appointing guardians or settling disputes when necessary.'

Finally, the court is at least as prone, if not more so, to making its own value judgements about these cases as are physicians. In raising certain issues about advance directives but not others, the court imposes its own values upon patients. As one judicial opinion (cited by Lo et al., 1990, p. 1231) put it: 'Courts are not the proper place to resolve the agonizing personal problems that underlie these cases. Our legal system cannot replace the more intimate struggle that must be borne by the patient, those caring for the patient, and those who care about the patient.'

8 Biomedical Technology: Towards Health for All?

The Relevance of 'Scientific Advance'

Rights to Scientific Benefit Including Health Care in Context: United Nations, National Governments and Policies, the Physician–Patient Dialogue

The 1948 United Nations Universal Declaration of Human Rights states, as previously noted, that 'Everyone has a right to a standard of living adequate for the health and well-being of himself and his family, including medical care and necessary social services.' Access to the 'benefits of scientific advance' is also among the 'rights' listed in that declaration. This was elaborated in the International Covenant of Economic, Social and Cultural Rights adopted on 10 December 1966 by the UN General Assembly, at the same time that it adopted its International Covenant of Civil and Political Rights. Article 12 of the Economic, Social and Cultural Rights Covenant 'recognizes the right of everyone to the enjoyment of the highest attainable standard of physical and mental health'.

Both covenants entered into force in 1976. By their twenty-fifth anniversary, 10 December 1991, that on Civil and Political Rights had been ratified by 101 UN Member States, and that on Economic, Social and Cultural Rights by 105 Member States. The Western world has considered civil and political rights to be indicators of democracy. However, major Western European nations have ratified the Economic, Social and Cultural Rights Covenant, and committed themselves to provide universal access to basic health care for their citizens as a human right. But the USA, which has not ratified either covenant, officially regards 'human rights' in terms of corrective justice, as limited to redressing wrongs committed against specific individuals. It does not recognize distributive justice, the allocation of resources, as a right. This it relegates to policy-making. Further, the US government considers that rights in order to be legally valid must be enforceable by judicial action and there is no way to legally enforce the right to an adequate standard of living. A first step in this direction would be to define a measurable standard of minimum health care for the industrialized democracies with advanced economies, which is consistent with the human rights declaration.

211

Opposing the US view is the official UN position, that human rights are interdependent and indivisible. The two categories are of equal importance and a practical distinction cannot be clearly made between civil and political rights and economic, social and cultural rights (United Nations DPI/NGO/SB/91/37 – not an official record or press release). This position is embodied in Article 28 of the Universal Declaration of Human Rights: 'Everyone is entitled to a social and international order in which the rights and freedoms set forth in this Declaration can be realized.'

A significant 'benefit' of scientific advance is high-technology medicine. Perhaps the most difficult problem which this poses is how to achieve just or equitable access to it. For the peoples of the developing world this is an abstract question; they know little about the new technologies and, although they are learning rapidly, the likelihood of their personal access in case of illness is so remote as to be non-existent. Biological science and biomedical applications continue to flow mainly from the academic and industrial laboratories of the industrialized West. While their allocation takes place within the context of national laws and health policies, the physician remains the essential intermediary between the laboratory and the patient. It is the knowledgeable and technically skilled physician who must finally decide whether or not to utilize a new procedure, device or drug with an individual patient. The physician's dialogue with patient and family forms the immediate context in which this decision is made. Jonsen (1990) summarizes the conflict inherent in the physician's role in his phrase, 'The Good Samaritan as Gatekeeper' (pp. 38–60). The compassionate and technically competent healer is simultaneously the one who does the allocating, who opens the door to the recipients of his or her limited services. This, then, becomes not solely a problem of ethics, politics or policy, it is one of conscience.

Health and High-technology Health Care as Human Rights

The technical competence of Western medical practitioners and the resources available to them reflect the years of national support for biomedical research since the Second World War, including the establishment of various types of national institutes of health. The bulk of extramural support in most industrialized democracies has been funnelled through academic health centres which produce technology-oriented physicians. But while the scientific benefits of this support have been enormous, the supply cannot meet the demand for them. As medical innovation continues, and supply catches up with demand in particular instances, it is likely that new technologies will create new demands.

High-technology medicine is 'the sum of all the advances in medical knowledge and technique that have been translated into improved diagnostic, therapeutic, and rehabilitative procedures during the past several decades' (Ginzberg, 1990a, p. 1820). This logically includes the organizational and supportive systems necessary to the use of all the medical and surgical procedures, drugs and devices which are part of contemporary medical care (Congress, 1978). These are all encompassed, by inclusion or exclusion, in the national health plans which have been adopted by the world's advanced industrial economies except for the USA. US medical practice, despite growing attempts at regulation and systems such as Medicare, Medicaid and the Veterans' Administration which partially cover significant population sectors, remains in 1993 an essentially *laissez-faire* activity with large numbers of people left with no provisions for health care at all.

'Health for All by the Year 2000'

The possibility of health in a particular society is not primarily a function of the availability of biomedical technology. It depends, fundamentally, upon how the society is organized to ensure its members' healthy development and to protect them against disease, injury and deficit. The primary prerequisite for child and adult health, after all, is to be born with an intact central nervous system to loving, wanting parents with the knowledge and available services allowing them to manage their own fertility, protect their offspring prenatally, and provide the conditions for their optimal development. This prerequisite, and the interests of the disadvantaged persons who constitute the bulk of the human race, require basic literacy to help them understand how to care for themselves, adequate shelter, clean water, and a standard of nutrition sufficient to ensure growth and development. Health promotion and disease prevention which allow the full fruition of latent capacities for everyone, regardless of parentage, culture and socio-economic status, begin with the technologies of safe, effective family planning and perinatal care, of inoculation against infectious disease, and antibiotics. These attitudes are embodied in the UN World Health Organization's aim for the end of the twentieth century, articulated at its 1978 Assembly in Alma Ata: 'Health for all by the year 2000'. 'Health for all' does not involve general availability of the advanced technology so central to modern medicine, but focuses instead on a less expensive goal, largely achievable by organizing available human resources and low-technology biomedicine. This goal is the provision of primary health care. The scientific advances upon which it depends stem mainly from epidemiology, family planning, maternal and child health, the prevention and treatment of malnutrition and infectious disease, and the recognition and treatment of mental illness masked by physical complaints. They also depend in some measure upon an understanding of human behaviour as it bears on the adherence of individual patients to prescribed regimens. This is 'low-technology' knowledge applicable to the world's predominantly resource-poor populations with limited health care personnel.

Despite reservations about deflecting scarce human and financial resources to technologically oriented health research, however, it seems likely that applied biomedical science will continue as a major element of modern society. Its actual significance for individual patients at any given time depends upon its availability and distribution. The most significant future elements may be those based on the identification of genes associated with particular diseases or defects (see Chapter 5). As noted in Chapter 2, biomedical science in the past has also contributed to major demographic changes, and continues to increase the length and quality of individual human life. This last benefit, however, is not equally distributed among the world's peoples. For most of them 'rights' to the possible benefits of biomedical science do not even exist as unfulfilled claims. The actual availability of these benefits requires not only their presence in the society, but sufficient awareness of them to fuel desire, and sufficient ability and personal capacity to obtain them. These last depend upon individual status. This is tied to privilege within one's own community, and the ability to go elsewhere in the world to obtain medical care when it is not available at home. The interests of those most remote from decision-makers, the most disadvantaged or least powerful members of a society, tend to be submerged when publicly funded public policy, including that bearing on health, is being formulated (Rawls, 1971).

Beyond these concerns the rapid advances of biomedical technology are changing the industrial societies of the world, their perceptions of the nature and rights of human beings, and the expectations of their citizens for care and respect. From this base they are already exporting ideas, expectations and technology to the less developed world. On the one hand, the expenditure of scarce funds on high-technology medical centres and training high-technology physician specialists in the Third World detracts from more essential investment in preventive and primary health care. On the other hand, the consumer movement is also being exported from the industrialized democracies to the rest of the world. Even the newly formed mental health associations, established under the aegis of the World Federation for Mental Health, are contributing to an informed and educated world citizenry, which is essential to the achievement of WHO's goal of 'health for all'. These mental health associations, members of WFMH, are pioneers in the health consumer movement, and are engaged in the tasks not only of moving their governments towards effective action, but of educating themselves and their neighbours about every aspect of health care and patients' rights.

Populations with Inadequate Access to Health Care

Persons of Low Status

Access to medical care in most communities is linked, however indirectly, to one's status in the community ranked on a variety of bases. In most industrialized nations discrimination or selective neglect in allocating medical resources have been most obvious with regard to persons in the lowest socio-economic strata, who suffer disproportionately from illness, injury, developmental deficit and disability. Within the lowest socio-economic stratum the likelihood of suffering and deprivation is greatest for children, women, the elderly, refugees and migrants, and members of other minority groups (ethnic, religious, political) with blocked or diminished access to sources of societal power. In the USA, about 33 million people lack health insurance, including 10–12 million children (Harvey, 1990). However, 'health care alone cannot entirely redress the conse-quences of the poverty, poor education, limited access to fertility services, unaffordable child care, and limited employment oppor-tunities that afflict women with low incomes' (Guyer, 1990, p. 2265).

Migrants, Refugees and Minorities

Contemporary migrants include large numbers of refugees who have typically been subject to severe and repeated trauma and loss, both in their home countries and in transit. Their culturally alien, minority status combined with lack of knowledge, skills and confidence, result, furthermore, in rejection by the host society. Vulnerable to illness, and without the supports of a familiar context, including language, they are targets of discrimination, excluded from full participation in the cultural process of their new society and access to the benefits available to its native members. This 'cultural exclusion' (Brody, 1966) is also directed in some measure against rural–urban migrants, especially in developing countries with a deep gulf between countryman and city dweller. Migrants of the lowest socio-economic status from the drought-stricken rural Brazilian north-east into Rio de Janeiro, suffering from overwork, fatigue, undernutrition and chronic disabling illnesses, and housed in unhygienic *favela* shacks without running water or indoor toilets, found it extremely difficult to develop viable connections with the new community, including its health system. Their capacity to find work and begin the slow process of upward mobility was significantly less than that of migrants with greater socio-economic advantages, especially those coming into Rio de Janeiro from other urban centres (Brody, 1973a).

The diseases, illness-related behaviour and help-seeking efforts of refugees and other migrants from the less developed world, and the minorities with the lowest socio-economic status in the developed nations, reveal the consequences of limited literacy, general education and access to employment opportunities. Their attempts to cope and adjust also reflect, especially for recent migrants, the consequences of development in contexts in which docility or avoidance in the face of authority is rewarded. Fear, unfamiliarity with the social system, and preference for familiar folk and traditional approaches to diagnosis and treatment make it difficult for many to utilize available medical help. As part of their collectivist orientation, attributing high value to the interdependence of individual, family, lineage and state, many from the Third World have the habit of agreement with heads of families which extends to community leaders and other holders of authority. Potential patients are not only uninformed; they have the habit of automatic agreement with authoritative professionals who are separated from them by a wide socio-economic gulf as well as command of specialized knowledge. This makes them vulnerable to incentives to participate in health programmes which include access to otherwise unobtainable material goods and thus have a subtly coercive nature. This appeared, for example, to be the case for young Indian males volunteering to be vasectomized in return for transistor radios (Brody, 1976). Similarly, as noted in Chapter 4, one-time payments to persons recruited as sources of kidneys for transplant into more affluent people can be interpreted as coercive in nature.

In the USA the two major minority groups identified as significantly health deprived are African–American and Hispanic (a term which loosely covers people from a variety of national and cultural origins). In June 1991 a meeting was held to review the Tuskegee project following the course of untreated syphilis in African–American men (see Chapter 1) and examine its long-term effect on the relationships between the US medical establishment and the African–American population. There, the US Secretary of Health and Human Services noted, 'Every year since 1984, while the health status of the general population has increased, black health status has actually declined . . . across the board.' While poverty was cited as a significant part of the problem, including the black infant mortality rate twice that for whites and a life expectancy for blacks six years less than for whites, prejudice and discrimination were also invoked. Cited as evidence was organized medicine's acceptance of the Tuskegee study the data from which have been incorporated into the medical mainstream. This led ethicist Arthur Caplan to state, 'Informed consent is a privileged man's protection' (Wilkerson, 1991c). However, there is some evidence that for poor, minority persons such information can make a difference. This comes from a study made to identify obstacles to organ transplantation in the US African–American population in order to understand why, although more than 50 per cent of end-stage renal disease patients in the south-eastern USA are black, less than 10 per cent of kidney donors are black. Five principal reasons for the reluctance of blacks to grant permission for organ donation were identified. These were: 'a lack of awareness of the status of organ transplantation and of the urgent need for organs by blacks; religious beliefs and misperceptions; distrust of the medical establishment; fear of premature declaration of death if a donor card has been signed; and a preference among black donors for assurance that the organs will be given preferentially to black donors' (Callender et. al., 1991, p. 442). After two-hour interviews with 40 black men and women concerning the issue every participant, including the 90 per cent who had previously been unwilling, agreed to sign an organ-donor card. Since that time a variety of approaches, designed specifically for this population, have been undertaken with apparent success.

Hispanics are the fastest growing minority subgroup in the USA and, overall, more likely to live in poverty, be unemployed or underemployed, and have little education and no private insurance. Among the illnesses for which they are at increased risk are diabetes, hypertension, tuberculosis, AIDS, alcoholism, cirrhosis, specific cancers and violent deaths. Proportionate to their representation in the population there are few Hispanic health providers (Council on Scientific Affairs, AMA, 1991). Proposed remedial measures are mainly non-specific, focusing on general issues of health insurance (mandated for employers, for example) and poverty relief. It does appear important, however, to differentiate the overall group into those from specific nationalities, such as Puerto Rican, Mexican, and so forth, in order to approach such health risks as substance abuse, smoking and obesity. It is also suggested that significant increases in the training of Hispanic health care providers will be important (Ginzberg, 1991).

Age-defined Minorities

Adolescents can also be regarded as members of a minority group with blocked access to societal power (Brody, 1968). Many suffer double jeopardy as they are, additionally, members of ethnic minority groups. The rights of minors *vis-à-vis* parents and guardians, including access to the benefits of science and technology, and to privacy, are continuing matters of debate in most of the world's societies. Among the debated issues regarding health care are informed consent; medication for presumed 'conduct disorders'; availability of and privacy regarding contraception, pregnancy termination, and treatment of sexually transmitted diseases; the requirement of being a witness against adult offenders in open court; and the definition of what constitutes a 'minor'.

Although the developed world is seeing for the first time a class of affluent, healthy persons over the age of 65, the population of older people worldwide still constitutes a minority in terms of access to societal power and its benefits. Further, the older population does have real impairments. In the USA, 23 per cent of those 65 years of age and older are disabled in one or more aspects of self-care, and more than 40 per cent of those 75 years of age and older have some degree of dementia (Lonergan, 1991). It is estimated that 43 per cent of those who have reached 65 years of age will need nursing-home care at some time during the remainder of their life, and that about 55 per cent of these will be in a nursing home for one year or more (Kemper and Murtaugh, 1991).

Major recommendations for research bearing on older people's right of access to care include increasing knowledge of behavioural and social factors in health and disease and helping them maintain their social as well as biological health (Lonergan and Krevans, 1991). Significant social issues relevant to justice in health care for older people include a loss of respect for them as self-determining individuals. This encompasses failure to involve them in informed-consent procedures for medical care; diminishing opportunities for independent functioning even though they may be capable; and lost opportunities for continuing employment forcing them to be dependent upon relatives or institutions. Modernization and the disintegration of the extended family also threaten the traditionally respected role of the elderly and, particularly in a youth- and technology-oriented society, increase the spectre of 'agism' as a form of anti-minority discrimination. Kane and Kane (1991) make the point that in the USA the 'current orthodoxy and rules for licensure' of nursing homes have generated 'an expensive form of professionally based services, each with its own professional aides'; this has restricted the options for frail elderly people, burdening them with the need for expensive oversight. They 'should have the right to take considered risks' (p. 628).

The Control of Health Care: Medical Power and Consumerism

Just access to technology-based health care, or the equitable distribution of scarce resources, cannot be considered in separation from the societal prerogatives of the physicians who are, in effect, gatekeepers controlling access to care.

Medical Authority

Medical power is based on culture and tradition as well as society; often charismatic, it proclaims itself in the language of an independent, autonomous, self-policing and self-perpetuating liberal profession. Its most fundamental claims, however, are rooted in the authority of the state which supports its training, licenses it, and permits its practitioners to invade the minds and bodies of their fellow citizens. As noted in Chapter 2, the almost universal public acceptance of contemporary medicine's monopoly on the definition, diagnosis and treatment of disease is reminiscent of the earlier, sacrosanct status of state religions (Freidson, 1970). To this may now be added its functional control of, and entrepreneurial involvement in, biomedical technology.

A graphic example of medical power to restrain others, deprive them of freedom, or grant liberties in association with validating the sick role, has been the abuse of psychiatry in totalitarian states (see Chapter 6). In the industrialized democracies physicians are also empowered to restrict freedoms on official grounds of public health or societal well-being. Here too, psychiatric commitment, an exercise of state-granted medical power, is the most obvious example of an act which can be rationalized both in terms of individual protection and the public health. New health threats and new screening technologies are expanding state power in this respect. Mandatory screening for AIDS, for example, is on the way to being added to older immunization and reporting procedures prescribed on public health grounds. Right to privacy concerns, already present with regard to state interference with reproductive freedom, and mass screening of low-risk populations for drug abuse, now encompass new technologies for predicting psychological or biological life courses. These can encourage a 'self-fulfilling prophecy', as well as official limitation of life opportunities on hereditarian or related grounds.

More commonplace manifestations of socially mandated medical power are granting excuses for absence from school, work or military service, or certifying someone as eligible for military duty or employment in hazardous or socially sensitive jobs. More subtle are the everyday, almost automatic and gently persuaded, clinical decisions made by physicians without adequate, fully informed, reflective discussion with patient or family.

Technological Medicine and the Competing Allegiances of Physicians to Patient or Society

Most of the new technologies amplify the social power of physicians and increase the likelihood of paternalistic decision-making in so far as they require mastery of esoteric knowledge and skills not readily available to most citizens. The enhanced perception of the modern clinician as a healer with semi-magical powers, sometimes in the instrumental cloak of a super-engineer, facilitates the aggressive marketing of his wares. The oversupply of expensive medical technology in industrialized urban areas is based in part on competition between hospitals trying for prestige as well as economic reasons to offer the most complete and up-to-date services. This has been especially marked with regard to imaging and organ transplantation. The USA uses more expensive technological interventions than either Britain or France (Payer, 1989).

This new availability of powerful technologies, even of unproved effectiveness, blurs the borderline between the twin allegiances of physicians: to their individual patients and to the society which enfranchises them. The situation is exemplified by a terminally ill patient with whom the physician wants to try a previously unavailable, scarce, expensive technological resource for which no controlled trials have yet shown clear benefits. In an earlier era, with no last-minute hopes to hold out, there would have been no conflict between a duty to society and one to the patient. In the present technological era a duty to society recognizes that the cost involved (for this patient with a very limited probability of survival) reduces the resource pool to be applied to others with higher survival likelihoods; even more drastically, it reduces funds which could be applied to less expensive preventive activities. The traditional duty to the patient, however, requires that all physicians should do everything possible for the patients for whom they are responsible. A classic instance would, hypothetically, pit high-dose chemotherapy with autologous bone marrow transplantation (with a 10 per cent treatment mortality and a high likelihood of complications and side-effects and limited life expectancy at best) for a breast cancer patient with liver and bone metastases, against using the money to treat patients with a better outlook, or devoting it to systematic mammography screening (Eddy, 1991). In the abstract, 'When one group [in society] receives a disproportionate amount of resources compared with another group, society suffers in the sense that the aggregate health of all of its individuals – measured by such indexes as mortality rates, morbidity rates, and life expectancies – is lower than would occur with a more even distribution' (Eddy, 1991, p. 1449). The blurring in allegiances or duties is extended by the competitive marketing of health care organizations, especially as they control increasingly expensive machines and facilities, so that allegiance to society (versus that to a patient) becomes confused with allegiance to one's organization or institution. When physicians are involved in prescribing or utilizing procedures and products in which they have a personal financial–entrepreneurial interest, an interest in the product or procedure (high-technology imaging, for example) tends to be weighed in the direction of higher fees and profit-making; an interest in the patient must be in the direction of reduced expenses as well as therapeutic efficacy recognizing the patient as a self-reflective person with subjective needs.

Consumerism in Medicine

Arrayed against the forces of technologically enhanced medical paternalism are those of consumerism (Haug and Lavin, 1983). Fundamental to a humane interpretation of society's interest in the employment of health-related technology is the balance between the paternalism of medical service providers, reinforced on the side of state or societal interests, and the self-determining, autonomy-seeking values of consumers of medical service. The help-seeker, *en route* to becoming a patient or client, is, as a 'consumer', a buyer who challenges medical knowledge and decisions, and wants to participate in so far as is possible in decisions affecting his or her own future. The consumer articulates rights of justice, autonomy and beneficence, and expects the physician to honour them. One idealized view states: 'In contemporary American culture, it is appropriate for doctor and patient to meet as equals, with the former rendering expert advice and the latter bearing ultimate responsibility for deciding whether or not to follow that advice' (Katon and Kleinman, 1981).

This ideal seems less achievable as the power of paternalism is enhanced by accumulating technology. Even without advanced technology, the anxious, dependent, disabled, unknowledgeable patient can never be the psychological equal of the healer possessing the golden secret which, it is hoped, will afford relief. But if the healer possesses technology that promises better health care most consumers in modern industrialized societies seem to want it. At the same time, it is not rational to believe that patients perceive the use of invasive procedures in a manner identical to the physician. The view, for example, 'that the current rates of use of invasive high-technology medicine could well be higher than the patients want is based on the hypothesis that, particularly when risks must be taken to reduce symptoms or improve the quality of life, patients tend to be more averse to risks than physicians' (Wennberg, 1990, p. 1203). This view is supported by patients' more conservative treatment preferences when confronted with their options regarding benign prostatic hypertrophy. It has also been argued (see Menzel, 1990, below) that patients are capable of making rational choices if they are given all the available information about the risks, benefits and comparative efficacy of various high- and low-technological approaches to their medical problems. Perhaps it would be more accurate to say that choices can be made in the course of dialogue and consultation and that a major goal in the high-technology medical era should be to improve communication between doctor and patient. The cognitively intact patient's informed, reflective participation should be a *sine qua non* for decision-making about the use of major technologies, particularly those about which predictions are difficult and which embody possible hazards. 'Rational choices . . . depend on attitudes about risks and benefits – how patients view their predicaments' (Wennberg, 1990, p. 1202).

Unintended Harms from New Biomedical Technologies

Indirect Cultural Consequences

Chaper 2 discussed the unintended, and often unmonitored, impact of advancing biomedical technology upon the value structure of society. The methods, modes and styles of technology transfer, including the selection of devices for transfer, require careful attention to social and cultural appropriateness in relation to existing values, as well as the possibility of exploitation of traditional by modern societies. They also require attention to unintended harmful technical–medical consequences.

Among the unintended social costs of advancing biomedicine are those from the treatment of mental disease as indicated in Chapter 6. For example, the population of persons diagnosed as schizophrenic has increased its reproductive rate in consequence of new drugs enabling them to live in the community (Arnhoff, 1975). Thus, the gene pool is changing in ways which may result in larger numbers of disease-vulnerable individuals.

A less apparent risk of a narrow biomedical orientation to research on health care is that of omitting subjective and other human factors from consideration when investigators depend primarily on survey data or technical measurements, including behavioural rating scales and telephone interviews. Obtaining data which include the subjective reality of informants in relation to their socio-cultural context requires ethnographic participant-observation (Brody, 1981b; Brody and Newman, 1981). The importance for biomedical clinician–scientists of private as well as public knowledge was foreshadowed by the eighteenth-century philosopher, Giambattista Vico. Believing that there is 'a sense in which we could know more about our own and other men's experiences – in which we [act] as participants, indeed as authors, and not as mere observers', the distinction he drew was between 'outer' and 'inner' knowledge (Berlin, 1976).

Direct Biomedical Consequences

With regard both to individuals and populations the human rights issue is how to maximize the benefits and minimize the harms coming from biomedical science and technology. An undramatic but significant example concerns the impact of saturating populations with drugs intended to destroy or change the nature of bacteria or viruses. Thus, Levy (1990) has pointed to the impact of prescribing antibiotics on the development of strains of drug-resistant organisms and the importance of reducing reservoirs of resistance genes: 'Those who prescribe and use antibiotics need to develop a greater respect for their long-range ecologic effects' (p. 337).

Another example concerns the conversion of innovative treatments to standard therapy. While the use of experimental therapies is restricted by legal and ethical norms, once a therapy becomes standard it can be regarded as obligatory. For example, parents who refuse to consent to its use for their children may become legally liable on grounds of medical neglect.

Market forces as well as justice considerations may encourage physicians to label a new approach as non-experimental (Lantos and Frader, 1990, p. 409). Many insurance companies will not pay for experimental treatments so patients who cannot afford to pay may have reduced access, and producers wishing for a rapid return on investments must await approval of their product. In an atmosphere in which physicians recommend 'last chance' quasi-experimental treatments to psychologically competent patients for whom early death has been predicted, this has had personally devastating consequences. An instance would be a patient's acceptance of a medical recommendation for a new form of bone marrow transplant combined with anti-cancer drugs, only to be refused by the hospital providing the treatment unless they could pay the large sum which insurance will not cover. Lack of coverage is based on categorization of the treatment as 'experimental'. Such patients and their families, understanding that the success of the treatment is uncertain, feel, none the less, that their only chance at continuing life has been denied. The fact that denial is on financial grounds is particularly difficult to accept in a culture which attaches high value to the egalitarian ideal. Part of the problem lies in the lack of generally accepted criteria for removing the treatment from the 'experimental' category. Frequently specified requirements include: 'a minimal number of treated patients whose cases have been reported, a threshold for rate of cure or improvement in the quality of life, or a randomized trial that establishes a benefit over conventional therapy' (Newcomer, 1990, p. 1702).

The Impact of Biomedical Technology on Less Developed Countries

Technological Development and Social Inequality

The 1985 UNESCO-sponsored resolution (Appendix 1) noted that scientific advance should not increase 'economic and cultural disparities among social and national groups'. This warning was stimulated in part by the aggressive marketing of international health care and pharmaceutical corporations in the less developed world, and an awareness that competitive promotion of biomedical technologies is influenced more by short-term, profit-oriented market interests than concern for long-term social development. Marketing practices can actively disturb plans for orderly community development with health care facilities and health improvement as a central feature. Inhabitants of the less industrialized world are also at risk of harm from the unprepared introduction of high technology into their low-technology settings. They have been used as secondary markets for pharmaceuticals when newer products are directed to primary markets in the industrial nations; it has been suggested that trials of new contraceptives carried out on Third World women could be considered exploitative. Many procedures, drugs and devices exported to developing nations are not relevant to or may even be contraindicated for disorders with cultural roots. Or they may destroy naturally occurring support groups or inhibit necessary intra-country development. It is clear that individual and community targets of aggressive First World marketing in the less developed world need advocates. In every instance the goal is to empower the group or the patient, to enable the community or the affected individual, to share intelligently in the decisions which will affect their lives. In the developing world a few health consumer organizations, prominently mental health associations, are just beginning to act as mechanisms for reducing anxiety and dependence upon paternalistic medical authority, and reducing vulnerability to aggressive marketing.

Need for a Research Base in Developing Countries

The UN warnings do not take into account the absence in many countries of the fundamental conditions for the simplest primary health care: political stability, access to existing modern science and technology, and capacity for research including the evaluation of treatment efforts. Only 5 per cent of global health research expenditures are concerned with the developing countries, which contribute 93 per cent of the world's premature mortality (Commission on Health Research for Development, 1990). Direct transfer of First World scientific knowledge and technology to the Third is considered 'inappropriate and ineffective'; 'the solution lies in building the capacity of developing countries to conduct and act on their own research in the areas most pertinent to the health of their citizens' (Evans, 1990, p. 913). Research necessary to determine how to use severely limited resources must be context-specific.

Technology Transfer and Modernization

The introduction of medical technology into traditional healing contexts may disrupt naturally occurring or traditional support structures. Family responsibilities and trusting relationships with local healers can be diminished. In some such settings families and healers have worked together with Western-trained physicians. A number of international health organizations, including WHO, are interested in the integration of biomedical and folk healing personnel and methods, sometimes in association with the delivery of mental health services in primary health care settings. It is also recognized, however, that traditional healing practices may have little therapeutic value, and, in some instances, can even damage the victim.

One little-noted consequence of medical modernization is loss of the traditional acceptance of death as part of life. This is an aspect of a context in which even pain and illness are understood as serving necessary functions (Pedersen et al., 1984). Healers in traditional cultures look for the sources of an afflicted individual's difficulties in social context, ancestral lineage and cosmologies (Brody, 1973a). They place less emphasis than biomedical practitioners in industrialized nations on solving specific problems or curing discrete illness. The continuing search for what their own transplanted healers can offer, as well as inability to cope with a more complex social system, influences the underutilization of conventional medical facilities by migrants and other ethnic minority persons living in industrial, urbanized society. Many customary practices of Western medicine, including the autopsy, are antithetical to the values and beliefs of migrants from a number of other cultures.

Technological Upgrading of Hospitals

There are many reasons for the transfer of high-technology medical devices to existing hospitals in both industrialized and developing nations. One is the understandable desire to upgrade the quality of services offered; this is driven in part by humanitarian concerns and in part by physicians' wishes to be in the forefront of the techno-logical medicine they were trained to practice. Another is the hospital's need in an era of market-oriented health care to be competitive with other hospitals for paying patients; many of these are supported by insurance coverage which pays larger fees for hospital than for office-based procedures. In the developing world, in which the upgraded sections of the hospital are available only to a tiny proportion of the ruling class or the urban population, and the impetus for modernization often comes from a totalitarian leader, these factors may be complicated by a wish to enhance national prestige. In all countries the appearance of new technologies leads to increased investment in specialized hospital units in which they may be used.

The technological upgrading of hospitals has had major functional consequences. These begin with the anticipation that the new devices and procedures will become available; individual as well as institutional desires for the new possibilities, such as organ trans-plant units, ICUs, advanced imaging devices, or IVF capabilities, may interfere with the community functions of particular hospitals, and create constituencies which can disturb the orderly distribution of health care facilities. In most European countries the hospital was traditionally a nursing institution in which 'doctors practised medicine for their patients'. The accelerating incorporation of technology has been 'a very important *de facto* stimulus for the integration of medicine into the hospital'. This includes expanded staffs; since increasingly sophisticated apparatus is no longer within the budget of the individual physician, increasing numbers of doctors and paramedical workers (the latter provided by the hospital) must be involved in operating the equipment (Schutyser, 1988, p. 49).

On the other hand, the 'schizophrenic separation', that is, the 'historic dualism of medicine versus hospitals' with its separation of charges, services and personnel, has, in some instances, become more complicated in ways which impair both health care delivery and the job satisfaction of some categories of care-givers. The charge per hospitalized day has gone up for everyone, and methods of third-party payment have required new attention to the very concept of the 'hospitalized patient' (Schutyser, 1988, p. 41).

There is a high regional variation in the use of the specialized technology in which US hospitals have made major investments (Wennberg et al., 1989). They are equipped to deal with common conditions by expensive, usually surgical, means. More than half of US inpatient surgery is accounted for by angina pectoris, benign prostatic hypertrophy, gallstones, arthritis of the hip, conditions of the uterus, and low back pain. Yet there are other common, less invasive treatments for these conditions that are consistent with contemporary standards of care (Wennberg, 1990). Some US areas in which there are relatively few hospital beds appear to have no higher mortality or morbidity rates than those elsewhere which have many hospital beds for the treatment of similar patients. 'The rules governing the use of hospitals' for serious, surgically treatable conditions are 'determined more by behavioral accommodations to the available supply than by recognized medical theory' (Wennberg, 1990, p. 1203). At the same time, the limited available data concerning local variations within a single US state in the use of coronary angiography, carotid endarterectomy and upper gastrointestinal tract endoscopy do not indicate that they are due to inappropriate use (Leape et al., 1990).

Medical Entrepreneurialism, Health Care Costs and Just Availability

The Competitive Development and Marketing of Biomedical Technologies

The allocation of scarce technology-based treatments, the facilities in which they are applied, and the trained personnel necessary to use them, pose a more immediate problem for the developed than the less developed world; ultimately, however, the health care models of the First World and their exported versions have an impact on the prospects for rational, sustainable community development in the latter. To the degree that effective health care in an agrarian village, or even a non-industrial urban economy, must be integrated into community life, and must be based on prevention and primary service delivery, the high-technology model of an industrial urban health care industry is inappropriate.

In a capitalist society without a national health care system, such as the USA, competition for partial government insurance subsidies has been a factor in the transformation of a locally based medical practice into a health care industry. More significant, however, has been the rise of medical entrepreneurialism including technological product development in all the industrial democracies. In the USA this has been associated in part with the new insurance schemes, but more fundamentally with the accelerated federal support for research and

physician training since the Second World War. Biomedical entrepreneurial activity and commercial competition have driven the costs
of services to patients up, not down. Competitive, aggressive
marketing (extending in the USA even to health maintenance
organizations (HMOs) designed to provide low-cost, prevention-
oriented services) has not only added advertising expenses to already
hard-pressed budgets, but stimulated demand beyond need and
resulted in wasteful duplication. Their high operating costs have
even caused HMOs, originally designed to provide comprehensive
care, to limit the time which physicians can spend with patients.

As in the case of any business depending upon product development and marketing, much of the hospital and physician demand for
new technologies (passed on to patients) is supplier-induced. The
crucial determinants of rising US health costs have been 'the basic
incentives in the health care system, especially its financing arrangements' including new demands for investment created by advances
in science and technology (Starr, 1982, p. 384). The costs of using the
new technologies, that is to say, their operating expenses, appear less
important than their role in the for-profit, competitive marketing,
investment-seeking features which modern medicine now shares
with typical business-oriented corporate entities. Within medicine
these have driven up the costs of hospital employees, medical fees,
and hospitals which must constantly seek new resources. 'New
forms of technology and insatiable demand' for their use

> are not the fundamental causes of cost inflation, nor are overuse,
> inefficiency, duplication, or excessive overhead expenses. They are
> . . . the manifestations of a system that has built-in incentives for waste
> and inflation. . . . The present health care environment . . . en-
> courages . . . physicians and hospitals to be expansive rather than
> conservative in providing medical services. Aggressive marketing, not
> the prudent use of resources is the prevailing imperative. . . . In an
> open-ended competitive system with more and more new physicians,
> new forms of technology, and new health care facilities entering the
> market, it is inevitable that costs will continue to escalate despite
> targeted restrictions on the delivery of certain services (Relman, 1990a,
> p. 912).

As suggested above, the significance of third-party payers, private
and public, in this equation is related to the post-Second World War
marketing context which evolved at the same time. This period in the
USA has been described as a period of health care 'destabilization' in
which government-sponsored Medicare for the elderly, Medicaid for
the indigent poor, and other public and private third-party payers
played a major part, initiating a drastic upward swing in medical care
costs, strengthening the financial autonomy of hospitals as insti-

tutions and the power of hospital administrators, with a concomitant weakening of the social power of physicians (Ginzberg, 1990b). It has also been argued, however, that the most significant impact of third-party payers is in insulating both patients and health care providers from the true cost of using high-technology medicine, compounded as fee schedules pay more for identical technology-based procedures when they are performed in hospitals rather than in private offices (Starr, 1982). These distorted prices encourage overuse of hospitalization, tests, technology-based instrumentation and procedures, and surgery.

In the US fee-for-service system, the economic incentives, as well as 'a fascination with technology', also encourage more doctors to enter specialities than the society needs, and fewer to go into general primary care or family medicine. 'The obvious defect is the absence of any restraint . . . the outcome of a long history of accommodation to private physicians . . . hospitals and insurance companies', an 'institutional phalanx . . . blocking any form of control or any alternative form of organization that would have threatened their domination of the market' (Starr, 1982, pp. 385–7).

On the other side of the argument are those who, while recognizing the role of medical entrepreneurship in increasing costs, are 'convinced that the paradigm of the competitive market cannot be applied to health care' in an affluent economy in which insurance plays a major role (Ginzberg, 1990b, p. 40). 'High tech is the driving force of contemporary medicine that is committed to continuing sophistication and change as a result of ongoing basic and clinical biomedical research and its application through new technology to the treatment of patients' (Ginzberg, 1990a, p. 1820). Much of this, such as hypothermic anaesthesia needed for specialized surgery, for example, of cerebral aneurysms, will be applicable to relatively few patients. With regard to more widely applicable technologies, 'Commercialized health care, like any other commercial activity, generates increased consumption, thereby adding to total expenditures. We cannot expect to control costs if public policy encourages commercial enterprise in health care and if professional organizations take no stand against entrepreneurialism by practitioners' (Relman, 1990b, p. 992).

Market competition also has a more direct impact on physicians, their patients and the relationship between them. One impact is through the accelerated attempt by insurance companies to identify persons who are not vulnerable to or apt to have undiagnosed, or presymptomatic chronic, or severe disabling illness. As noted in Chapter 2, predictive screens are now capable of excluding some such potentially expensive patients from financially pressed hospitals (Nelkin and Tancredi, 1989). At the level of personal choice, 'competition will increase pressures on sicker subscribers toward adverse selection of more comprehensive plans, and insurers will attempt to skim the cream of healthy subscribers into lower-cost coverage' (Menzel, 1990, pp. 132–4). The effect of being uninsured in the USA (compounded, of course, with the impact of poverty and marginal status) is revealed in the finding that uninsured patients had a significantly higher risk of in-hospital mortality at the time of admission than did the privately insured, and were less likely to have normal results on tissue pathology biopsy reports (Hadley et al., 1991). The fact that they were less likely to undergo high-cost or high-discretion procedures suggests the possible role of financial capacity in the use of the procedures.

In the USA the transformation of medicine into an industry has also fostered the rise in malpractice suits, with huge judgements rendered against physicians. These have increased the costs of practice, both through the purchase of malpractice insurance and the pressure to order large volumes of laboratory tests in order to fulfil the necessities of 'defensive medicine'.

Corporate Medicine and Health Care Costs

The human rights impact of science and technology is determined by those who control it commercially as well as politically. This includes the scientists, clinicians and other specialists who are engaged in the tasks of discovering and developing it, applying it in the clinic, interpreting and disseminating public knowledge about it and, through membership on ethics committees, making rules concerning its use. Linkages between physicians, medical schools, hospitals, pharmaceutical and medical equipment manufacturers and suppliers, insurance companies, the military establishment, and other government agencies all feed the development of a for-profit entrepreneurial spirit within the health care industry. The hypothetical cost-reducing and service-enhancing value of competition between providers has been destroyed in other ways.

Fuelled by these interconnections, and financial infusions from third-party payers, the 1970s in the USA saw the rise of corporations, often involving chains of institutions, to sell health services to patients for a profit (Starr, 1982, pp. 428–9). Relman had earlier described this 'new medical industrial complex' as 'the most important health care development of the day' (1980). He distinguished the new for-profit businesses such as hospitals, dialysis centres, and home care companies from the older firms selling drugs, insurance and equipment.

Corporate medicine with its progressively concentrated managerial power increased its effective monopoly on facilities. In the

presence of monopoly neither insurers nor patients can find alternatives; this encourages 'diminishingly beneficial and increasingly
expensive marginal services' (Menzel, 1990, pp. 134–6), permits
higher charges to those whose insurance or private means can pay
them, and promotes cost-shifting for others. Through patented
research, corporations have been able to maintain high prices for new
products. The expense of developing, marketing and maintaining
new technologies, and of training personnel to use them, has further
contributed to high selling prices, not only for surgical instrumentation and other equipment but for prescription drugs; many poor
persons in the USA who are not covered by health insurance must
choose between buying prescribed medications and buying food. In
many other countries the drugs are not available at all except to the
small, wealthy elites who may obtain them elsewhere.

The corporate transformation of health care signalled another
change in the values of medicine as well as its organization. The new
chains of investor-owned hospitals, directed by centralized corporate
management with no ties to a particular community, and aimed
single-mindedly at making a profit, were a marked contrast to the
traditional free-standing, community-based hospitals, with strong
medical staff participation in their operation (Starr, 1982). In order to
make their profits hospital chains must admit patients not needing
hospitalization, overuse heavily reimbursed technological services,
and duplicate expensive equipment with costs recoverable through
insurance. Since they are focused on the profitable, privately insured
sector of the health care market, diagnosis and treatment in their
facilities is effectively allocated on the basis of ability to pay, except
for procedures and patients with advertising or public relations
value. This means that patients who cannot afford them are
transferred to overloaded public and teaching hospitals, which, with
no way to recover their costs, may be driven into insolvency.

The Allocation of High-technology Reparative Medical Care

Respect for the Individual and 'Health for All' in Cost-conscious Society

As noted above, the classic dilemma for most attempts at just dealing,
including the equitable allocation of health care, is that of reconciling
allegiance to and respect for the individual with the overall welfare of
society. The latter requires socially efficient, including cost-effective,
use of resources; in the case of health, this means effective utilization
of low-cost, low-technology, readily available maintenance and
preventive care measures. In terms of scarcer resources it requires an
allotment policy which is culturally congruent, that is to say, it must
support the prevailing values of the society. In totalitarian or

autocratic societies it may be important for political reasons to conserve resources so that the mass of the population can receive free basic health care while high-technology life preservation is neither available nor expected. In these settings the allotment of benefits to the leader and the elite, including the privilege of going elsewhere in the world for technologically advanced treatment, is taken for granted. Preserving the life of the maximum member of society fits the official value system. Similarly, in theocratic societies, major resources are used to preserve the lives of the religious elite or those designated by it.

In the Western industrialized democracies privilege also accrues to the powerful, but this does not fit the culturally accepted stereotype. The prevailing value, to the contrary, is egalitarian. But whether, even with the best of goodwill, this value can be translated into equal access to life-preserving technologies is problematic. It is even possible that, despite continuing reiteration of the ideal, the prevailing tendency is away from egalitarianism. The evidence suggests a popular drift towards utilitarian thinking which tends to favour productivity, efficiency and social well-being in selecting candidates for the assignment of scarce life-preserving resources (Kilner, 1990, p. 28). While this is described as most marked in such Western nations as the USA and the UK, it has also been observed in other countries, such as Kenya, apparently through values implicit in the educational system – thus people are viewed more in terms of social usefulness than intrinsic worth (Kilner, 1990). However, neither utilitarian values, nor status attributes such as education, social position and ability to pay, fit the explicit values of the Western democracies; in these cultures they are not acceptable as deliberately arrived at bases for access to limited resources.

An examination of 'the poor and the puzzle of equality' (Menzel, 1990, p. 116) indicates the persistence of the dilemma, as it emphasizes the impossibility of achieving the kind of strict medical egalitarianism which might fit the society's shared values. High-technology resources for diagnosis, reparative and life-sustaining treatment, as well as those desired but not needed, such as IVF, have become almost prohibitively expensive. The discrepancies between personal need or desire and overall societal welfare, and between the personal and social costs and benefits of biomedical technologies, are rooted in the overall social context in which individual care and the individual doctor–patient relationship are embedded. This is why, without changing the broader socio-economic context of health care, 'medical egalitarianism' cannot be achieved. 'If we . . . stick to our egalitarian convictions, we end up in the seemingly insane situation of funding million-dollar-per-life-saved technologies for the poor while we let them live as paupers otherwise' (Menzel, 1990, p. 117).

This is why the WHO vision of 'health for all' is confined to the simplest primary care, and to the prevention of ill health and disease through non-technological public health measures. Even in the industrialized nations where public tax-supported research has made a private biomedical technology industry possible, the literal provision of equal access to high-technology care, utilized most often by the elderly, would inevitably raise the level of spending to a point which would preclude investment in preventive care for the young, and maintenance care for working adults. That is why most national health systems do not offer, or severely ration (under a variety of disguises), expensive technological care such as renal dialysis or organ transplants.

'Rationing' in Response to Inequalities in Health Care Allocation

Various definitions of health care rationing follow that of Aaron and Schwartz (1984). The essential point is that all patients do not receive, or more directly stated are systematically denied, care which would be expected to be beneficial to them. Even in the absence of deliberate and systematic denial, however, *de facto* rationing of most aspects of technical health care, including access to mass-produced antibiotics or immunization, exists in every country of the world. Where access is not based on ability to pay it is limited by lack of social power, geographically available facilities, knowledge about how to utilize the social system, the presence of competing folk-medical beliefs, or even the active interference of particular governments with international health relief efforts.

The industrialized democracies are just beginning to recognize the importance of utilizing their existing knowledge of low-technology preventive health care which should reduce the eventual incidence of disease requiring high-technology repair or life preservation. WHO's emphasis on primary health care as the means for achieving 'health for all by the year 2000' underscores this. The growing US concern with primary health care, particularly its preventive aspects, is seen, for example, in studies indicating that the main barriers to early and regular prenatal care associated with more favourable pregnancy outcome are not financial (Piper et al., 1990). They appear, rather, to be unhealthy behaviours (such as smoking, substance abuse, poor nutrition) potentially under the pregnant woman's own control, and a fragmented health care system which interferes with easy access to it. Stimulated by an expanding population of children who may achieve less than optimal development, and the examples of basic health care coverage in other industrialized democracies, a proposal has been made to provide health insurance to all US children and pregnant women (Harvey, 1990).

Most discussions of health care rationing in the industrialized democracies, however, concern general access to technology-based medicine. They are especially intense in North America, Europe and Oceania, where the media and the public have developed an accelerating interest in the availability of quasi-experimental procedures and the fate of those asking for them as a 'last chance at life'. Even insured patients are facing explicit denial of certain expensive high-technology services, such as organ transplants. When support is denied because insurance companies will not cover treatments regarded as experimental, surgical teams, sometimes with research motivations, and the hospitals in which they work, may be pressed to donate their services without pay – in which case the costs are silently shifted to others who are able to pay. The preferred answer to the ethically loaded question of individual patient selection for a drastically limited resource varies with the socio-economic system and the culture. In the free-choice, self-improvement, nature-mastering US culture the prevailing faith of the dominant elite is in rapid medical progress leading to universal high-quality care, and the eventual conquest of every disease. But this faith exists in a country with no comprehensive fiscally autonomous national health system and a capitalistic health industry. In this setting the culturally determined ideal is, almost paradoxically, to make publicly supported technological resources available to all. The unfortunate consequence is that, where such support does become available for treatment not covered by insurance, and for a person without the money to afford it, it is often a response to impulsive emotional appeal. Obviously, this is an erratic, unpredictable and inherently unjust way to allocate a scarce resource. Similarly, for most of the modern era, indigent patients coming to metropolitan emergency rooms before the advent of the high-cost health industry could always count on the best care available to any other patient. But in the current market-oriented health industry many emergency services threatened with financial collapse are turning patients away; other indigent help-seekers may not receive the same care as those who are able to pay depending upon the locality in which they happen to be at the time.

In the nationalized systems of such countries as the UK, organized in terms of set fiscal allocations, planning for care within the budget is accepted as simply precluding the possibility of some high-technology procedures; others, such as renal dialysis, are generally not a practical option. A small private sector does, however, allow access outside the national system to the affluent, powerful and mobile who could go to another country for their medical repair if necessary.

In some welfare-oriented or liberal socialist economies, with heavy taxation, the most complex high-technology treatment is unavailable, but there does exist easy access to basic care, and a reasonable level of medical competence. Publicly supported technical care, which does not generally include the most expensive, state-of-the-art procedures, usually coexists with a small private practice sector to which a small proportion of the people have access. Again, a private market, and the possibility of obtaining care outside the country, are viable options for those with sufficient means.

In other, especially totalitarian, nations with much-vaunted publicly supported health care, the readily available service is largely of a rescue, first aid, or primary nature; in these countries shortages of sterilizing equipment, needles for parenteral therapy, essential drugs such as antibiotics, adequately trained personnel, and even lack of basic amenities such as hot water, may lead to unnecessary morbidity or mortality, and more technically sophisticated care is difficult to obtain. Most regimes which advertise their health systems as political achievements accept as given a gross inequality between what is available to the population at large and to high government officials and others with status and privilege, including that of going abroad for medical treatment.

Rationing, Resource Allocation and Patient Selection for Treatment

The most obvious alternative to medical egalitarianism is to deliberately ration, allocate, positively select or selectively restrict resources used to promote and preserve life and health. Official patient selection proposals for specific scarce life-preserving procedures are typically made on the basis of categorical standards produced by some government body arrived at through a consensus of presumed financial, medical, legal and ethical 'experts'. Age is an example of one such categorical criterion.

Resource allocation is inherent both in national health systems and private insurance coverage. There is no totally satisfactory solution to the problem of selecting individual recipients for scarce life-saving medical resources. Leading examples are major interventions such as organ, including bone marrow, transplants, or complex surgery requiring large, expensive specialist teams and operating room support.

When needed elements are limited at their source and new supplies depend upon the availability of other human bodies, as in the case of transplantable organs, the choice of someone to save always means that another person is left to die. Where supplies are not so clearly limited, as in the case of major surgery, teams are able to choose between equally pressing priorities; the patient must then be able to survive until their time and operating facilities are available. Cost and the interest of involved specialists become major factors.

Most of the frequently discussed social criteria for deliberate patient selection, such as usefulness to or responsibility for others, or power and affluence, do not fit their accepted value systems, and would not, therefore, be chosen by responsible committees in the industrialized democracies. The only selection criteria with some promise of cultural acceptance are medical. The criterion of medical benefit, 'according to which only those who satisfy minimum standards regarding likelihood, length and quality of benefit should receive treatment' (Kilner, 1990, p. 223) appears to underlie other criteria with the greatest potential for widespread support. It can be useful as a basis for resisting demands for useless treatment (see Chapter 7). Two other criteria are those of ability to prevent imminent death by the technological intervention, and the more debatable one of relative likelihood of benefit *vis-à-vis* other candidates. After such specific criteria the most widely acceptable approach appears to be random selection, in a form of lottery (Kilner, 1990).

Individual patient selection criteria have been less widely argued for more routinely applied technologies than for the assignment of more acutely life-preserving procedures. These 'routine' technologies, perhaps overused, include carotid endarterectomies, hysterectomies and Caesarean sections; diagnostic devices such as nuclear magnetic resonance imaging, mammography, CAT or PET scans; and less expensive instrumental exploration such as gastrointestinal endoscopy. In these cases the rationing focus is less on individual criteria for assigning treatment than on structural change through manipulating the capacity of the medical system. This means reducing the number of hospital beds, the number of specialist physicians wedded to particular technologies, and the numbers of technician employees. 'Efforts to micromanage the doctor–patient relationship and teach physicians to practice cost-effective care did not really address the issue of capacity' (Wennberg, 1990, p. 1204). Rationing in the USA is unlikely to control costs unless its 'inherently inflationary and wasteful health care system' is dealt with (Relman, 1990a, p. 913).

The most widely discussed 'alternative' to rationing is 'cost-containment', itself a form of rationing. Cost-containment measures include limits for public insurance coverage. US cost-containment measures directed to either hospitals or physicians have elicited doubtful and often angry responses. Legal measures have been aimed at enforced physician participation in health insurance plans (Grumet, 1989). Administratively costly peer review organizations and 'managed care' with intrusive enquiries, 'micromanaging' and denial of specialist referrals or practitioner-recommended hospital admission, are among the many challenges to the autonomy of physicians and their roles in forming health care policy. It has been suggested that cost-containment measures will succeed 'only in shifting services to private offices and outpatient facilities . . . and in encouraging marketing and other entrepreneurial efforts to protect providers' revenues' (Relman, 1990b, p. 991).

Age as a Criterion for Rationing

It was only late in the period after the Second World War that the USA created its first national plan aimed specifically at improving the health care of older persons. However, since health care has been perceived as suffering a financial crisis, 'in a remarkable reversal of recent history age has been proposed as a criterion for withholding medical care' (Levinsky, 1990, p. 1813). US ethicists Callahan (1987), Daniels (1988) and Veatch (1988),

> argue that limits on health care for the elderly are justifiable because each citizen, throughout a lifetime, would benefit if funds now used to extend life at its end were redirected to earlier stages of life. . . . Each person would be entitled to a fair share of national health care expenditures as a person's lifetime 'health care budget' (Levinsky, 1990, p. 1814).

This kind of 'fair share' rationing recognizes the support accorded to the elderly earlier in their lives, up to the point where, as they reach some unspecified age, it is curtailed. By logical extension just allocation based on a 'lifetime health care budget' implies a medical care priority inversely related to age throughout life (Veatch, 1988). It would also suggest (without recognizing the scientific unfeasibility of compartmentalizing this kind of investigation) an end to public funding of research and health care on diseases most frequently encountered in old age (Callahan, 1990). Restrictions based upon other categorical divisions such as gender or ethnicity could not be considered just in this sense since they would have to be imposed at birth.

Callahan (1990) proposes that those who are still comparatively young be prepared, after full guarantees of 'decent palliative (but not life-extending) treatment' to support 'a democratically achieved, self-imposed future limitation on their public entitlement to expensive high-technology medical care' (p. 194). His point is that, while the elderly have a moral claim on health care, it does not include an unlimited effort to extend their lives 'regardless of cost and regardless of the burdens it can impose on the young' (p. 195). This position is based in part on indications that newly emerging forms of technology will drive up the costs of health care for the elderly in the future: 'It is a fallacy to infer from the success of earlier efforts all but eliminating lethal infectious disease that there will be similar success with the present chronic degenerative diseases of the elderly' (p. 194). US government insurance coverage for mammograms, for example, may be restricted on grounds of age. This is not a life-preserving procedure and the restriction is justified on clinical rather than pure cost-containment grounds: it was concluded that past the age of 65 this kind of preventive diagnostic screening is unnecessary or ineffective. But such measures emphasize the need for intensified programmes of technology assessment (see below).

Age as a criterion for rationing expressed in the withholding of aggressive treatment tends to become confounded with the disease-based impairment of the quality of life. A decision not to dialyse or to perform CPR on a demented older person, for example, could be supported on the basis of lost cognitive capacity, often associated with a predictably rapid downhill course. Under these circumstances, where family members often tend to agree with the decision not to treat, the patient may have earlier indicated a wish not to be resuscitated or sustained by technical methods at a stage when cognitive facilities and a sense of self in relation to others has eroded. Survival data without reference to quality of life are unclear. Thus, while post-CPR survival of 'chronically ill older people' after out-of-hospital discharge has been estimated at only 1 per cent (Murphy and Matchar, 1990, p. 2105), it has been suggested that the outcome is largely independent of age up to the ninth decade of life (Longstreth et al., 1990). Further, the limited evidence at hand suggests that a majority of persons who have survived the intensive care unit experience would want it again even if it offered them only a brief period of additional life (Danis et al., 1988). In this instance, as in many others, it appears that more adequate assessment is indicated.

Age rationing of biomedical technologies is an aspect of the problem of aggressive versus supportive care in situations in which supportive care alone, that is, failure of aggressive intervention, leads predictably to early death (see Chapter 7). Dialysis is a prime instance of supportive care which may afford many years of productive life, but 30 per cent of European dialysis centres have excluded patients older than 65 (Prottas et al., 1983). In 1972 the US Congress amended the Social Security Act to provide an entitlement to Medicare (government health insurance for people over 65) for persons with end-stage renal disease (ESRD) regardless of age. Thus, since 1973 Medicare has covered a major proportion of the costs of caring for end-stage renal failure, primarily dialysis, and this takes care of most Americans. In 1991 nearly 150 000 US patients with ESRD were receiving these benefits. A study committee of the US Institute of Medicine estimates that in the year 2000 approximately 240 000 patients will be enrolled (Levinsky and Rettig, 1991). It notes that there are some ineligible persons, concentrated disproportion-

ately among the poor and minorities, and recommends that entitlement be extended to all US citizens and resident aliens who have
ESRD. It also believes that kidney transplantation should be
encouraged, and recommends that patients receiving such transplants be granted a life-time entitlement (in contrast to their present
three years). Despite these recommendations the available data
suggest that reductions in federal reimbursement payments have led
to shortened dialysis times for US patients which are directly
correlated with increased mortality, giving the USA the highest
mortality rate among dialysis patients among the developed nations
(Berger and Lowrie, 1991).

In the UK, as discussed earlier, implicit rationing of high-
technology health support, exemplified by renal dialysis, on the basis
of age is carried out largely through the compliant silence of general
practitioners who do not make the necessary referrals. It is also
accomplished through a deliberate failure to invest in large numbers
of expensive high-technology facilities. Thus, proportionally less
than 20 per cent of the number of patients treated in US hospital
intensive care are referred to intensive care units in the UK (Aaron
and Schwartz, 1984). The average person over the age of 65 who
depends upon the national health system is glossed over with regard
to renal dialysis, as well as kidney transplants or comparable
procedures. Questioning patients and families may be told that the
desired treatment would be ineffective. This leads some observers to
believe that, in this instance, the practitioner's need to choose
between allegiance to the patient's individual interest and that of the
state's need for cost-effectiveness is resolved by possible self-
deception as well as deceiving the patient: 'Instead of "commitment
to the patient" the British speak of "clinical freedom" and "the right
of the doctor to act as he thinks is best for an individual patient".' For
the practitioner, however, these represent 'the same essential conflict
with [clinical] efficiency. . . . To avoid [this] conflict they will deny,
for example, that renal dialysis would do any good for the elderly
patient. Such denial often amounts to willing deception of the patient
or a slide in standards of care' (Menzel, 1990, p. 8; see also, Maynard
and Ludbrook, 1980, p. 29; Aaron and Schwartz, 1984, p. 101; and
Miller and Miller, 1986, all cited by Menzel).

Opposing the arguments for age as a criterion for health care
rationing is the view that resources should be allocated on an
individual rather than a categorical basis; this lays particular stress on
a patient's ability to benefit from them. Categorical criteria for
treatment are inevitably crude in the sense that they do not take
account of the individual variations which constitute the norm in
clinical medicine. Categorical approvals or disapprovals for applying
technology, such as life support or organ transplantation, cannot

weigh the costs versus the potential benefits in the individual patient concerned (Relman, 1990b). They may even prevent treatment in cases where the benefits are worth the costs. This can only be accomplished by a personalized, case-by-case system involving dialogue between patient and/or surrogate, and the treating physician. An example is

> not being allowed to prescribe kidney dialysis for a model seventy-year-old with no other problems. Admittedly, dialyzing patients older than sixty-five may generally be inefficient, but if we deny treatment in this particular case, efficiency-motivated rationing will have partially defeated itself. Here both individual patient welfare and larger efficiency favor treatment (Menzel, 1990, p. 7).

The intertwining of individual patient welfare and the 'larger efficiency' is illustrated by the question: 'Would it benefit society to persuade its Picassos to accept their deaths from treatable illnesses as part of a natural process for the good of the community?' (Levinsky, 1990, p. 1815).

Patient Participation in Allocation Decisions: the Lack of Data Necessary to Make Rational Decisions

A less categorical approach to allocating expensive technological resources fits the Kantian emphasis on respect for the individual, and places less responsibility in the hands of impersonal committees or physicians. It takes into account contemporary consumerism's emphasis on participation by patients and potential patients in their own health decisions. This approach is most conceivable in the context of capitalist society with fee-for-service health care. Here, the desired care would be available to anyone properly referred through medical channels, and able to pay the price through current private means, or government or employer-supported insurance. It may be less viable under monolithic national health plans which offer only restricted options, as in the case of the UK's implicit age rationing. Yet individual, although less broad-ranging, decision-making can also be exercised with a limited range of choices. The problem in both cases, especially with regard to more routine high-technology procedures, is that the data on the basis of which rational choices may be made are inadequate. We do not yet know, for example, just 'what the level of demand would be if patients were fully informed of their options and the probabilities of the various outcomes were presented to them. . . . Outcomes research provides this opportunity for the first time' (Wennberg, 1990, p. 1203). It seems likely that 'current rates of use of invasive high-technology medicine could well be higher than patients want . . . when risks must be taken to reduce symptoms or improve the quality of life, patients tend to be more averse to risks than physicians' (Wennberg, 1990, p. 1203). The 'rational' decision, under conditions limited not by personal affluence but by actual availability, would involve the collaborative (doctor and patient) assessment of possible risks (including pain, death and disability) versus possible benefits of the available procedure. This is, essentially, an estimate of probable outcome.

The increasing public interest in living wills or advance directives suggests that a majority of people might be willing to forgo resuscitation and intensive life support if they were chronically ill and impaired in the last stages of life. However, a prior decision to forgo such support if it offers a chance at additional active engagement with life is more difficult. A young 'prudent buyer' estimating his or her future health status would, presumably, make decisions designed to maximize healthy longevity rather than extend the final, perhaps incapacitated, period of life (Daniels, 1988). Further, if consumers planning for their futures actually knew what is involved they might 'knowingly consent to leaner packages of health care' (Menzel, 1990, p. 132). This would, presumably, reflect the worth which they attribute to the omitted items (such as insurance coverage for organ transplantation). It could be the basis for a rational decision to save money for other purposes by buying health insurance which does not cover the extreme high-technology care necessary to ensure survival under catastrophic circumstances. The 'rational decision' under these circumstances is one for 'prior consent to less than maximum health security for one's future'. It concerns possibly needed life-preserving as well as life-saving interventions at some time in the future. But, despite reluctance to be salvaged in an impaired state, this is not a conflict-free solution. The moral legitimacy of obtaining 'persons' presumed consent to risk to justify policies that later happen to work to their disadvantage' is arguable (Menzel, 1990, p. x). Argument is also possible about the valid definition of 'maximum health security' in terms of one's idiosyncratic life history, feelings and values. In this context a discussion of 'medical egalitarianism' (Menzel, 1990, pp. 116–31) recognizes the need to distinguish between health care that is, and is not, worth what it costs in relation to the likelihood of survival and quality of life. Rational persons with limited means usually make informed choices about where to invest them in order to obtain a maximum quality of life. They are thus less likely than the affluent to invest in coverage which would recognize a future, hypothetical, need for very expensive or debatably effective life-sustaining or therapeutic procedures. In giving prior consent for insurance which does not cover high-technology life support, the subscribers do their best to predict their later feelings about being kept alive with intensive technology, and the restrictions and diminished quality of life which it entails.

This rational concept does not take account of the wish to live which continues to drive much human behaviour even under conditions of extreme deprivation, disability and illness. It is, furthermore, impossible to project one's self accurately into the future, especially with regard to a wish for an optimal chance to survive in the event of physiological catastrophe which leaves one's brain and reflective capacities intact, and carries no risk of later social incapacity. This might be the case in a relatively young adult suffering severe automobile or aeroplane crash injuries, or an expanding cerebral aneurysm, who could be saved with organ transplants, or brain surgery under hypothermic conditions, or who might survive on a life-support system until definitive treatment is available. This could also be true for many active, socially involved, productive people of advanced age who suffer from organ system failure. 'It is easy to underestimate the ability of some elderly persons to endure treatment when their lives are at stake' (Kilner, 1990, p. 223). Nor can 'prior consent' deal with the likelihood that biomedical advances will continue at an accelerating pace and that accurate predictions about available treatments are, in fact, not possible. This is not a definitive argument against 'prior consent'. It may be taken simply as recognition of the hazardous nature of life, and the unpredictability both of hazardous events and biomedical innovation.

Increased knowledge by the individual help-seeker, combined with personalized interaction between patient and physician, is stressed here as the desirable, humane course. In contrast are rigid, categorical forms of resource rationing, solutions which depend upon restrictions imposed and enforced by governmental agencies with no role or only a minor role for patient and physician. Ultimately important in the argument for control from above is the view that strict standards of efficacy should be used to reduce or eliminate the use of technologies which, though demonstrably effective, are not financially affordable (Callahan, 1990). This view could be supported by the obvious appeal to guilt and a sense of the absurd: 'Can we ever rest in good conscience if private hospitals sell dramatic headline-grabbing technologies to well-off clients while such procedures are excluded from government programs for the poor?' (Menzel, 1990, p. 116). In the USA the Oregon state legislature did decide, in consequence of budgetary constraints, to take the hotly debated, deplored, difficult, but socially rational decision to transfer Medicaid funding for organ transplantation to a preventive care programme.

The Assessment of Health Technology in Order to Make Rational Decisions

The importance of technology assessment for rational choices by consumers and practitioners is indicated above. In accordance with a person-centred orientation it should include, in so far as is possible, the patients' own views of the personal utility of undergoing the treatment in question. Such assessment is essential for makers of health policy, and is increasingly used, sometimes over the objections of care providers and manufacturers, for quality assurance and cost-containment (Relman, 1980; Banta and Thacker, 1990). Outcome studies are especially important in a competitive, market-oriented health industry in which medical equipment and hospitals are bought and sold and medical practitioners earn major fees through performing hospital-based procedures. It has been estimated that the use of new technologies and the overuse of those already available have contributed approximately 50 per cent of the increases in the cost of US health care (Institute of Medicine, 1985). A major health insurance company, Blue Cross/Blue Shield, has estimated that more than $6 billion are spent each year in the USA on unnecessary tests (Banta and Thacker, 1990).

The utility assessment of biomedical technology for policy purposes has other, less apparent, significance achieved through a multi-step procedure. For example, the conclusion that biopsy side-effects should be weighed against the poor magnetic resonance scanning identification of nodal involvement in prostatic cancer (Rifkin et. al., 1990) implies 'that the next logical step is part of a third-stage assessment: a comprehensive analysis of how the two techniques should be used in the care of patients with prostate cancer' (Fuchs and Garber, 1990, p. 675).

Another illustration is the case of cystic fibrosis (see Chapter 5). In this instance it is necessary not only to confirm that a new test detects the mutation, but to estimate its sensitivity and specificity in various populations, evaluate its ethical implications as a general population screen, follow up with regard to family decisions about what to do regarding a foetus that has tested positive, and, in general, to make a social as well as financial cost–benefit assessment (Fuchs and Garber, 1990, p. 673).

A national report on health care in the USA (Pepper Commission, 1990) reflects not only the market-oriented context of US medicine, but the fact that high-technology medicine is 'normative' (as it is in other industrialized societies), with both utilization trends and opinion polls indicating that the American people favour it (Ginzberg, 1990a, p. 1822). In this context the commission emphasizes the 'unnecessary and inappropriate' use (p. 40) of technology by physicians. It estimates that as few as 15–20 per cent of contemporary clinical interventions in the USA have been scientifically shown to produce unambiguous benefits which outweigh whatever harm they might do. This fits an earlier Office of Technology Assessment estimate (Congress, 1978) that only 10–20 per cent of medical practices are supported by randomized clinical trials.

> Unless we make a major investment in new trials of the safety, cost and relative effectiveness of the drugs, tests, procedures and operations we now employ so generously, and unless we systematically collect and analyze the results of our clinical experience . . . we will remain tied to the inflationary spiral of expanding technology (Relman 1990b, p. 992).

The Pepper Commission notes the lack of systematic knowledge about indications for and results of technology use, which is revealed in major regional and city-to-city variations. These include variations, some noted above, in the frequency of procedures such as Caesarean section, hysterectomy, carotid endarectomy, coronary bypass surgery, angioplasty, cardiac pacemaker implantation, coronary angiography and upper gastrointestinal endoscopy. All appear to have contributed to overinvestment in hospital and clinic facilities in which to carry them out. The crucial point, again, is the suggestion that significant proportions of these high-technology procedures are performed in order to recoup investments; while there is no evidence that they are harmful, it is not clear what proportion of them produce actual medical benefit for the patient. If this is true they waste limited resources, deprive others of needed care and pose risks to the patients involved. Following the appearance of the commission's report debate has been carried to the US public via the popular media. The question has been clearly posed as to whether or not medical, including dental, technology is being used prematurely with fundamentally commercial motivations, without adequate risk assessment and at considerable expense, by private practitioners and groups for general screening as well as treatment. The presentations also make it clear that regardless of the lack of data to support the use of these technologies many patients, allied with their doctors, want them and invest their availability with high emotional significance. Among the procedures discussed in this vein have been positive emission tomography, PET scans used for general disease screening, lasers for treating ischaemic arterial disease, and various electromyographic devices for treating and monitoring the progress of mandibulo-temporal joint disorders. A general point of conflict is between patients and their doctors on the one hand who want the technologies, and insurance companies on the other who refuse to pay for them on the grounds that they are still experimental, unproven and lack adequate risk–benefit assessment.

It is apparent that an intensified technology-assessment programme is essential to provide data on the basis of which patients and
their physicians and policy-makers can make rational decisions, and
scarce health care resources can be justly utilized. Such a programme
should provide for periodic reassessment of techniques as new data
about safety and efficacy become available, new indications emerge,
or the intervention is used differently. An example is the declining
level of radiation exposure which makes mammography more
attractive as a screening test (Fuchs and Garber, 1990). It is equally
apparent that patients, potential patients and families ('consumers'
of health care services), as well as professionals, should be informed
about the results of the assessment programme. Without such
knowledge they will be in no position to make rational choices for
themselves or to engage in constructive dialogue with their care-
givers.

'Human Rights' and Health Require Social and Individual Responsibility

The Concerns of Free Citizens

The educated, literate citizens of the industrialized democracies
constitute the ultimate key to global 'health for all' in the future. This
does not discount the role of those who inhabit the developing world,
which includes many who live under totalitarian governments. It
simply recognizes that most of the scientific 'benefits', access to
which the UN regards as a 'right' for all the world's inhabitants, come
from the hospitals and research laboratories of the industrialized
democracies. Most of the people living in these countries understand
that the fundamental maintenance and preventive health care upon
which a nation depends, encompassing reproductive and developmental care in their broadest sense, does not depend upon advanced
biomedical technology. They realize that it is their knowledge about
their own behavioural contributions to personal health, and their
society's experientially honed low-technology, maintenance and
preventive health knowledge and skills which should be first
exported to the developing world as it creates its own context-specific
research capacities. Beyond these understandings, however, they
are intensely interested in the progress of technological medicine as it
might apply immediately to them, their families and friends. But they
are less concerned with the threat to essential humanhood and
human rights from non-coital reproduction, genetic research, or
organ transplantation, than with accessible medical care. Most want
biomedical research to continue producing the devices and pro-

cedures which have so drastically reduced the incidence of pre-mature death from all causes, decreased the likelihood of disability, and increased longevity. They are increasingly aware of the possible hazards of high-technology medicine, but they want it to continue, and to be more easily available to all.

What Would Citizens support?

Citizens of the industrialized democracies, knowledgeable about the expanding cornucopia of technological diagnostic and reparative devices, are able to appreciate their privileges as 'prudent buyers' of health care (Daniels, 1988), and to understand the rationality of 'prior consent' to resource limitation (Menzel, 1990). It seems doubtful, however, that as consumers with high expectations, regardless of current economic status, they would be willing to foreclose at the outset access to any of the potential advantages of technological society, including the possibility of long and vigorous life. Neither prior consent, nor prudent buying in young adulthood, would be regarded as totally satisfactory ways of achieving life-time justice in the allocation of scarce medical resources. Nor would an enlightened citizenry be likely to support limiting the biomedical research which has produced the knowledge basic to most advances in longevity and the quality of individual lives.

On the other hand an informed public might be expected to support improved assessment of technology, including individual subjective responses to it, in the interests of making rational choices, and of public dialogue about the new biomedical frontiers. It would probably support limitations upon the competitive, free-market development and selling of medical devices and pharmaceuticals in the interests of reducing medical costs. It might also find it salutary to promote public debate about resource allocation rather than suffer the intermittent appeals of tragic individuals seeking organ transplants or complex last-chance surgery for themselves or their children.

This view recognizes the functioning of the concerned citizen as a whole person rather than just a patient. The opportunity to partici-pate as a citizen in shaping the policy context of health care, and collaboratively with one's own physician in decisions about one's own health care, are aspects of the health care system's commitment to the whole individual as a sentient, self-determining, self-legislating person, rather than as someone simply in the role of patient. At the level of the individual, the only solution to supporting the integrity of patients and physicians as whole persons, as citizens apart from their specific roles in the medical system, is to involve both in a flexible system of decision-making in which input is in part 'prior' and in part current in the context of the medical care system.

Beyond Technology Assessment – Rationing and/or Cost-containment?

Any rational decision about the benefits of biomedical technology, especially its just availability to physicians and the general public, bears directly on its human rights aspects. A valid decision about assigning a treatment or procedure can only be based on repeated risk–cost–benefit assessments of all the drugs, devices and procedures used in contemporary medicine, including the supporting staff necessary to use them. Without such information, shared with the public and specifically with patients, the decision may be driven by wishful thinking, clinical hunches, or unidentified personal factors such as the physician's wish to engage in the forefront of technological medicine or a parent's desire for continued futile treatment of a fatally defective infant. This means that a massively increased and continuing programme of assessing the personal, medical, social and financial efficacy, benefits, hazards and risks of biomedical technology is a necessary prerequisite to attempts to ration or otherwise allocate its use. It is apparent, however, as many observers have pointed out (for example, Callahan, 1987), that some biomedical technologies which prove to be effective, to have major benefits, and minimum hazards and risks, will also be too expensive to be generally affordable. 'Unless we are prepared to spend an unconscionable proportion of our resources on health care . . . we cannot possibly afford every medical advance that might be of benefit' (Levinsky, 1990, p. 1812).

Under these circumstances an initial step in cost-containment must be to make the new technologies more affordable, in other words, less expensive, at the source. The competitive, market- and profit-oriented climate of contemporary medicine is the primary source of the flow of new unproven technologies with publicity-driven demand. The entrepreneurial and competitive development of newer biomedical technologies requires partners who supply and manage venture capital; it makes it necessary to pay back development costs and acquire profits for investors as well as originators; and it encourages their premature use and commercial exploitation by clinicians. If commercial monopolies on the development, sale and maintenance of new technologies are ended, and the corporate transformation of medicine is modified or in some measure undone, the costs to patients and individual physicians should be sufficiently decreased that their availability to those in need would increase. This would allow physicians to become more autonomous in their exercise of clinical judgement, and less burdened by either the profit motive or government regulations. Patients should more easily be able to work towards their own rational decisions in collaboration with their personal physicians and others about whether or not they want to invest in high-technology reparative medicine for their uncertain futures, or whether they want to utilize their limited resources in other ways.

Reducing expenses at the source is less emotionally involving than determining criteria for individual patient selection for scarce resources, but it is probably the most important and difficult task to be undertaken. Changing the business matrix of the contemporary health care enterprise need not diminish the rate of new scientific discovery. It could, however, diminish the rate at which technological applications of these discoveries are produced, unless publicly supported or private foundation laboratories undertake some of the engineering and other tasks of product development. On the other hand, the pressure to apply new technologies for commercial gain will be less and the possibilities of scientific stimulation greater in an open system with free knowledge sharing, not oriented to patents and profits. The achievement of this system, including more rational linkages between scientific discovery and economically feasible technological product development, is a task for governments and their judiciary and legal systems. Without such change, and with the continuing industrialization and corporate engulfing of medical care,

> there will be no way to control its costs except through much firmer regulation. A far better approach would be to restructure our health care system as a social service, managed primarily by non-entrepreneurial professionals working to deliver the best available care at an affordable price (Relman, 1990b, p. 992).

Service Delivery and the Primary Care Physician

Another set of change-producing tasks involves the service delivery systems. Current unlabelled rationing in the USA according to ability to pay and imposed inconvenience in collecting from private or public insurance agencies (Grumet, 1989) follows the basic assumptions of the economy (Murphy and Matchar, 1990). While many US prepaid, health maintenance organizations (HMOs) have been forced to drastically 'manage' their use of expensive procedures and specialist referrals, this activity is not inherent in the structure of an HMO. It is forced by profit-making pressure. If the pressure could be relieved an increased role for these physicians would be a potential strength in making high-cost procedures more affordable to those who truly need them. Primary care physicians under less time pressure could work collaboratively with the patient and family, as well as with technology- and procedure-oriented specialists, to determine which, if any, technologies or procedures are appropriate for a particular person, with a particular set of medical problems, living in a particular social context, at a particular point in his or her life trajectory.

High-technology medicine promotes the training of specialists who require expensive equipment and support staff, increasing hospital overheads, and, in turn, charge high prices for their services. This is an argument for increased emphasis on the training of primary care physicians and, as already initiated in the USA, for third-party payment based on the extent of patient contact in the physician's office rather than the use of technological procedures in hospitals. Emphasizing the role of primary care physicians suggests modifications in medical education. Part of the overall approach to change should be a re-emphasis on the traditional humane, individual orientation of doctors in an earlier era with a reorientation to persons rather than technology. This orientation has been drastically weakened by the acceleration of high-technology care, with the relegation of much intimate patient interaction to non-physician therapists.

But even with these changes some essential medical resources will always remain scarce; some are too inherently rare (such as human organs) for general access to ever be possible; others are too expensive to provide for many. In these instances demand will continue to outstrip supply, and the essentially insoluble problem of satisfactory allotment will remain until new solutions, such as synthetic or animal organs, are found. In centralized national health systems with limited resources physicians' adaptation to practice limitations may include unconscious denial of their significance as a way of preserving the illusion of professional autonomy and of behaving in the patients' best interests. In the Federal Republic of Germany, the United Kingdom, France and Sweden with clear-cut economic restrictions on the care which can be prescribed, physicians' assertions that their professional autonomy remains intact may reflect, as already indicated in the case of the UK, an element of self-deception. A less pejorative way of describing the link between practice regulations and physician behaviour is that economic and assessment-imposed limitations may become un-consciously incorporated into clinical judgements about the needs of individual patients (Freddi and Bjorkman, 1989).

The kinds of allotment problems encountered in an open, fee-for-service society, or even one with equal access privileges without the resources to fulfil them all, are not solved by categorical rationing. However, something similar to the practices described above may be involved in the use of institutional protocols for technology appli-cation in the USA. They limit the tendency to feel the application of any potentially life-preserving technology as a moral imperative. Although protocols are not intended as guides to 'rationing' or resource allocation they have contributed to this end.

Even without the drive for commercial profit the production of new medical technologies will continue, and will be matched by responsive demand. No universally satisfactory method of allocating individual life and death through the allocation of technology will be discovered. The best that can be done is to avoid categorical criteria for patient selection, and work, in so far as is possible, on an individual case-by-case basis. In this context it will be important to develop clinically based standards for appropriate resource use. Aggressive care, for example, of patients with poor prognoses may be seen as an inappropriate use of resources (Murphy and Matchar, 1990, p. 2104). Yet persons who make the presumed 'rational' prior decisions for limited benefits early in life should know that these decisions are not necessarily irreversible, and are subject to joint scrutiny with medical collaboration at any time.

Perhaps the most fundamental answer to the uneven 'right' to the benefits of science may lie in a cultural shift. Modern humankind's belief in science is accompanied by the expectation of its continued yield of wonders. Biological science, in particular, is invested with enormous power, intensified by the new genetic discoveries. The corollary is an increasing inability to accept the limitations of one's own biological make-up and mortality. New biotechnologies and new fantastic medical feats are presented through the media in a way which fuels continued expectation. The drive for new biological discovery is reminiscent of historical searches for the Fountain of Youth. But those quests exhausted all the searchers' resources and were, ultimately, in vain. Even contemporary science does not promise a disease-free life or immortality. No conceivable human society will have the resources to develop every promising bioscientific advance with a beneficial potential into a useful medical technology. 'Nor is there any reason to think we would automatically and proportionately increase our happiness and improve our general welfare by even trying to do so' (Levinsky, 1990, p. 1812).

It seems likely that, given the nature of human beings, the precarious nature of their existence, and their urgent claims for life, no generally satisfactory principle of fair and equitable distribution of life-preserving technologies will be discovered. That does not mean that the attempt at discovery should not continue. It does mean that rigid adherence to whatever principles are established, and whatever rules flow from them, will not fit the physician's requirement to be both compassionate and competent.

Appendix 1

United Nations Educational
Scientific and Cultural Organization

International Symposium of the Effects on Human Rights
of Recent Advances in Science and Technology
(Barcelona, Spain, 25–28 March 1985)

organized by
The International Social Sciences Council (ICSS)

Conclusions and Recommendations

A.   The symposium considered contributions of the following
disciplines: anthropology, biochemistry, biology, brain research,
clinical psychology, experimental psychology, genetics, law, mental
health, molecular biology, neuroscience, pharmacology, physiological psychology, and psychiatry.

The symposium agreed that:

1.   Advances in these disciplines are relevant to attaining a number
of human rights, which the following rights received major
consideration:

- *From the Universal Declaration of Human Rights*:

    'Article 5: No one shall be subjected to torture or to cruel,
    inhuman and degrading treatment or punishment.'

    'Article 26: Everyone has the right to education (. . .)'.

    'Article 27: Everyone has the right freely (. . .) to share in
    scientific advancement and its benefits.'

251

- *From the International Covenant on Economic, Social and Cultural Rights*:

  'Article 12.1: The State Parties to the present Covenant recognize the right of everyone to the enjoyment of the highest obtainable standard of physical and mental health.'

  'Article 13.1: The state Parties to the present Covenant recognize the right of everyone to education.'

  'Article 15.1: The State Parties to the present Covenant recognize the right of everyone (. . .) b) to enjoy the benefits of scientific progress and its applications.'

- *From the International Covenant on Civil and Political Rights*:

  'Article 7: No one shall be subjected to torture or to cruel, inhuman or degrading treatment or punishment. In particular, no one shall be subjected without his free consent to medical or scientific experiment.'

2.   Advances on research in biology and behaviour, especially in genetics and in the study of relations between brain and behaviour, are resulting in a revolution in human understanding. People are now able to look at themselves objectively, to do research in the social, cultural and psychological domains as well as the biological and physical, and to acquire the information and techniques needed to modify their own biology and physiology, their minds, and perhaps even their own evolution. These advances open up major opportunities for progress in achieving human rights, but they also allow some possibilities for abuses. In applying these advances, it is essential to ensure that the application decrease the economic and cultural disparities among social and national groups.

3.   It is important for Unesco to promote broad general education, not only about the benefits, for human rights, of applying discoveries but also about the dangers of withholding, abusing or preventing discoveries. This can best be done with a public that already has a good basic education, so this again stresses the importance of the right to such education. Since many of the benefits concern individual and social behaviour, basic education should include components on the behavioural and social sciences. Increased knowledge of what has been accomplished and what can reasonably be expected from research in neuroscience, behaviour, and related disciplines should heighten public support for research and applications.

4.   Support should be given to the right of all individuals to develop fully their intellectual capacities as prerequisites to attaining the highest obtainable standard of physical and mental health and to benefit from education. Particular attention should be paid to the vulnerability of the unborn during gestation and of the newborn until the end of the suckling period, especially regarding the normal differentiation of the Central Nervous System. The effects of malnutrition, environmental conditions, therapeutic treatments, alcohol, tobacco and drug addiction, etc. can irreversibly damage the brain and, therefore, impair the human rights of the child. It is the duty of parents and society to adopt the measures necessary to protect the integrity and full expression of every individual's personality.

5.   In the interest of achieving the highest level of physical and mental health, and of not depriving persons diagnosed as mentally ill of their liberty, autonomy, and rights to beneficent and just treatment, the following guidelines should be kept in mind:

   (i) adequate efforts should be made to establish reciprocal communication between patient and doctor;
   (ii) in the interest of justice, equal access to necessary treatment with neuroleptic drugs or other technological means should be a right within the overall context of the right to health. Mere resistance to such drug treatment should not be a reason for either compulsory administration without discussion or for medical abandonment of a patient in need of treatment and protection.

6.   Concerning genetic manipulations and artificial procreation, the responsibility for final decisions with regard to individual or family matters should be left to the individual and family and their chosen advisors, rather than to governmental agencies. Model laws and regulations could be provided by international bodies in order to reduce the impact of local political or ideological view points. The use of advances in this field shall not be restricted to the benefit of certain nations or social groups because this could impair the rights stated respectively in Article 12.1 and Article 15.1 paragraph (b) of the International Covenant on Economic, Social and Cultural Rights.

7.   On the basis of the reports presented at the symposium and the discussions, the symposium forwards to the Director-General five recommendations of the highest priority and five other recommendations that are also of major importance.

B.   *Recommendations of highest priority*

I.   *Promote human rights by seeking the broadest possible applications, on a worldwide basis, of scientific advances already tested in the fields discussed at this meeting.*

(a)   The human rights mentioned above should be promoted by seeking the broadest possible applications, on a worldwide basis, of well tested relevant scientific and technical advances in neuroscience, biological sciences, genetic manipulation, physiology and pharmacology, and behavioural and social sciences.

(b)   These advances should be applied in ways that will work towards the elimination of disparities between social, cultural and national groups in the enjoyment of human rights.

(c)   In order to ensure 1 and 2, we propose that:

> (i) the proceedings and recommendations of this symposium be given wide dissemination and reach both governments and relevant NGOs;
> (ii) follow-up meetings of concerned scientists should be scheduled on a regular basis in order to monitor the application of well-established scientific techniques for achieving human rights and to assess the value of recommendations made in the earlier conferences;
> (iii) an international conference be held to explore and analyze the causes of failures to apply such advances, both generally and to specific human groups or in specific regions. Reasons for such failures, including social and cultural factors, are to be determined as precisely and accurately as possible;
> (iv) based on these analyses, recommendations should be proposed to achieve greater progress in human rights.

II.   *Promote contributions of all disciplines represented at this symposium and of interdisciplinary teams to enhancement of human rights.*

(a)   This could be fostered through a systematic overview of these disciplines and their relevance for human rights, establishing an inventory of relevant areas of research in the various branches of basic and clinical biological and behavioural sciences.

(b)   This inventory could help to delineate future research orientations and create an awareness of the human rights issues involved in such research among these various scientific disciplines.

III. *Encourage awareness, responsibility and action for human rights on the part of scientists and clinicians in the disciplines considered at this symposium.*

Scientists and clinicians in the fields considered at this symposium should become more aware of the impact of their work on human rights; they must assume responsibility for the uses made of the findings and discoveries of their disciplines as these affect human rights; they must assume responsibility for informing the public about basic advances in knowledge and in technology and about potentialities for benefits and for possible abuses of these findings for human rights.

We recommend that the Director-General undertake both general and specific actions:

(a) to promote international exchange of information and collaboration for research and applications, coming from all the fields represented in this symposium, that will benefit human rights. Involving investigators from developing countries in research and application will help to ensure that problems of prime concern to these countries are studied and that methods of application suitable to their nationals are devised. This could be done partly by Unesco, and the recommendation could also be forwarded to ICSU, ISSC, CIOMS, CIPSH and other interested professional NGOs for implementation;

(b) to promote the application of scientific advances for the achievement of human rights and combat possible abuses by encouraging scientific and professional societies and relevant NGOs to take the following actions:

   (i) promote those human rights contained in the Universal Declaration of Human Rights, the related International Covenants, and to take effective measures to realize the provisions contained in the Declaration and Convention Against Torture and Other Cruel, Inhuman or Degrading Treatment or Punishment, as well as the UN Principles of Medical Ethics;

   (ii) explain to their members the relevance of their discipline and specialized activities for these human rights;

(c) to request that relevant NGOs (e.g., ICSU, ISSC, CIOMS, CIPSH, . . .) plan and sponsor an international conference on the responsibilities for human rights of scientists and clinicians in the disciplines considered at the present symposium. The conference should include representatives of these disciplines as well as experts in the fields of the social sciences. It should make recommendations for action by scientific and professional groups, relevant NGOs, and individual scientists. In particular:

(i) the proceedings and recommendations of the conference should be disseminated widely;

(ii) a network should be set up through which scientific and professional societies and other relevant NGOs can regularly exchange information and recommendations about this topic; and

(iii) regular conferences should be held to monitor the status and progress of responsibility of scientists in these regards;

(d) to promote in co-operation with WHO a canon of research ethics that will protect the rights of human subjects of research and the welfare of animal subjects, in the latter case imposing unjustified restrictions on research. For this purpose:

(i) have a compilation made from as many countries as possible, and from relevant scientific and professional societies and other relevant NGOs, of statutes, regulations, and codes dealing with the use of human subjects in scientific and medical research;

(ii) appoint an international committee to assess this compilation, the committee to include scientists of the relevant disciplines, physicians, jurists and experts in human rights. The results of the assessment should be given wide dissemination to governments and to relevant professional societies and NGOs. The committee may also make recommendations, including the recommendation that model statutes and/or codes be drafted and made available for consideration by national governments, scientific and professional societies and NGOs;

(iii) since the use of animal subjects is crucial to continuation of research for attainment of the human right to the highest levels of physical and mental health, encourage CIOMS to disseminate more widely the 'International Guiding Principles for Biomedical Research Involving Animals';

(iv) appoint an international committee as in (ii), the members to include scientists of the relevant disciplines, physicians, veterinarians and jurists.

IV. *Consider the impact of new reproductive technologies on the human rights of women.*

Since new reproductive technologies can have an impact on women's rights and because these issues most closely touch families and individuals, recommendation is made:

(a) to convene a meeting specifically on the new reproductive technologies, including strategies for assessment of technologies that affect women's rights (for example amniocentesis and selective abortion of female fetuses, new contraceptive technologies with potential for coercive use; etc.);

(b) to encourage NGOs to address this issue in their own forums;

(c) to disseminate scientifically exact information in ways planned to be accessible to all populations.

V. *Promote consideration of the human rights of patients and in particular promote standards for the use of neuroleptic drugs.*

In regard to the right to enjoy the highest obtainable standard of physical and mental health, patients are clearly a crucial group; and we therefore recommend to the Director-General that Unesco, in co-operation with WHO:

(a) obtain from relevant professional and scientific groups and other relevant NGOs material concerning codes and programs dealing with the rights of patients in relation to health professionals and health institutions and/or facilities;

(b) entrust the assessment of this compilation to an international committee with a view to show special concern for particularly vulnerable groups (e.g. pregnant women, fetuses, children, people defined as mentally ill, the ageing, the dying and prisoners). This committee would include representatives of the relevant disciplines (e.g. physicians, psychiatrists, clinical psychologists, nurses) as well as social scientists. It would make recommendations based on its assessment and evaluation. One possible recommendation would be either to draft model statutes and/or codes or to propose that such model statutes and/or codes be drafted, which would then be made available for consideration by governments, relevant professional and scientific organizations, and other relevant NGOs;

(c) widely disseminate to governments and relevant NGOs the proceedings and recommendations of such a committee.

C.   *Recommendations of major importance*

I.   *Promote research on topics and in areas of the world where improvement is clearly needed.*

For example promote research in co-operation with WHO to determine, among existing scientific and clinical methods, the most effective methods of therapy for various kinds of symptoms and complaints (such as anxiety, alcoholism, depression, drug abuse). Where no existing method is effective, promote research to find new methods. Where an existing method helps some but not all who suffer from a disorder, retain the existing method but promote research to find other therapies that will aid those not presently being treated effectively.

Promote research to find methods of application that are suitable for developing as well as developed countries, that is, that are inexpensive and that do not require many highly trained individuals or elaborate technology. Establish a network among governments and relevant NGOs to disseminate information about such effective and appropriate methods.

II.   *In the formulation of policies and the administration of programs in education and health, consult panels of experts in neuroscience and behavior and related disciplines.*

Many current questions in such fields as education and health require expertise that non-specialists do not possess. Administrators and professionals in such fields should be willing to take advice from panels of experts in neuroscience and behavior, and experts in these disciplines should be urged to perform the public service of participating in such panels. Furthermore, the experts undoubtedly have much to learn from those involved in practical administration and application.

III.   *Consider critically any calls to limit research particularly when it is claimed that the research would directly contravene human rights.*

Calls to limit research in neuroscience, behavior and related disciplines have been made either on the grounds that the research process itself could be harmful to the subjects or that the objectives of the research, such as gaining control over the human personality, should be restricted. Such calls run counter to academic freedom and to the right to share in scientific advancement. Furthermore, it is almost impossible to predict outcomes of research. Even research that is well-intended can be misapplied or can have unforeseen adverse side effects. The possible dangers of new research must be weighed against the heavy costs in ignorance and suffering being borne at present. We cannot progress in attaining the right levels of physical and mental health by remaining where we are. Ethical commissions, such as those established in the United States of America and France, are an excellent means of monitoring research.

IV.   *Promote basic research in order to ensure continued possibilities for benefiting human rights beyond what can now be envisaged.*

Basic long-term research in the disciplines considered at the present meeting must be promoted in order to ensure continued possibilities for benefiting human rights in ways that cannot now even be envisaged.

We recommend to the Director-General:

(a)   to present this view forcefully to governments and to relevant NGOs;

(b)   to call a conference to explore ways of presenting effectively to governments and to relevant NGOs the case for basic, longterm research in the disciplines represented at the present meeting.

V.   *Consider and assess the impact on human rights of current research on genetic manipulation and artificial procreation.* (In particular this bears on the stated right to marry and to found a family, Article 16 of the Universal Declaration of Human Rights and Article 23 of the International Covenant on Civil and Political Rights.)

For this purpose:

(a)   have a compilation made from as many nations as possible and from relevant scientific and professional societies and other relevant NGOs, of statutes, regulations and codes dealing with genetic manipulation and artificial procreation;

(b)   have this compilation and the general topic of genetic manipulation and artificial procreation assessed by an international committee chosen to include scientists of the relevant disciplines, physicians, and social scientists. The committee would investigate the following questions:

(i) with regard to artificial procreation, the utilization of those techniques that do not alter directly the genome (e.g. artificial insemination and 'in vitro' fertilization) may be allowed under regulations established at the national level (Ethical Commissions) in accordance with international guidance (for instance, recommendations by regional organizations concerning donors, surrogate mothers, storage and freezing periods of gametes and blastocysts, ovum differentiation period after fecundation, etc);

(ii) gene therapy is subject to the same considerations. Techniques that alter directly the human genome (cloning for example) and that could result in multiple identical offspring should be examined critically as imparing personal integrity and individuality. Indeed, artificial modification of the random process leading to the individual genetic endowment may run counter to individual personal integrity;

(iii) in cases of artificial procreation, the relations among the rights of the child, the rights of the procreators, the rights of the biological mother and those of the genetic one, the rights of the adoptive parents who nurture and educate the child, and the rights of the donors should be examined and clarified:

(iv) genetic manipulations in micro-organisms, non-human animals and plants should be undertaken only after authorization of Ethical or Expert Committees in order to avoid causing ecological effects that could impair the exercise of human rights.

Appendix 2

Universal
Declaration
of
Human Rights

ON 10 DECEMBER 1948, *the General Assembly of the United Nations adopted and proclaimed the Universal Declaration of Human Rights, the full text of which appears in the following pages. Following this historic act, the Assembly called upon all Member countries to publicize the text of the Declaration and to 'cause it to be disseminated, displayed, read and expounded principally in schools and other educational institutions, without distinction based on the political status of counties or territories'.*

Universal Declaration of Human Rights

Preamble

Whereas recognition of the inherent dignity and of the equal and inalienable rights of all members of the human family is the foundation of freedom, justice and peace in the world,

Whereas disregard and contempt for human rights have resulted in barbarous acts which have outraged the conscience of mankind, and the advent of a world in which human beings shall enjoy freedom of speech and belief and freedom from fear and want has been proclaimed as the highest aspiration of the common people,

Whereas it is essential, if man is not to be compelled to have recourse, as a last resort, to rebellion against tyranny and oppression, that human rights should be protected by the rule of law,

Whereas it is essential to promote the development of friendly relations between nations,

Whereas the peoples of the United Nations have in the Charter reaffirmed their faith in fundamental human rights, in the dignity and worth of the human person and in the equal rights of men and women and have determined to promote social progress and better standards of life in larger freedom,

Whereas Member States have pledged themselves to achieve, in co-operation with the United Nations, the promotion of universal respect for and observance of human rights and fundamental freedoms,

Whereas a common understanding of these rights and freedoms is of the greatest importance for the full realization of this pledge,

Now, therefore, THE GENERAL ASSEMBLY proclaims

this

UNIVERSAL DECLARATION OF HUMAN RIGHTS

as a common standard of achievement for all peoples and all nations, to the end that every individual and every organ of society, keeping this Declaration constantly in mind, shall strive by teaching and education to promote respect for these rights and freedoms and by progressive measures, national and international, to secure their universal and effective recognition and observance, both among the peoples of Member States themselves and among the peoples of territories under their jurisdiction.

Article 1

All human beings are born free and equally in dignity and rights. They are endowed with reason and conscience and should act towards one another in a spirit of brotherhood.

Article 2

Everyone is entitled to all the rights and freedoms set forth in this Declaration, without distinction of any kind, such as race, colour, sex, language, religion, political or other opinion, national or social origin, property, birth or status.

Furthermore, no distinction shall be made on the basis of the political, jurisdictional or international status of the country or territory to which a person belongs, whether it be independent, trust, non-self-governing or under any other limitation of sovereignty.

Article 3

Everyone has the right to life, liberty and the security of person.

Article 4

No one shall be held in slavery or servitude; slavery and the slave trade shall be prohibited in all their forms.

Article 5

No one shall be subjected to torture or to cruel, inhuman or degrading treatment or punishment.

Article 6

Everyone has the right to recognition everywhere as a person before the law.

Article 7

Are all equal before the law and are entitled without any discrimination to equal protection of the law. All are entitled to equal protection against any discrimination in violation of this Declaration and against any incitement to such discrimination.

Article 8

Everyone has the right to an effective remedy by the competent national tribunals for acts violating the fundamental rights granted him by the constitution or by law.

Article 9

No one shall be subjected to arbitrary arrest, detention or exile.

Article 10

Everyone is entitled in full equality to a fair and public hearing by an independent and impartial tribunal, in the determination of his rights and obligations and of any criminal charge against him.

Article 11

1. Everyone charged with a penal offence has the right to be presumed innocent until proved guilty according to law in a public trial at which he has had all the guarantees necessary for his defence.
2. No one shall be held guilty of any penal offence on account of any act or omission which did not constitute a penal offence, under national or international law, at the time when it was committed. Nor shall a heavier penalty be imposed than the one that was applicable at the time the penal offence was committed.

Article 12

No one shall be subjected to arbitrary interference with his privacy, family, home or correspondence, nor to attacks upon his honour and reputation. Everyone has the right to the protection of the law against such interference or attacks.

Article 13

1. Everyone has the right to freedom of movement and residence within the borders of each State.
2. Everyone has the right to leave any country, including his own, and to return to his country.

Article 14

1. Everyone has the right to seek and to enjoy in other countries asylum from persecution.
2. This right may not be invoked in the case of prosecutions genuinely arising from non-political crimes or from acts contrary to the purposes and principles of the United Nations.

Article 15

1. Everyone has the right to a nationality.
2. No one shall be arbitrarily deprived of his nationality nor denied the right to change his nationality.

Article 16

1. Men and women of full age, without any limitation due to race, nationality or religion, have the right to marry and to found a family. They are entitled to equal rights as to marriage, during marriage and at its dissolution.
2. Marriage shall be entered into only with the free and full consent of the intending spouses.
3. The family is the natural and fundamental group unit of society and is entitled to protection by society and the State.

Article 17

1. Everyone has the right to own property alone as well as in association with others.
2. No one shall be arbitrarily deprived of his property.

Article 18

Everyone has the right to freedom of thought, conscience and religion; this right includes freedom to change his religion or belief, and freedom, either alone or in community with others and in public or private, to manifest his religion or belief in teaching, practice, worship and observance.

Article 19

Everyone has the right to freedom of opinion and expression; this right includes freedom to hold opinions without interference and to seek, receive and impart information and ideas through any media and regardless of frontiers.

Article 20

1. Everyone has the right to freedom of peaceful assembly and association.
2. No one may be compelled to belong to an association.

Article 21

1. Everyone has the right to take part in the government of his country, directly or through freely chosen representatives.
2. Everyone has the right of equal access to public service in his country.
3. The will of the people shall be the basis of the authority of government; this will shall be expressed in periodic and genuine elections which shall be by universal and equal suffrage and shall be held by secret vote or by equivalent free voting procedures.

Article 22

Everyone, as a member of society, has the right to social security and is entitled to realization, through national effort and international co-operation and in accordance with the organization and resources of each State, of the economic, social and cultural rights indispensable for his dignity and the free development of his personality.

Article 23

1. Everyone has the right to work, to free choice of employment, to just and favourable conditions of work and to protection against unemployment.

2.   Everyone, without any discrimination, has the right to equal pay for equal work.

3.   Everyone who works has the right to just and favourable remuneration ensuring for himself and his family an existence worthy of human dignity, and supplemented, if necessary, by other means of social protection.

4.   Everyone has the right to form and to join trade unions for the protection of his interests.

Article 24

Everyone has the right to rest and leisure, including reasonable limitation of working hours and periodic holidays with pay.

Article 25

1.   Everyone has the right to a standard of living adequate for the health and well-being of himself and of his family, including food, clothing, housing and medical care and necessary social services, and the right to security in the event of unemployment, sickness, disability, widowhood, old age or other lack of livelihood in circumstances beyond his control.

2.   Motherhood and childhood are entitled to special care and assistance. All children, whether born in or out of wedlock, shall enjoy the same social protection.

Article 26

1.   Everyone has the right to education. Education shall be free, at least in the elementary and fundamental stages. Elementary education shall be compulsory. Technical and professional education shall be made generally available and higher education shall be equally accessible to all on the basis of merit.

2.   Education shall be directed to the full development of the human personality and to the strengthening of respect for human rights and fundamental freedoms. It shall promote understanding, tolerance and friendship among all nations, racial or religious groups, and shall further the activities of the United Nations for the maintenance of peace.

3.   Parents have a prior right to choose the kind of education that shall be given to their children.

Article 27

1. Everyone has the right freely to participate in the cultural life of the community, to enjoy the arts and to share in scientific advancement and its benefits.
2. Everyone has the right to the protection of the moral and material interests resulting from any scientific, literary or artistic production of which he is the author.

Article 28

Everyone is entitled to a social and international order in which the rights and freedoms set forth in this Declaration can be fully realized.

Article 29

1. Everyone has duties to the community in which alone the free and full development of his personality is possible.
2. In the exercise of his rights and freedoms, everyone shall be subject only to such limitations as are determined by law solely for the purpose of securing due recognition and respect for the rights and freedoms of others and of meeting the just requirements of morality, public order and the general welfare in a democratic society.
3. These rights and freedoms may in no case be exercised contrary to the purposes and principles of the United Nations.

Article 30

Nothing in this Declaration may be intercepted as implying for any State, group or person any right to engage in any activity or to perform any act aimed at the destruction of any of the rights and freedoms set forth herein.

Appendix 3

Declaration of Human Rights
and Mental Health

(October 1989)

This Declaration, marking the 40th anniversary of the World Federation for Mental Health founded on the 21st of August 1948 and of the United Nations Universal Declaration of Human Rights proclaimed on the 10th December of 1948, was first adopted on 17 January 1989 as the Declaration of Luxor: Human Rights for the Mentally Ill during the Federation's 40th Anniversary Congress at Luxor, Egypt. The present revision recognises the Federation's concern not only with people defined as mentally ill, but also with those vulnerable to or at risk of mental and emotional illness or distress. It recognises that human rights transcend political, social, cultural and economic boundaries and apply to the human family as a whole. It was adopted by the Federation's Board of Directors on the 26th of August 1989 on the occasion of the Federation's biennial World Congress for Mental Health convened in that year at Auckland, New Zealand.

Declaration of Human Rights
and Mental Health

(Preamble)

Whereas the 1948 founding document of the World Federation for Mental Health entitled 'Mental Health and World Citizenship' regards mental health as involving an 'informed, reflective, responsible allegiance to mankind as a whole,' built 'on free consent' and 'respect for individual and cultural differences,'

Whereas persons publicly labelled or professionally diagnosed, treated or confined as mentally ill, or suffering from emotional distress, share, in the words of the 1948 United Nations Universal Declaration of Human Rights, 'the inherent dignity' and 'the equal and inalienable rights of all members of the human family' and, in the words of the 1948 founding document of WFMH, the 'common humanity' of persons everywhere,

Whereas the World Health Organization defines health as 'a state of

269

complete physical, mental, social and moral well-being and not merely the absence of disease or infirmity,'

Whereas a diagnosis of mental illness by a mental health practitioner shall be in accordance with accepted medical, psychological, scientific and ethical standards and difficulty in adapting to moral, social, political or other values in itself shall not be considered a mental illness; and, whereas, persons have, nonetheless, been at times and continue to be inappropriately labelled, diagnosed, treated or confined as mentally ill,

Whereas severe mental illness not only impairs an individual's capacity for work, love and play, but impairs, as well, the life of his or her family and community and places a continuing burden of care upon society,

Whereas WFMH has endorsed the principle of user or consumer involvement in the planning, management and operation of mental health services.

Whereas WFMH affirms the fundamental rights and freedoms set out in the 1948 United Nations Universal Declaration of Human Rights and its subsequent human rights instruments,

Whereas WFMH recognizes that while implementing these principles requires note of the cultural, economic, historical, social, spiritual, and other circumstances of particular societies, minimum basic standards of human rights, transcending the limits of political and cultural groupings, shall be observed at all times,

Now, therefore, the Board of Directors of the WORLD FEDERATION FOR MENTAL HEALTH proclaims this

DECLARATION OF HUMAN RIGHTS
AND MENTAL HEALTH

as a common standard for all peoples and all nations and all members of the human family.

Article 1

Mental health promotion is a responsibility of governmental and nongovernmental authorities, as well as the intergovernmental system, especially in times of crisis. In keeping with the WHO definition of health and recognizing the WFMH concern with optimal function, health and mental health programs shall contribute both to the development of individual and family responsibility for personal and group health and to promoting the highest possible quality of life.

Article 2

The prevention of mental or emotional illness or distress is an essential component of any mental health service system. Education in this respect shall extend to all health care providers as well as the public. Preventive efforts also require attention beyond the confines of the mental health care system to include optimal circumstances for development, beginning with family counseling, prenatal and perinatal care, and continuing throughout the life cycle with adequate general health care, opportunities for education, employment and social security. High priority shall be given to research on the prevention of mental disease, illness and ill health.

Article 3

The prevention of mental or emotional illness and distress and the care of those suffering from them requires cooperation between intergovernmental, governmental and nongovernmental health, science, and social welfare systems as well as educational institutions. Such cooperation shall include community involvement and the participation of professional and voluntary mental health associations and consumer and self-help groups. It will extend to research, education, planning and all necessary aspects of the problems which may arise as well as the provision of direct services.

Article 4

The fundamental rights of persons who are labelled, or diagnosed, treated or defined as mentally or emotionally ill or distressed, shall be the same as those of all other citizens. These include the right to coercion-free, dignified, humane and qualified treatment with access to medically, psychologically and socially indicated technology; freedom from discrimination regarding equitable access to therapy or inequitable restraint on grounds of political, socio-economic, cultural, ethnic, racial, religious, gender or age status, or sexual orientation; the right to privacy and confidentiality; the right to protection of personal property; the right to protection from physical or psychological abuse; the right to protection from professional or nonprofessional neglect and abandonment; and the right, for every person, to adequate information about his or her clinical status. The right to treatment shall include hospitalization and outpatient or psychosocial treatment as appropriate, with the safeguards of accepted medical, ethical and legal opinion, and for involuntarily committed patients the rights of impartial representation, review and appeal.

Article 5

All mentally ill persons have the right to be treated under the same professional and ethical standards as other ill persons. This must include efforts to promote the greatest degree of self-determination and personal responsibility on their part. Treatment shall be in settings valued and accepted by the community, in the least intrusive manner, and under the least restrictive circumstances possible. It shall be beneficent in the sense of being carried out in the patient's best interest, not that of the family, community, professionals or the state. Treatment for persons whose capacities for self-management have been impaired by illness shall include psychosocial rehabilitation aimed at reinstating skills for living and shall take account of their needs for housing, employment, transportation, income, information and continuing care after hospital discharge.

Article 6

All populations include vulnerable groups at particular risk for mental or emotional illness or distress. Members of such groups require special preventive as well as therapeutic attention and concern for the protection of their health and human rights. They include victims of natural disaster, community and other violence including war, and of collective abuse including state sponsored abuse; and those vulnerable because of residential mobility (migrants, refugees), age (infants, children and elderly people), minority status (ethnic, racial, sexual, socio-economic), loss of civil rights (soldiers, prisoners) and health status. Life crises such as bereavements, family disruption and unemployment also place persons at risk.

Article 7

Inter-sectoral collaboration is essential to protect the human and legal rights of those who are or have been mentally or emotionally ill or at risk of mental ill health. All public authorities must recognize an obligation to respond to major mental health related social problems, as well as to the mental health consequences of catastrophic conditions. Public responsibility shall include the provision of specialized mental health services, whenever possible within the context of primary care facilities, and public education regarding mental health and illness and ways of supporting or coping with them.

Article 8

Nothing in this Declaration may be interpreted as implying for any State, group or person any right to espouse any belief or engage in any activity leading to the destruction of any of the rights or freedoms set forth herein.

References

Aaron, H. and Schwartz, W. (1984), *The Painful Prescription: Rationing Hospital Care*, Brooking Institution: Washington, DC.

Abelson, P. (1990), 'The asbestos removal fiasco' (Editorial), *Science*, 347:1017.

Al-Hasani, S., Diedrich, K., van der Ven, H. et al. (1987), 'Cryo-preservation of human oocytes', *Human Reproduction*, 2: 695–700.

American Psychiatric Association (1978), *Report of the Task Force on Electroconvulsive Therapy of the American Psychiatric Association*, No. 14, American Psychiatric Association: Washington DC.

Anderson, C. (1989), 'DNA evidence questioned: Bronx judge rules lab failed to use accepted techniques', *Am. Bar. Assoc. Journ.*, 75: 18–19.

Andrews, M., Muasher, S., Levy D. et al. (1986), 'An analysis of the obstetric outcome of 125 consecutive pregnancies conceived in vitro and resulting in 100 deliveries', *Am. J. Obstet. Gyn.*, 154: 848–54.

Angell, M. (1988), 'Ethical imperialism? Ethics in international collaborative clinical research', *New Engl. J. Med.*, 319: 1081–3.

Angell, M. (1990a), 'Prisoners of technology: the case of Nancy Cruzan', *New Engl. J. Med.*, 322: 1226–8.

Angell, M. (1990b), 'New ways to get pregnant', *New Engl. J. Med.*, 323: 1200–2.

Angell, M. (1991), 'A dual approach to the AIDS epidemic', *New Engl. J. Med.*, 324.

Angier, N. (1990), 'Vast, 15-year effort to decipher genes stirs opposition', *New York Times*, 5 June, pp. C1 and C12.

Annas, G. (1979), 'Artificial insemination: beyond the best interests of the donor', *Hastings Cent. Rep.*, 4: 14–15.

Annas, G. (1987), 'Transferring the ethical hot potato', *Hastings Cent. Rep.* 17: 20–1.

Annas, G. (1988), 'Life, liberty and the pursuit of organ sales', pp. 378–420, in Annas, G. (ed.), *Judging Medicine*, pp. 378–420, Humana Press: Clifton, NJ.

Annas, G. (1990), 'Nancy Cruzan and the right to die', *New Engl. J. Med.*, 323: 670–3.

Annas, G. (1991), 'The health care proxy and the living will', *New Engl. J. Med*, 324: 1210–13.

Annas, G. and Elias, S. (1989), 'The politics of transplantation of human fetal tissues', *New. Engl. J. Med.*, 320: 1079–82.

Annas, G. et al. (1990), 'Bioethicists' statement on the US Supreme Court's Cruzan decision', *New Engl. J. Med.*, 323: 686–7.

Anonymous (1989), 'It's over, Debbie', *JAMA*, 259: 272.

APHA (1992), 'The nation's health', May–June.

Appelbaum, P. and Roth, L. (1983), 'Patients who refuse treatment in medical hospitals', *JAMA*, 250: 1296–1301.

Arkin, H. (1984), 'Forcible administration of antipsychotic medication', *JAMA*, 252: 2620–1.

Arnhoff, F. (1975), 'Social consequences of policy toward mental illness', *Science*, 188: 1277–81.

Arras, J. and Shinnar, S. (1988), 'Anencephalic newborns as organ donors: a critique', *JAMA*, 259: 2284–5.

Asch, R., Ellsworth, L., Balmaceda, J. et al. (1984), 'Pregnancy after translaparascopic gamete intrafallopian transfer' (letter), *Lancet*, 3 November: 1034–5.

Balter, M. (1991), 'How Europe regulates its genes', *Science*, 252: 1366–8.

Banta, H. and Thacker, S. (1979), 'Asssessing the costs and benefits of electronic fetal monitoring', *Obstet. Gynecol. Surv.*, 34: 627–42.

Banta, H. and Thacker, S. (1990), 'The case for reassessment of health care technology: once is not enough', *JAMA*, 264: 235–40.

Barinaga, M. (1989), 'Manic depression gene put in limbo', *Science*, 246: 886–7.

Barnes, D. (1987), 'Defect in Alzheimer's is on chromosome 21', *Science*, 235: 846–7.

Baron, M. (1989), 'The genetics of manic depressive illness' (abstract), *Journ. Nerv. and Ment. Dis.*, 177: 645.

Barry, M. (1988), 'Ethical considerations of human investigation in developing countries: the AIDS dilemma' ('Sounding Board'), *New Engl. J. Med.*, 319: 1083–5.

Basler, B. (1991), 'Kidney transplants in China raise concern about sources', *New York Times*, 3 June, p. 1.

Bayer, R. (1991), 'Public health policy and the AIDS epidemic: an end to HIV exceptionals?', *New Engl. J. Med.*, 324: 1500–4.

Bechtold, F. (1989), 'The admissibility of scientific evidence: DNA print identifications', *Stetson Law Review*, 19: 245–72.

Becker, G. and Nachtigall, R. (1986), 'Infertility as a chronic illness', American Anthropological Association, Annual Meeting, Philadelphia, December.

Becker, H. (1966), 'Ethics and clinical research', *New Engl. J. Med.*, 74: 1354–60.

Becker, M. (1990), 'Can employers exclude women to protect children?', *JAMA*, 264: 2113–17.

Bellagio Declaration (1989), *Overcoming Hunger in the 1990s*, Rockefeller Foundation Study and Conference Center: Bellagio, Italy. (Copies obtainable from the Alan Shawn Feinstein World Hunger Program, Brown University, Box 1831, Providence, RI, 02912 USA.)

Benda Report (1985), Report of the Commission on In-vitro Fertilization, Genome Analysis and Gene Therapy, Bonn.

Benrubi, G. (1992), 'Euthanasia – the need for procedural safeguards', *New Engl. J. Med.*, 326: 197–9.

Benson, P., (1984), 'Informed consent: drug information disclosed to patients prescribed antipsychotic medication', *J. Nerv. Ment. Dis.*, 172: 642–53.

Berger, E. and Lowrie, E. (1991), 'Mortality and the length of dialysis', *JAMA*, 265: 909–10.

Berger, P., Berger, B. and Kellner, H. (1974), *The Homeless Mind: Modernization and Consciousness*, Random House, Vintage Books: New York.

Berkowitz, A. (1989), Letter to the editor, *Science*, 246: 874.

Berlin, I. (1976), *Vico and Herder: Two Studies in the History of Ideas*, Viking: New York.

Blakeslee, S. (1990), 'Ethicists see omens of an era of genetic bias', *New York Times*, 27 December.

Blumstein, J. (1989), 'Government's role in organ transplantation policy', *J. Health Politics, Policy and Law*, 14: 5–39.

Bonnie, R. (1982), 'The psychiatric patient's right to refuse medication: a survey of the legal issues', in Doudera, A. and Swazey, J. (eds), *Refusing Treatment in Mental Health Instituitions – Values in Conflict*, AUPHA Press: Ann Arbor and Washington, DC.

Bouchard, T., Lykken, D., McGue, M. et al. (1990), 'Sources of human psychological differences: the Minnesota study of twins reared apart', *Science*, 250: 223–8.

Bowler, P. (1989), *The Mendelian Revolution: The Emergence of Hereditarian Concepts in Modern Science and Society*, Johns Hopkins University Press: Baltimore.

Brett, A. and Grodin, M. (1991), 'Ethical aspects of human experimentation in health services research', *JAMA*, 265: 1854–7.

Brody, E. (1958), 'Superego, introjected mother and energy discharge in schizophrenia: contribution from the study of anterior lobotomy', *J. Am. Psa. Assoc.*, 6: 481–91.

Brody, E. (1966), 'Cultural exclusion, character and illness', *Am. J. Psychiat.*, 122: 852–8.

Brody, E. (ed.) (1968), *Minority Group Adolescents in the United States*, Williams and Wilkins: Baltimore.

Brody, E. (1973a), *The Lost Ones: Social Forces and Mental Illness in Rio de Janeiro*, International Universities Press: New York.

Brody, E. (1973b), 'On the legal control of psychosurgery', (Editorial), *J. Nerv. Ment. Dis.*, 157: 151–3.

Brody, E. (1975a), 'The freedom of medical information', *JAMA*, 233: 145–6.

Brody, E. (1975b), 'The right to know: on the freedom of medical information', *J. Nerv. Ment. Dis.*, 161: 73–81.

Brody, E. (1975c), 'Rights, privileges and obligations: the physician as bioethicist', in *Anthropology and Society*, pp. 19–26, Anthropological Society of Washington: Washington DC.

Brody, E. (1976), 'Reproductive Freedom, Coercion and Justice: Some Ethical Aspects of Population Policy and Practice', *Social Science and Medicine*, 10: 553–7.

Brody, E. (1981a), *Sex, Contraception and Motherhood in Jamaica*, Harvard University Press: Cambridge, Mass.

Brody, E. (1981b), 'The clinician as ethnographer: a psychoanalytic perspective on the epistemology of fieldwork', *Culture, Medicine and Psychiatry*, 5: 273–301.

Brody, E. (1983), 'Mental health: more than the absence of illness', *Am. J. Soc. Psychiat.*, 3: 21–4.

Brody, E. (1985), 'Patients' rights: a cultural challenge to Western psychiatry', *Am. J. Psychiat.*, 142: 58–62.

Brody, E. (1987a), *Mental Health and World Citizenship. The View from an International Non-governmental Organization*, Hogg Foundation for Mental Health: Austin.

Brody, E. (1987b), 'Reproduction without sex – but with the doctor', *Law, Medicine and Health Care*, 15: 152–5.

Brody, E. (1988a), 'Culture, reproductive technology and women's rights: an intergovernmental perspective', *J. Psychosom. Ob. Gyn.*, 9: 199–205.

Brody, E. (1988b), 'Patients' rights: science, ethics and the law in international perspective', in Bell, S. (ed.), *Legal and Consumer Issues in Mental Health Law*, Vol. I, Proceedings of the Mental Health Foundation 'Conference '87', Mental Health Foundation of New Zealand: Auckland.

Brody, E. (1989a), 'New horizons for liaison psychiatry: biomedical technologies and human rights', *Am J. Psychiat.*, 146: 293–5.

Brody, E. (1989b), 'Biomedical technology and women's rights', in Van Hall, E. and Everaerd, W. (eds), *The Free Woman: Women's Health in the 1990s*, pp. 34–46, Parthenon Publishing Group: Carnforth, Lancs.

Brody, E. (1990a), 'Women's rights and the medical use of fetal tissue: an international perspective', *Rhode Island Med. J.*, 2: 53–8.

Brody, E. (1990b), *Human Rights Aspects of Transactions in Body Parts and Human Fetuses*, SHS-90/WS/6, Division of Human Rights and Peace, UNESCO: Paris.

Brody, E. (1990c), *Psychoanalytic Knowledge*, International Universities Press: Madison, Conn.

Brody, E. (1990d), 'The new biological determinism in socio-cultural context', *Australia and New Zealand Journal of Psychiatry*, 24: 464–9.

Brody, E. and Klein, H. (1980), 'The intensive care nursery as a small society: its contribution to the socialization and learning of the pediatric intern', *Paediatrician*, 9: 169–81.

Brody, E. and Newman, L. (1981), 'Ethnography and psychoanalysis: comparative ways of knowing. *J. Am. Acad. Psychoanalysis*, 9: 17–32.

Brody, E. and Newman, L. (1983), 'Psychosocial apects of personal fertility regulation', in Dennerstein, L. and Burrows, G. (eds), *Handbook of Psychosomatic Obstetrics and Gynaecology*, pp. 353–72, Elsevier Biomedical Press: New York.

Brody, E. and Redlich, F. (eds) (1952), *Psychotherapy with Schizophrenics*, International Universities Press: New York.

Brody, E. and Rosvold, H. (1952), 'Influence of prefrontal lobotomy on social interaction in a monkey group', *Psychosomat. Med.*, 14: 406–15.

Buergenthal, T. (1989), 'International human rights law and institutions', in *Right to Health in the Americas: A Comparative Constitutional Study*, pp. 3–16, Pan American Health Organization: Washington, DC.

Callahan D. (1987), *Setting Limits: Medical Goals in an Aging Society*, Simon and Schuster: New York.

Callahan, D. (1990), *What Kind of Life: The Limits of Medical Progress*, Simon and Schuster: New York.

Callender, C., Hall, L., Yeager, C., Barber, J., Dunston, G. and Pinn-Wiggins, V. (1991), 'Organ donation and blacks: a critical frontier', *New Engl. J. Med.*, 325: 442–4.

Carman, J., Wyatt, E., Fleck, R. et al. (1984), 'Neuroleptic compliance in schizophrenic outpatients', *Psychiatric Hospital*, 15: 173–8.

Cassel, C. and Meier, D. (1990), 'Morals and moralism in the debate over euthanasia and assisted suicide', *New Engl. J. Med*, 323: 750–2.

Cassell, E. (1978), 'What is the function of medicine?', in McMullin, E. (ed.), *Death and Decision*, Westview Press for AAAS: Boulder, Col.

Cawte, J. (1974), *Medicine is the Law: Studies in Psychiatric Anthropology of Australian Tribal Societies*, University Press of Hawaii: Honolulu.

Cefalo, R. and Engelhardt, H. (1989), 'The use of fetal and anencephalic tissue for transplantation', *J. Med. and Philosophy*, 14: 25–43.

Chapman, C. and Talmadge, J. (1971/1977), 'The evolution of the right to health concept in the United States' (*Pharos*, 14: 30–51), in

Reiser, S., Dyck, A. and Curran, W. (eds), *Ethics in Medicine: Historical Perspectives and Contemporary Concerns*, pp. 553–72, MIT Press: Cambridge, Mass.

Charo, R. (1991), 'A political history of RU–486', in Hanna, K. (ed.), *Biomedical Politics*, pp. 43–93, National Academy Press: Institute of Medicine, Washington DC..

Cherfas, J. (1991), 'Transgenic crops get a test in the wild', *Science*, 251: 878.

Childress, J. (1987), 'Some moral connections between organ procurement and organ distribution', *J. Contemp. Health Law and Policy*, 3: 85–110.

Childress, J. (1989), 'Ethical criteria for procuring and distributing organs for transplantation', *J. Health Politics, Policy and Law*, 14: 87–113.

Cohen, C. (1979), 'Medical experimentation on prisoners', in Robison, W. and Pritchard, M. (eds), *Medical Responsibility: Paternalism, Informed Consent, and Euthanasia*, Humana Press: Clifton, NJ.

Colledge, M., van Geuns, H. and Svensson, P. (1986), *Migration and Health: Towards an Understanding of the Health Needs of Ethnic Minorities*, WHO Regional Office for Europe: Copenhagen.

Commission on Health Research for Development (1990), *Health Research: Essential Link to Equity in Development*, Oxford University Press: New York.

Confino, E., Tur-Kaspa, I., DeCherney, A. et al. (1990), 'Transcervical balloon tuboplasty: a multicenter study', *JAMA*, 264: 2079–82.

Congress of the United States Office of Technology Assessment (1978), *Assessing the Efficacy and Safety of Medical Technologies*, OTA-H-75, US Government Printing Office: Washington, DC.

Congress of the United States Office of Technology Assessment (1984), *Human Gene Therapy – A Background Paper*, OTA-BA-266, US Government Printing Office: Washington, DC.

Congress of the United States Office of Technology Assessment (1985), *Reproductive Health Hazards in the Workplace*, OTA-BA-266. US Government Printing Office: Washington, DC.

Congress of the United States Office of Technology Assessment (1987), *Life-Sustaining Technologies and the Elderly: Summary*, US Government Printing Office: Washington, DC.

Congress of the United States Office of Technology Assessment (1988a), *Biology, Medicine and the Bill of Rights:, Special Report*, US Department of Commerce, National Technical Information Service: Springfield, Va.

Congress of the United States Office of Technology Assessment (1988b), *Institutional Protocols for Decisions about Life-Sustaining*

Treatments: Special Report, US Government Printing Office: Washington, DC.

Congress of the United States Office of Technology Assessment (1988c), *Infertility: Medical and Social Choices*, OTA-BA-358, US Government Printing Office: Washington, DC.

Congress of the United States Office of Technology Assessment (1988d), *The Role of Genetic Testing in the Prevention of Occupational Disease*, US Government Printing Office: Washington, DC.

Congress of the United States Office of Technology Assessment (1990), *Genetic Monitoring and Screening in the Workplace*, US Government Printing Office: Washington, DC.

Cooper, D. (1989), Letter to the editor, *Science*, 246: 873–4.

Coppens, M. (1991), 'Assisted suicide and euthanasia' (correspondence), *New Engl. J. Med.*, 324: 1434–5.

Corea, G. (1985), *The Mother Machine: Reproductive Technologies from Artificial Insemination to Artificial Wombs*, Harper & Row: New York.

Council of Europe (1978), *The European Convention on Human Rights*, Directorate of Press and Information: Strasbourg.

Council of Europe (1986), *Parliamentary Assembly Report of Human Embryos and Foetuses for Diagnostic, Therapeutic, Scientific, Industrial and Commercial Purposes: Draft Recommendations*, Doc. 5615, 1 September.

Council of Europe (1988), Final Text of the Third Conference of European Health Ministers, app. II, at 13 (Paris Conference of European Health Ministers, 16–17 November 1987). Reprinted in 39 *Internat. Dig. Health Legis.*, 274, 277.

Council of Europe, Ad Hoc Committee of Experts on Bioethics (CAHBI) (1986), *Provisional Principles on the Techniques of Human Artificial Procreation and Certain Procedures Carried Out on Embryos in Connection with Those Techniques*, Secretariat Memorandum, prepared by the Directorate of Legal Affairs.

Council on Ethical and Judicial Affairs, AMA (1991), 'Guidelines for the appropriate use of do-not-resuscitate orders', *JAMA*, 265: 1868–71.

Council on Ethical and Judicial Affairs, AMA (1992), 'Decisions near the end of life', *JAMA*, 267: 2229–33.

Council on Scientific Affairs, AMA (1991), 'Hispanic health in the United States', *JAMA*, 265: 248–52.

Council on Scientific Affairs, AMA (1991), 'Gynecologic sonography: Report of the ultrasonography task force', *JAMA*, 265: 2851–5.

Cravens, H. (1978), *The Triumph of Evolution: American Scientists and the Heredity–Environment Controversy, 1900–1941*, University of Pennsylvania Press: Philadelphia.

Curran, W. (1987), 'Compulsory drug testing: the legal barriers', *New Engl. J. Med.*, 316: 318–21.

Curran, W. (1991), 'Beyond the best interests of a child: bone marrow transplantation among half-siblings', *New Engl. J. Med.*, 324: 1818–19.

Daes, E. (1986), *Principles, Guidelines and Guarantees for the Protection of Persons Detained on Grounds of Mental Ill-Health or Suffering from Mental Disorder*, United Nations (E/CN.4/Sub.2/1983/17/Rev.1): New York.

Daniels, N. (1988), *Am I my Parents' Keeper? An Essay on Justice between the Young and the Old*, Oxford University Press: New York.

Danis, M., Patrick, D., Southerland, L. et al. (1988), 'Patients' and families' preferences for medical intensive care', *JAMA.*, 260: 787–802.

Danis, M., Southerland, L., Garrett, J. et al. (1991), 'A prospective study of advance directives for life-sustaining care', *New Engl. J. Med.*, 324: 882–8.

Devereux, G. (1956), 'Normal and abnormal: the key problem of psychiatric anthropology', in *Some Uses of Anthropology: Theoretical and Applied*, pp. 23–48, Anthropological Society of Washington: Washington DC.

deWachter, M. (1989), 'Active euthanasia in the Netherlands', *JAMA*, 262: 3316–19.

Dickson, E. (1989), 'Europe tries to untangle laws on patenting life', *Science*, 243: 1002–3.

Doolittle, R. (1991), 'Biotechnology – the enormous cost of success', *New Engl. J. Med.*, 324: 1360–2.

Dorozynski, A. (1991), 'Privacy rules blindside French glaucoma effort', *Science*, 252: 369–70.

Doukas, D. (1991), 'Family consent to orders not to resuscitate' (letter), *JAMA*, 265: 355.

Dowie, M. (1988), *'We Have a Donor.' The Bold New World of Organ Transplanting*, St Martin's Press: New York.

Drane, J. (1984), 'Competency to give an informed consent: a model for making clinical assesssments', *JAMA*, 252: 925–7.

Dworkin, G. (1976), 'Autonomy and behavior control', *Hastings Center Rep.*, 6: 23–8.

Ecological Society of America (1989), *Ecology*, 70: 298.

Economic and Social Council (1969), Resol. 1672 (LII), United Nations: Geneva.

Eddy, D. (1991), 'The individual vs. society: is there a conflict?', *JAMA*, 265: 1446–50.

Edmunds, L. (1989), 'The long wait for a new life', *Johns Hopkins Magazine*, 4: 37–44.

Eisenstadt, S. (1983), Continuities and tradition in the shaping of contours of modern societies: remarks on a program of research', *Bulletin*, Israeli Academic Center in Cairo, Issue No. 2, Spring.

Elias, S. and Annas, G. (1986), 'Social policy considerations in non-coital reproduction', *JAMA*, 255: 62–8.

Elias, S. and Annas, G. (1987a), *Reproductive Genetics and the Law*, Year Book Press: Chicago.

Elias, S. and Annas, G. (1987b), 'Routine prenatal screening', *New Engl. J. Med.*, 317: 1407–9.

El Periodico (1990), 20 April, p. 33, Barcelona, Spain.

Emanuel, E. (1991), *The Ends of Human Life: Medical Ethics in a Liberal Polity*, Harvard University Press: Cambridge, Mass.

Engelhardt, H., Jr. (1989), personal communication (letter), 14 April.

Engelhardt, H., Jr. (1991), *Bioethics and Secular Humanism: The Search for a Common Morality*, Trinity Press International: Philadelphia.

Evans, J. (1990), 'Essential national health research: a key to equity in development', *New Engl. J. Med.*, 323: 913–15.

Evans, R., Orians, C. and Ascher, N. (1992), 'The potential supply of organ donors: an assessment of the efficiency of organ procurement efforts in the United States', *JAMA*, 267: 239–46.

Fabrega, H. (1987), 'Psychiatric diagnosis: a cultural perspective', *N. Nerv. Ment. Dis.*, 175: 383–94.

Faden, R. and Beauchamp, T. (1986), *A History and Theory of Informed Consent*, Oxford University Press: New York.

Farwell, J., Lee, J., Hirtz, D., Sulzbacher, S., Ellenberg, J. and Nelson, K. (1990), 'Phenobarbital for febrile seizures – effects on intelligence and on seizure recurrence', *New Engl. J. Med.*, 322: 364–9.

Fisher, S. and Apfel, R. (1985), *To Do No Harm: DES and the Dilemmas of Modern Medicine*, Yale University Press: New Haven.

Fluss, S. (1991), 'Commerce in human organs: the international response', *World Health Forum*, 12: 307–10.

Forsythe, D. (1989), *Human Rights and World Politics*, second edition, revised (first edition, 1983), University of Nebraska Press: Lincoln and London.

Frances, A., Pincus, H., Widiger T. et al. (1990), 'DSM-IV: work in progress', *Am. J. Psychiat.*, 1417: 1439–48.

Freddi, G. and Bjorkman, J. (eds) (1989), *Controlling Medical Professionals: The Comparative Politics of Health Governance*, Sage Publications: Newbury Park, Calif.

Freeman, W. and Watts, J. (1942), *Psychosurgery*, Charles C. Thomas: Springfield.

Freidson, E. (1970), *Profession of Medicine: A Study of the Sociology of Applied Knowledge*, Dodd, Mead: New York.

Friedmann, T. (1989), 'Progress toward human gene therapy', *Science*, 244, 16 June: 1275–81.

Fuchs, V. and Garber, A. (1990), 'The new technology assessment', *New Engl. J. Med.*, 323: 673–7.

Fuenzalida-Palma, H. (1990), 'Organ transplantation: the Latin American legislative response', *Bulletin*, Pan American Health Organization, 24: 469–79.

Gallup Organization (1985), 'Attitudes Toward Contraception', Unpublished Report to the American College of Obstetricians and Gynecologists: Princeton, NJ.

Gewirth, A. (1984), 'An epistemology of human rights', in Paul, E., Miller, F. and Paul, J. (eds), *Human Rights*, pp. 1–24, Basil Blackwell: Oxford.

Gibbard, A. (1984), 'Utilitarianism and human rights', in Paul, E., Miller, F. and Paul, J. (eds), *Human Rights*, pp. 92–102, Basil Blackwell: Oxford.

Ginzberg, E. (1990a), 'High-tech medicine and rising health costs', *JAMA*, 263: 1820–2.

Ginzberg, E. (1990b), *The Medical Triangle: Physicians, Politicians and the Public*, MIT Press: Cambridge, Mass.

Ginzberg, E. (1991), 'Access to health care for Hispanics', *JAMA*, 265: 238–41.

Glover, J. (1989), *Ethics of New Reproductive Technologies*, (The Glover Report to the European Commission), Northern Illinois University Press: De Kalb.

Golding, M. (1981), 'Justice and rights: a study in relationship', in Shep, E. (ed.), *Justice and Health Care*, pp. 23–36, D. Reidel: Dordrecht, Holland.

Golding, M. (1984), 'The primacy of welfare rights', in Paul, E., Miller, F. and Paul, J. (eds), *Human Rights*, pp. 119–36, Basil Blackwell: Oxford.

Gonzalez, N. (1983), 'Science is sciencing' (Editorial), *Science*, 219: 4583.

Gorovitz, S., Jameston, Al, Macklin, R., O'Connor, J., Perrin, E., St Clair, B. and Sherwin, S. (eds) (1976), *Moral Problems in Medicine*, pp. 123–42, Prentice-Hall: Englewood Cliffs, NJ.

Gostin, L. (1986), *Institutions Observed: Towards a New Concept of Secure Provision in Mental Health*, King Edward's Hospital Fund for London: London.

Gostin, L. (1987a), *Human Rights in Mental Health: Japan*, Report of an international mission to Japan, 1987, WFMH, WHO, Harvard University International Collaborating Center on Health Legislation, American Society of Law and Medicine: Boston.

Gostin, L. (1987b), 'Human rights in mental health: a proposal for five international standards based upon the Japanese experience', *Internat. J. Law and Psychiat.*, 10: 353–68.

Graves, J. (1971), *The Conceptual Foundations of Contemporary Relativity Theory*, MIT Press: Cambridge, Mass.

Grobstein, C. (1988), *Science and the Unborn: Choosing Human Futures*, Basic Books: New York.

Grumet, G. (1989), 'Health care rationing through inconvenience: the third party's secret weapon', *New Engl. J. Med.*, 321: 607–11.

Gutheil, T. and Appelbaum, P. (1983), ' "Mind control", "synthetic sanity", "artificial competence" and genuine confusion: legally relevant effects of antipsychotic medications', *Hofstra Law Rev.*, 12: 77–120.

Guyer, B. (1990), 'Medicaid and prenatal care: necessary but not sufficient', *JAMA*, 264: 2264–5.

Guyer, R. and Koshland, D. (1989), 'The molecule of the year', *Science*, 246: 1543–6.

Hackler, J. and Hiller, C. (1990), 'Family consent to orders not to resuscitate: reconsidering hospital policy', *JAMA*, 264:1281–3.

Hadley, J., Steinberg, E. and Feder, J. (1991), 'Comparison of uninsured and privately insured hospital patients: condition on admission, resource use and outcome', *JAMA*, 265: 374–9.

Hallowell, A. (1965), 'Hominid evolution, cultural adaptation and mental dysfunctioning', in de Reuk, A. and Porter, R. (eds), *Transcultural Psychiatry*, Little Brown: Boston.

Haney, A., Hughes, C., Whitesides D. et al. (1987), 'Treatment-independent, treatment-associated, and pregnancies after additional therapy in a program of in vitro fertilization and embryo transfer', *Fertility and Sterility*, 47: 634–8.

Hansen, J. and Sladek, J. (1989), 'Fetal research', *Science*, 246: 775–9.

Harvey, B. (1990), 'A proposal to provide health insurance to all children and all pregnant women', *New Engl. J. Med.*, 323: 1216–20.

Hastings Center (1987), *Guidelines on the Termination of Life-Sustaining Treatment and the Care of the Dying*, Hastings Center: Briarcliff Manor, New York.

Haug, M. and Lavin, B. (1983), *Consumerism in Medicine: Challenging Physician Authority*, Sage Publications: Beverly Hills.

Hegel, G.W.F. (1807), *Phänomenologie des Geistes*, Meiner, 1952: Hamburg.

Hellman, S. and Hellman, D. (1991), 'Of mice but not men: problems of the randomized clinical trial', *New Engl. J. Med.*, 324: 1585–9.

Hillman, A., Eisenberg, J., Pauly, M. et al. (1991), 'Avoiding bias in the conduct and reporting of cost-effectiveness research sponsored by pharmaceutical companies', *New Engl. J. Med.*, 324: 1362–5.

Hoeffel, J. (1990), 'The dark side of DNA profiling: unreliable scientific evidence meets the criminal defendant', *Stanford Law Review*, 42: 465–538.

Hogness, J. and Van Antwerp, M. (eds) (1991), *The Artificial Heart: Prototypes, Policies and Patients*, National Academy Press: Washington, DC.

Hohfeld, W. (1964), *Fundamental Legal Conceptions*, Yale University Press: New Haven.

Hollingshead, S. and Redlich, F. (1958), *Social Class and Mental Illness*, Wiley: New York.

Holtzman, N. (1988), 'Recombinant DNA technology, genetic tests and public policy', *Am. J. Human Genetics*, 42: 624–32.

Hufford, D. (1992), 'Parnanormal experiences in the general population' (commentary), *J. Nerv. Ment. Dis.*, 180: 362–8.

Human Fetal Tissue Transplantation Panel (1988), *Report of Consultants to the Advisory Committee to the Director, National Institutes of Health*, NIH: Bethesda.

Humphry, D. (1991), *Final Exit: The Practicalities of Self-Deliverance and Assisted Suicide for the Dying*, Hemlock Society: Eugene, Oreg.

Ijesselmuiden C. and Faden R. (1992), 'Research and informed consent in Africa – another look', *New Engl. J. Med.*, 326: 830–4.

Ingelfingen, F. (1973), 'Bedside ethics for the hopeless cases', *New Engl. J. Med.*, 289: 914–15.

Inkeles A. (1969), 'Making man modern: on the causes and consequences of individual changes in six developing countries', *Am. J. Sociol.*, 75: 208–25.

Inkeles, A. and Smith, D. (1974), *Becoming Modern*, Harvard University Press: Cambridge, Mass.

Institute of Medicine (1985), *Assessing Medical Technologies*, National Academy Press: Washington, DC.

International Collaborative Group (1982), 'Circulating cholesterol level and risk of death from cancer in men aged 40 to 69 years: experience of an international collaborative group', *JAMA*, 248: 2853–9.

International Union of United Auto, Aerospace and Agricultural Implement Workers of America, UAW v. *Johnson Controls Inc.*, 111 s.Ct. 1196, 113 L. ed. 2d. 158, 59 U.S.L.W. 4209 (20 March 1991).

Jacobsen, C. (1936), 'Studies of cerebral functions in primates. I: The function of the frontal association areas in monkeys', *Comp. Psychol. Monogr.*, 13: 1.

Jones, E. and Forrest, J. (1992), 'Contraceptive failure rates based on the 1988 National Survey of Family Growth in Family Planning Perspectives, January/February'. Reported in *APHA*, May–June 1992.

Jonsen, A. (1988), 'Transplantation of fetal tissue: an ethicist's viewpoint', *Clinical Research*, 36: 215–19.

Jonsen, A. (1990), *The New Medicine and the Old Ethics*, Harvard University Press: Cambridge, Mass.

Joseph, S. (1987), 'The biotechnology revolution: a primer for non-scientific faculty', *Faculty Voice*, April, University of Maryland: College Park.

Kahn, P. (1992), 'Germany's gene law begins to bite', *Science*, 253: 524–6.

Kane, R.L. and Kane, R.A. (1991), 'A nursing home in your future?', *New Engl. J. Med.*, 324: 627–9.

Kant, I. (1785), *Foundations of the Metaphysics of Morals*, Transl. L. Beck from *Grundlegung Zur Metaphysik der Sitten*, Library of Liberal Arts, 1959: Indianapolis.

Kasiske, B., Neyland, J., Ruggio, R., Danoviitch, G., Kahana L., Alexander, S. and White, M. (1991), 'The effect of race on access and outcome in transplantation', *New Engl. J. Med.*, 324: 302–7.

Kass, L. (1985), 'The end of medicine and pursuit of health', in Kass, L., *Toward a More Natural Science*, pp. 157–86, Free Press: New York.

Katon, W. and Kleinman, A. (1981), 'Doctor–patient negotiation and other social science strategies in patient care', in Eisenberg, L. and Kleinman, A. (eds), *The Relevance of Social Science for Medicine*, D. Reidel: Dordrecht, Holland.

Kemper, P. and Murtaugh, C. (1991), 'Lifetime use of nursing home care', *New Engl. J. Med.*, 324: 595–600.

Kendler, K., Heath, A., Martin, N. et al. (1987), 'Symptoms of anxiety and symptoms of depression: same genes, different environments?', *Arch. Gen. Psychiat.*, 44: 451–7.

Kidd, K. (1989), 'Genetic linkage studies of schizophrenia' (abstract), *J. Nerv. and Ment. Dis.*, 177: 645.

Kilner, J. (1990), *Who Lives? Who Dies? Ethical Criteria in Patient Selection*, Yale University Press: New Haven and London.

Kittrie, N. (1971), *The Right to be Different: Deviance and Enforced Therapy*, Johns Hopkins Press: Baltimore. Penguin, 1973: New York.

Klerman, G. (1989), Introduction to Section 17, 'Mood Disorders', in *Treatments of Psychiatric Disorders: A Task Force Report of the American Psychiatric Association*, Vol. 3, pp. 1726–44, American Psychiatric Association: Washington, DC.

Kluckhohn, C. (1944), *Mirror for Man*, McGraw-Hill: New York.

Kolata, G. (1991), 'More babies being born to be donors of tissue', *New York Times*, 4 June, p. 1.

Kolder, V., Gallagher, J. and Parsons, M. (1987), 'Court-ordered obstetrical interventions', *New Engl. J. Med.*, 316: 1192–6.

Koshland, D., Jr. (1986), *Biotechnology: The Renewable Frontier*, American Association for the Advancement of Science: Washington, DC.

Koshland, D., Jr. (1989), 'Sequences and consequences of the human genome', (Editorial), *Science*, 246: 189.

Kracke, W. (1976), 'The complementarity of social and psychological forms and the leader as mediator', presented, Annual Meeting American Anthropological Association, Washington, DC, 12 November.

Kracke, W. (1979), 'Dreaming in Kogwohic: dream beliefs and their psychic use in an Amazonian Indian culture', *Psychoanalytic Study of Society*, 8: 119–71, International Universities Press: New York.

Krimsky, S. (1992), 'Tomatoes may be dangerous to your health', *New York Times*, 1 June, p. A17.

Kristof, N. (1991), 'Parts of China forcibly sterilizing the retarded who wish to marry', *New York Times*, 15 August, p. A1.

Krumholz, A., Fisher, R. and Lesser, R. (1991), 'Driving and epilepsy: a review and reappraisal', *JAMA*, 265: 622–6.

Kuhn, T. (1975), *The Structure of Scientific Revolutions*, second edition, enlarged (first edition, 1970), University of Chicago Press: Chicago.

Laborie, F. (1987), 'Looking for mothers, you only find fetuses', in Shallone, P. and Steinberg, D.L. (eds), *Made to Order. The Myth of Reproductive and Genetic Progress*, pp. 48–57, Pergamon Press: Oxford and New York.

Lantos, J. and Frader, J. (1990), 'Extracorporeal membrane oxygenation and the ethics of clinical research in pediatrics', *New Engl. J. Med.*, 323: 409–13.

Lappe, M. (1972/1977), 'Moral obligations and the fallacies of "genetic control" ', originally published in 1972, reprinted in Reiser, S., Dyck, A. and Curran W. (eds), *Ethics in Medicine: Historical Perspectives and Contemporary Concerns*, pp. 356–63, MIT Press: Cambridge, Mass.

Leape, L., Park, R., Solomon, D. et al. (1990), 'Does inappropriate use explain small-area variations in the use of health-care services?', *JAMA*, 263: 669–72.

Lehrman, D. (1988), *A Summary: Fetal Research and Fetal Tissue Research*, Association of American Medical Colleges: Washington, DC.

Leikin, S. (1987), 'Children's hospital ethics committees: a first estimate', *Am. J. Dis. Child.*, 141: 954–8.

Levine, R. (1981), 'Psychoanalytic theory and the comparative study of human development', in Monroe, R. and Whiting, B. (eds), *Handbook of Cross-Cultural Human Development*, Garland STMPM Press: New York.

Levinsky, N. (1990), 'Age as a criterion for rationing health care', *New Engl. J. Med.*, 322: 1813–16.

Levinsky, N. and Rettig, R. (1991), 'The Medicare end-stage renal disease program: a report from the Institute of Medicine', *New Engl. J. Med.*, 324: 1143–8.

Levran, D., Dor, J., Rudak, E. et al. (1990), 'Pregnancy potential of human oocytes – the effect of cryopreservation', *New Engl. J. Med.*, 323: 1153–6.

Levy, S. (1990), 'Starting life resistance-free', *New Engl. J. Med.*, 323: 335–7.

Lidz, C., Meisel, A., Zerubavel, E., Carter, M., Sestak, R. and Roth, L. (1984), *Informed Consent: A Study of Decision Making in Psychiatry*, Guilford Press: New York.

Lillich, R. (1990), 'Transplanting organs from living donors: an international regime or trade free enterprise?', *Finnish Yearbook of International Law*, 1: 510–27.

Lo, B. (1987), 'Behind closed doors: promises and pitfalls of ethics committees', *New Engl. J. Med.*, 317: 46–50.

Lo, B., Rouse, F. and Dornbrandt, L. (1990), 'Family decision-making on trial: who decides for incompetent patients?', *New Engl. J. Med.*, 322: 1228–32.

Lock, M. and Honde, C. (1990), 'Reaching consensus about death: heart transplants and cultural identity in Japan', in Weisz, G. (ed.), *Social Science Perspectives on Medical Ethics*, pp. 99–120, Kluwer Academic Publishers: Boston.

Lonergan, E. (ed.) (1991), *Extending Life, Enhancing Life: A National Research Agenda on Aging*, National Academy Press: Washington, DC.

Lonergan, E. and Krevans, J. (1991), 'A national agenda for research on aging', *New Engl. J. Med.*, 324: 1825–8.

Longino, H. (1990), *Science as Social Knowledge: Values and Objectivity in Scientific Inquiry*, Princeton University Press: Princeton, NJ.

Longstreth, W.T. Jr., Cob, L.A., Fahrenbruch, C.E. and Cofass, M.K. (1990), 'Does age affect outcomes of out-of-hospital cardiopulmonary resuscitation?', *JAMA*, 264: 2109–10.

Lumsden, C. and Wilson, E. (1981), *Genes, Mind and Culture*, Harvard University Press: Cambridge, Mass.

Luria, D. (1989), letter to the editor, *Science*, 246: 873.

MacKenzie, J. (1991), 'Whose choice is it anyway?', *New York Times*, 28 January, p. A22.

Macklin, R. (1983), 'Treatment refusals: autonomy, paternalism and the "best interest" of the patient', in Pfaff, D.W. (ed.), *Ethical Questions in Brain and Behavior: Problems and Opportunities*, pp. 41–56, Springer Verlag: New York.

Marshall, E. (1991), 'Artificial heart: the beat goes on', *Science*, 253: 501–3.

Marx, J. (1990), 'Dissecting the complex diseases' ('Research News'), *Science*, 247: 1540–2.

Massachusetts General Hospital, Critical Care Committee (1976), 'Optimum care for hopelessly ill patients', *New Engl. J. Med.*, 295: 362–4.

Maynard, A. and Ludbrook, A. (1980), 'What's wrong with the NHS?', *Lloyds Book Review*, 138 (October): 27–41, quoted in Menzel, 1990, op. cit.

Mayor, F. (1985), 'Genetic manipulation and human rights', presented, International Symposium on Biomedical Technology and Human Rights, ISSC/UNESCO, Barcelona, March.

McCune, J., Namikawa, R., Kaneshima, H. et al. (1988), 'The SCID-hu mouse: murine model for the analysis of human hemato-lymphoid differentiation and function', *Science*, 241: 1632–9.

McKusick, V. (1989), 'Mapping the Human Genome' (The Passano Lecture), University of Maryland, September.

Medearis, D. and Holmes, L. (1989), 'On the use of anencephalic infants as organ donors', *New Engl. J. Med.*, 321: 391–3.

Mental Health Act Commission (1985), *Consent to Treatment*, Ministry of Health: London.

Menzel, P. (1990), *Strong Medicine: The Ethical Rationing of Health Care*, Oxford University Press: New York.

Merz, B. (1987), 'Matchmaking scheme solves Tay–Sachs problem', *JAMA*, 258: 2636–9.

Meyers, D. (1985), *Inalienable Rights: A Defense*, Columbia University: New York.

Miles, S., Singer, P. and Siegler, M. (1989), 'Conflicts between patients' wishes to forgo treatment and the policies of health care facilities', *New Engl. J. Med.*, 321: 48–50.

Miller, B. (1981), 'Autonomy and the refusal of lifesaving treatment', *Hastings Center Rep.*, ll: 22–8.

Miller, F. and Miller, G. (1986), 'The painful prescription: a Procrustean perspective', *New Engl. J. Med.*, 314: 1383–5.

Miller K. and Inkeles A. (1974), 'Modernity and acceptance of family limitation in four developing countries', *J. Soc. Issues.*, 30: 167–88.

Mohs, R., Breitner, J., Silverman, J. and Davis, K. (1987), 'Alzheimer's disease: morbid risk among first degree relatives', *Arch. Gen. Psychiatry*, 44: 405–8.

Moniz, E. (1937), *Tentatives Opératoires dans le Traitement de Certaines Psychoses*, Masson & Cie: Paris.

Moss, A. and Siegler, M. (1991), 'Should alcoholics compete equally for liver transplantation?', *JAMA*, 265: 1295–1301.

Moss, D. (1988), 'DNA – the new fingerprints', *Am. Bar Assoc. Journ.*, 5: 66–70.

Muller, H. (1990), 'Genetic diagnosis and screening of children and adults: postnatal genetic testing', Ad Hoc Committee of Experts on Bioethics, Council of Europe, photocopied for Restricted Distribution, 29 May.

Murphy, D. (1988), 'Do-not-resuscitate orders: time for reappraisal in long-term care institutions', *JAMA*, 260: 2098–101.

Murphy, D. and Matchar, D. (1990), 'Life-sustaining therapy: a model for appropriate use', *JAMA*, 264: 2103–8.

Murphy, E. (1988), 'Psychiatric implications', in Hirsch, S. and Harris, J.

(eds), *Consent and the Incompetent Patient: Ethics, Law and Medicine*, pp. 65–73, Gaskell (Royal College of Psychiatrists): London.

Nadel, A., Green, J., Holmes, L. et al. (1990), 'Absence of need for amniocentesis in patients with elevated levels of maternal serum alpha-fetoprotein and normal ultrasonographic examinations', *New Engl. J. Med.*, 323: 557–61.

National Commission for the Protection of Human Subjects of Biochemical and Behavioral Research (1979), *Report and Recommendations: Psychosurgery*, 2 Volumes, Government Printing Offices: Washington, DC.

National Institute of General Medical Sciences (1986), *The New Human Genetics: How Gene Splicing Helps Researchers Fight Inherited Diseases*, National Institutes of Health: Bethesda, Maryland.

National Institutes of Health (1984), *Consensus Statement: Diagnostic Ultrasound Imaging in Pregnancy*, US Department of Health and Human Services: Washington, DC.

National Women's Consultative Council (1986), *Manufacturing Babies: What Reproductive Technologies Mean to Women*, Australian Government: Canberra.

Neilson, J. (1986), 'Implications for ultrasonography in obstetrics', *Birth*, 13: 11–15.

Nelkin, D. and Tancredi, L. (1989), *Dangerous Diagnostics: The Social Power of Biological Information*, Basic Books: New York.

Newcomer, L. (1990), 'Defining experimental therapy – a third-party payer's dilemma', *New Engl. J. Med.*, 323: 1702–4.

Newman, L. (1985), *Women's Medicine*, Rutgers University: New Jersey.

Newman, L. (1989), 'Reproduction and technology', in Van Hall, E. and Everaerd, W (eds), *The Free Woman: Women's Health in the 1990s*, Parthenon Publishing Group, Carnforth, Lancs.

Newman, L. (1991), 'Historical and cross-cultural perspectives on abortion', in Stotland N. (ed.), *Psychiatric Aspects of Abortion*, American Psychiatric Press: Washington, DC.

Nichols, E. (1988), *Human Gene Therapy*, Harvard University Press: Cambridge, Mass.

Nietzsche, F. (1882), *The Gay Science*, transl. W. Kaufman, Random House, 1974: New York.

Nightingale, E. and Goodman, M. (1990), *Before Birth: Prenatal Testing for Genetic Disease*, Harvard University Press: Cambridge, Mass.

Norman, C. (1989), 'Maine case deals blow to DNA fingerprinting' ('Research News'), *Science*, 246: 1556–8.

Notzon, F., Placek, P. and Taffel, S. (1987), 'Comparison of national cesarean-section rates', *New Engl. J. Med.*, 316: 386–9.

Nyberg, D., Maloney, B. and Pretorius, D. (eds) (1990), *Diagnostic ultrasound of fetal anomalies: text and atlas*, Year Book: Chicago.

Oberman, M. (1989), letter to the editor, *JAMA*, 262: 2093–4.

Okin, R. (1984), 'Brewster vs. Dukakis: Developing community services through use of the consent decree', *Am. J. Psychiat.*, 141: 786–9.

Osler, M. and David, H. (1987), *Sexuality and Family Planning for the Mentally Ill*, Danish Family Planning Association: Copenhagen.

Paradis, N. (1991), 'Family consent to orders not to resuscitate', (letters), *JAMA*, 265: 354–5.

Paris, J., Crone, R. and Reardon, F. (1990), 'Physicians' refusal of requested treatment: the case of Baby L', *New Engl. J. Med.*, 322: 1012–15.

Parliamentary Assembly of the Council of Europe (1983), *Biotechnology Law Report*, Recommendation 934 (1982) on Genetic Engineering, pp. 17–18.

Parsons, T. (1951), 'Illness and the role of the physician: a sociological perspective', *Am. J. Orthopsychiat.*, 21: 452–60.

Passamani, E. (1991), 'Clinical trials – are they ethical?', *New Engl. J. Med.*, 324: 1589–92.

Patton, P., Williams, T. and Coulam, C. (1987), 'Microsurgical reconstruction of the proximal oviduct', *Fertil. Steril.*, 47: 35–9.

Payer, L. (1989), *Medicine and Culture*, Holt: New York.

Peabody, J., Emery, J. and Aswal, S. (1989), 'Experience with anencephalic infants as prospective organ donors', *New Engl. J. Med.*, 321: 344–50.

Pearsall, A. (1989), 'DNA printing: the unexamined "witness" in criminal trials', *California Law Review*, May: 665–703.

Pedersen, P., Sartorius, N. and Marsella, A. (1984), *Mental Health Services, the Cross-Cultural Context*, Sage Publications: Beverly Hills.

Pellegrino, E. (1985), 'Health policy, ethics and human values', in Bankowski, Z. and Bryant, J. (eds), *Health Policy, Ethics and Human Values. An International Dialogue*, pp. 7–17, Council for International Organizations of Medical Sciences: Geneva.

Pepper Commission: US Bipartisan Commission on Comprehensive Health Care (1990), *A Call for Action*, Final Report, US Government Printing Office: Washington, DC.

Perez-Stable, E. (1991), 'Cuba's response to the HIV epidemic', *Am. J. Public Health*, 81: 563–7.

Perlez, J. (1992), 'In Rwanda, births increase and the problems do, too', *New York Times*, 31 May, p. 1.

Petrie, A. (1952), *Personality and the Frontal Lobes: An Investigation of the Psychological Effects of Different Types of Leucotomy*, Routledge & Kegan Paul: London.

Pichot, P. (1967), 'Criticism of psychiatry', (The Adolph Meyer Lecture), *Psychiatria Clinica*, 9: 133–47.

Pichot, P. (1983), *A Century of Psychiatry*, Editions Roger Dacosta: Paris.

Piper, J., Ray, W. and Griffin, M. (1990), 'Effects of Medicaid eligibility expansion on prenatal care and pregnancy outcome in Tennessee', *JAMA*, 264: 2219–23.

Plomin, R. (1989), 'Behavioral genetics' (abstract), *J. Nerv. Ment. Dis.*, 177: 645.

Plomin, R. (1990), 'The role of inheritance in behavior', *Science*, 248: 183–8.

Pollack, A. (1991), 'Both heart drugs are effective; doctors prescribe the costly one. Genentech pushes its medicine with a hard sell', *New York Times*, 30 June, p. A1.

Powledge, T. (1989), 'Toward the year 2005', AAAS Observer, Suppl. to *Science*, 3, November, No. 8., p. 1.

President's Commission for the Study of Ethical Problems in Medicine and Biomedical and Behavioral Research (1982), *Splicing Life*, US Government Printing Office: Washington DC., Stock No. 83–600504.

President's Commission for the Study of Ethical Problems in Medicine and Biomedical and Behavioral Research (1983), *Deciding to Forego Life-Sustaining Treatment*, US Government Printing Office: Washington, DC

Prottas, J. (1989), 'The organization of organ procurement', *J. Health Politics, Policy and Law*, 14: 41–55.

Prottas, J., Siegel, M. and Sapolsky, H. (1983), 'Cross-national differences in dialysis rates', *Health Care Financing Review*, 4: 91–103.

Quill, T.E. (1991), 'Death and dignity – a case of individualized decision-making', *NEJM*, 324: 691–4.

Rabkin, M., Gillerman, G. and Rice, N. (1976), 'Orders not to resuscitate', *New Engl. J. Med.*, 295: 364–6.

Randall, T. (1991), 'Key to organ donation may be cultural awareness', *JAMA*, 265: 176–7.

Rawls, J. (1971), *A Theory of Justice*, Belknap Press of Harvard University Press: Cambridge, Mass.

Raymond, C. (1989), 'Where are the children of the "Dirty War"? Science seeks answers for their relatives', *JAMA*, 261: 1389–93.

Regelson, W., Loria, R. and Kalimi, M. (1990), 'Beyond "abortion": RU–486 and the needs of the crisis constituency', *JAMA*, 264: 1026–7.

Reilly, P. (1991), *The Surgical Solution: A History of Involuntary Sterilization in the United States*, Johns Hopkins University Press: Baltimore.

Reinhart, J. and Kemph, J. (1988), 'Renal transplantation for children: another view', *JAMA*, 260: 3327–8.

Relman, A. (1980), 'The new medical–industrial complex', *New Engl. J. Med.*, 303: 963–70.

Relman, A. (1990a), 'The trouble with rationing', *New Engl. J. Med.*, 323: 911–13.

Relman, A. (1990b), 'Reforming the health care system', *New Engl. J. Med.*, 323: 991–2.

Remick, R. and Maurice, W. (1978), 'ECT in pregnancy', *Am J. Psychiatry*, 135: 761–2.

Renteln, A.D. (1990), *International Human Rights: Universalism versus Relativism*, Sage: Newbury Park.

Ribes, B. (1978), *Biology and Ethics*, UNESCO: Paris.

Rifkin, J. (1983), *Algeny*, Viking: New York.

Rifkin, J. (1987), 'Patenting new forms of animal life. Is nature just a form of private property?', *New York Times*, 26 April, Section III, p. F2.

Rifkin, M., Zerhouni E., Gastsonis C. et al. (1990), 'Comparison of magnetic resonance imaging and ultrasonography in staging early prostate cancer: results of a multi-institutional cooperative trial', *New Engl. J. Med.*, 323: 621–6.

Rigter, H., Borstilers, E. and Leenen, H. (1988), 'Euthanasia across the North Sea', *BMJ*, 297: 1593–5.

Roberts, L. (1989), 'Ecologists wary about enironmental releases' ('Research News'), *Science*, 242: 1141.

Roberts, L. (1990), 'CF screening delayed for a while, perhaps forever' ('Research News'), *Science*, 247: 1296–7.

Roberts, L. (1992), 'DNA fingerprinting: Academy reports', *Science*, 256: 300–1.

Roheim, G. (1950), *Psychoanalysis and Anthropology*, International Universities Press: New York.

Roper Organization of New York City (1988), *The 1988 Roper Poll on Attitudes Toward Active Voluntary Euthanasia*, National Hemlock Society: Los Angeles.

Rosenthal, E. (1991), 'Technique for early prenatal test comes under question in studies', *New York Times*, 10 July, p. C11.

Rosenzweig, M. (1985, revised 1989), 'Implications of Research in Neuroscience and Behavior for Human Rights', presented, UNESCO/ISSC Symposium on Biomedical Technology and Human Rights, Barcelona, March 1985.

Ross, C. and Joshi, S. (1992), 'Paranormal experiences in the general population', *J. Nerv. Ment. Dis.*, 180: 357–61.

Rothman, D. (1991), *Strangers at the Bedside: A History of how Law and Bioethics Transformed Medical Decision Making*, Basic Books: New York.

Royal College of Obstetricians and Gynaecologists Working Party on

Routine Ultrasound Examination in Pregnancy (1984), Royal College of Obstetricians and Gynaecologists: London.

Rymer, C. (1989), 'Evidence – admissibility of genetic fingerprinting in criminal cases', *Suffolk University Law Review*, 23: 167–74.

Saazi-Kemppainen, A., Karjapainen, O., Ylastulo, P. and Hainonen, O. (1990), 'Ultrasound screening and perinatal mortality: controlled trial of systematic one-stage screening in pregnancy. The Helksinki Ultrasound Trial', *Lancet*, 336 (8712): 387–91.

Sachdev, P. and Lonergan, C. (1991), 'The present status of akathisia', *J. Nerv. Ment. Dis.*, 179: 381–91.

St George-Hyslop, P. et al (1987), 'The genetic defect causing familial Alzheimer's disease maps on chromosome 21', *Science*, 235: 885–90.

Sakel, M. (1938), *Pharmacological Treatments of Schizophrenia*, Nervous and Mental Disease Publishing Co.: New York.

Sauer, M., Paulson, R. and Lobo, R. (1990), 'A preliminary report on oocyte donation extending reproductive potential to women over 40', *New Engl. J. Med.*, 323: 1157–60.

Schermerber v. California (1966), 384 US 757.

Schiedermayer, D.L. (1981), 'The decision to forego CPR in the elderly patient', *JAMA*, 260: 2089–97.

Schmidt, W. (1989), 'Risk to fetus ruled as barring women from jobs', *New York Times*, 3 October.

Schuck, P. (1989), 'Government funding for organ transplants', *J. Health Politics, Policy and Law*, 14: 169–190.

Schutyser, K. (1988), 'The Role of Technology in the Development and Structure of the Hospital', *Journal International Hospital Federation*, 24: 40–44.

Schutz, A. (1962), *Collected Papers Volume I, The Problem of Social Reality*, Nijhoff: The Hague.

Sehgal, A., Galbraih A., Chesney M., Schoenfeld, P., Charles G., and Lo B. (1992), 'How strictly do dialysis patients want their advance directives followed?', *JAMA*, 267: 59–63.

Sensky, T. (1988), 'Measurement of the quality of life in end-stage renal failure' (letter to the editor), *New Engl. J. Med.*, 319: 1353.

Shalev, C. (1992), quoted in, 'Surrogate mothers: saviors or victims', *Tel Aviv University News*, Spring p. 4.

Shapiro, M. (1988), letter to the editor, *JAMA*, 260: 1239–40.

Shear, M., Ball, G., Fitzpatrick, M. et al. (1991), 'Cognitive–behavioral therapy for panic: an open study', *J. Nerv. Ment. Dis.* 179: 468–472.

Shewmon, D., Capron, A., Peacock, W. and Schulman, B. (1989), 'The use of anencephalic infants as organ sources: a critique', *JAMA*, 261: 1773–81.

Silove, D. (1990), 'Biologism in psychiatry', *Australian and New Zealand Journal of Psychiatry*, 24: 461–3.

Silvestre, L., Dubois, C., Renault, M., Resvani, Y., Baulieu, E. and Ulman, A. (1990), 'Voluntary interruption of pregnancy with Mifepristone (RU–486) and a prostaglandin analogue: a large-scale French experience', *New Engl. J. Med.*, 322: 645–8.

Simon, G. (1991), 'Letter to the Editor', *Science*, 252: 629–30.

Singer, P. and Wells, L. (1985), *Making Babies: The New Science and Ethics of Conception*, Scribner's Sons: New York.

Singer, P.A. and Siegler, M. (1990), 'Euthanasia – a Critique', *NEJM*, 322: 1881–3.

Sjogren, B. (1989), 'Autonomy in decision-making in prenatal diagnosis', in Van Hall, E. and Everaerd, W. (eds), *The Free Woman: Women's Health in the 1990s*, Parthenon Publishing Group: Carnforth, Lancs.

Skerrett, P. (1990), 'Parallel track: where should it intersect science?', *Science*, 250: 1505–6.

Sladek, J. and Shoulson, E. (1988), 'Neural transplantation: a call for patience rather than patients', *Science*, 240: 1386–8.

Sloan, J., Kellermann, A., Reay, D. et al. (1988), 'Handgun regulations, crime, assault, and homicide: a tale of two cities', *New Engl. J. Med.*, 319: 1256–62.

Sloan, J., Rivara, F., Reay, D. et al. (1990), 'Firearm regulations and rate of suicide: a comparison of two metropolitan areas', *New Engl. J. Med.*, 322: 369–73.

Smothers, R. (1992), 'Court gives ex-husband rights on use of embryo', *New York Times*, 1 June, p. A1.

Snowden, L. and Cheung, F. (1990), 'Use of inpatient mental health services by members of ethnic minority groups', *Am. Psychologist*, 45: 347–55.

Sokol, L., Beck, A., Greenberg, Wright, F. and Berchick, R. (1989), 'Cognitive therapy of panic disorder: a nonpharmacological alternative', *J. Nerv. Ment. Dis.*, 177: 711–16.

Spallone, P. (1989), *Beyond Conception: The New Politics of Reproduction*, Bergin and Garvey: Granby, Mass.

Spielberg, T. (1991), 'Assisted suicide and euthanasia' (correspondence), *New Engl. J. Med.*, 324: 1435.

Spital, A. and Spital, M. (1991), 'Euthanasia debate' (correspondence), *New Engl. J. Med.*, 324: 1771.

Sprung, C. (1990), 'Changing attitudes and practices in forgoing life-sustaining treatments', *JAMA*, 263: 2211–15.

Stanford University Medical Center Committee on Ethics (1989), 'The ethical use of human fetal tissue in medicine', *New Engl. J. Med*, 320: 1093–6.

Starr, P. (1982), *The Social Transformation of American Medicine: The Rise of a Sovereign Profession and the Making of a Vast Industry*, Basic Books: New York.

State v. *Superior Court in and for County of Puma* (1984), 691 P. 2d 1073 (Ariz.).

Steffen, G. (1991), 'Family consent to orders not to resuscitate' (letters), *JAMA*, 265: 354.

Stenson, S. (1989), 'Admit it! DNA fingerprinting is reliable', *Houston Law Review*, 26: 677–706.

Stephens, J., Cavanaugh, M., Gradie, M. et. al (1990), 'Mapping the human genome: current status', *Science*, 250: 237–44.

Steptoe, P. and Edwards, R. (1978), 'Birth after the reimplantation of a human embryo', *Lancet*, 2: 366.

Stone, A. (1984), 'The new paradox of psychiatric malpractice', *New Engl. J. Med.*, 311: 1384–7.

Stromberg, C. and Stone, A. (1983), 'A model state law on civil commitment of the mentally ill', *Harvard Journal of Legislation*, 20: 275–396.

Suddath, R., Christison, G., Torrey, E., Casanova, M. and Weinberger, D. (1990), 'Anatomical abnormalities in the brains of monozygotic twins discordant for schizophrenia', *New Engl. J. Med.*, 322: 789–94.

Sullivan, D. (1988), 'The incapable patient and the law', in Hirsch, S. and Harris, J. (eds), *Consent and the Incompetent Patient: Ethics, Law and Medicine*, pp. 1–7, Gaskell (Royal College of Psychiatrists): London.

Sundram, C. (1988), 'Informed consent for major medical treatment of mentally disabled people: a new approach', *New Engl. J. Med.*, 318: 1368–73.

Susman, V. and Addonizio, G. (1988), 'Recurrence of neuroleptic malignant syndrome', *J. Nerv. Ment. Dis.*, 176: 234–41.

Tande, C. (1989), 'DNA typing: a new investigatory tool', *Duke Law Journal*, April: 474–94.

Taylor C. (1989), *Sources of the Self: The Making of the Modern Identity*, Harvard University Press: Cambridge, Mass.

Taylor, N. and Schwartz, H. (1988), 'Neuroleptic malignant syndrome following amoxapine overdose', *J. Nerv. Ment. Dis.*, 176: 249–51.

Thacker, S. (1986), 'Research strategies for the use of imaging ultrasound as an obstetric screening tool', *Birth*, 13: 39–42.

Thornburgh v. *American College of Obstetrics and Gynecologists* (1986), 106 S. Ct. 2169.

Tomlinson, T. and Brody, E. (1990), 'Futility and the ethics of resuscitation', *JAMA*, 264: 1276–80.

Tormey, J. and Brody, E. (1978), 'Values and Ethics in Medicine', in Balis, G. et al. (eds), *The Behavioral and Social Sciences and the Practice of Medicine*, pp. 656–71, Butterworth: New York and London.

Trent, J. (1990), 'Thoughts on political thought: an introduction', *Internat. Pol. Sci. Rev.*, 11: 5–23.

Triandis, H. (1990), 'Cross-cultural studies of individualism and collectivism', in Berman, J. (ed), *Cross-Cultural Perspectives: Nebraska Symposium on Motivation 1989*, pp. 41–134, University of Nebraska Press: Lincoln.

Triandis, H., Bontempo, R., Betancourt, H. et al. (1986), 'The measurement of the etic aspects of individualism and collectivism across cultures', *Australian Journal of Psychology*, 38: 257–67.

Truog, R. and Fletcher J. (1989), 'Anencephalic newborns: can organs be transplanted before brain death?', *New Engl. J. Med.*, 321: 388–90.

Tuskegee Syphilis Study, Ad Hoc Advisory Panel, Final Report (1973/1977), in Reiser, S., Dyck, A. and Curran, W. (eds), *Ethics in Medicine: Historical Perspectives and Contemporary Concerns*, pp. 316–21, MIT Press: Cambridge, Mass. Originally published by the US Public Health Service, 1973.

UN Commission on Human Rights (1991), *Human Rights and Scientific and Technological Developments*, Report of the Working Group on the Principles for the Protection of Persons with Mental Illness and for the Improvement of Mental Health Care. Chairman-Rapporteur, H. Steel, E/CN.4/1991/39, 5 February 1991, Economic and Social Council: Geneva.

UNESCO (1985), *International Symposium on the Effects on Human Rights of Recent Advances in Science and Technology* (Barcelona, Spain, 25–28 March). Organized by the International Social Science Council. Conclusions and Recommendations, SHS-86/WS/39. Division of Human Rights.

UNESCO/ISSC/WFMH (1987), 'Reproductive Technologies and the Rights and Roles of Women', unpublished commissioned report by working group, Newman, L. and Brody, E. (Chairs), Division of Human Rights and Peace.

Uniform Anatomical Gift Act (UAGA) (1983), 8A U. L. A. 30–60, in *Uniform Laws Annotated*, West: St Paul.

Uniform Determination of Death Act (1980), #7189 of the Health and Safety Code, in *Uniform Laws Annotated*, 12: 310–13, West: St Paul.

United Nations (1945), *Charter of the United Nations*, Department of Public Information, United Nations: New York.

United Nations (1948), *Universal Declaration of Human Rights*, Department of Public Information, United Nations: New York.

United Nations (1959), *Declaration of the Rights of the Child*, General Assembly Resolution 1386 (XIV), 20 November, United Nations: New York.

United Nations (1966a), *International Covenant on Economic, Social and Cultural Rights*, United Nations: New York.

United Nations (1966b), *International Covenant on Civil and Political Rights*, United Nations: New York.

United Nations (1967), *Declaration on the Elimination of Discrimination against Women*, General Assembly Resolution 2263 (XXII), 7 November, United Nations: New York.

United Nations (1968), *The Proclamation of Teheran*, International Conference on Human Rights, 13 May. Human Rights and Scientific and Technological Developments, Resolution XI. UN No. E. 68. XIV. 2, United Nations: New York.

United Nations (1974), *Report of the Symposium on Population and Human Rights* (Amsterdam, 21–29 January 1974). Conference Background Paper, World Population Conference, Bucharest, Romania 19–30 August 1974, pp. 7–8. E/Conf./60/CBP/4, 19 March, United Nations: Geneva.

United Nations (1979), *Convention on the Elimination of All Forms of Discrimination against Women*, General Assembly Resolution 34/180, 18 December, United Nations: New York.

United Nations (1985a), *Declaration of Basic Principles of Justice for Victims of Crime and Abuse of Power*, Resolution 40/34. Adopted by the General Assembly 29 November.

United Nations (1985b), *The Nairobi Forward-Looking Strategies for the Advancement of Women*, Paragraph 29, United Nations: New York.

United Nations (1988), *Human Rights: Status of International Instruments*, Centre for Human Rights, United Nations: New York and Geneva.

United Nations (1989), *Convention on the Rights of the Child*, General Assembly Resolution 44/25, 20 November, United Nations: New York.

United Network for Organ Sharing (1989), *Report of the Ethics Committee* (approved by the Board of Directors), February, Richmond, Va.

United States (1987), *Official Gazette* of the US Patent and Trademark Office, 1077: 8. Cited in Bloomberg, C., Marylander, S. and Yaeger, P. (1987), 'Patenting medical technology', *New Engl. J. Med.*, 317: 565–7.

United States House of Representatives Bill G852, 11 April (1973a), To prohibit psychosurgery in federally connected health care facilities.

United States House of Representatives – Senate Joint Resolution No. 86: March (1973b), To suspend for two years federal support of projects involving psychosurgery.

United States Organ Transplantation Task Force (1986), *Organ Transplantation: Isssues and Recommendations*, Office of Organ Transplantation, Health Resources and Services Administration, Public Health Service, US Department of Health and Human Services: Washington, DC.

Van Hall, E. (1985), 'The gynaecologist and artificial reproduction', *J. Psychosom. Ob. Gyn.*, 4: 317–20.

Van Putten, T., May, P. and Marden, S. (1984), 'Response to antipsychotic medication: the doctor's and the consumer's view', *Am. J. Psychiat.*, 141: 16–19.

Veatch, R. (1981), *A Theory of Medical Ethics*, Basic Books: New York.

Veatch, R. (1988), 'Justice and the economics of terminal illness', *Hastings Center. Rep.*, 18: 34–40.

Veatch, R. (1989), *Death, Dying and the Biological Revolution. Our Last Quest for Responsibility*, revised edition, Yale University Press: New Haven and London.

Waddington, C. (ed.) (1969), *Towards a Theoretical Biology*, Aldine: Chicago.

Wald, N., Cuckle, H. and Nanchabal, K. (1990), 'Amniotic fluid acetylcholinesterase measurement in the prenatal diagnosis of open neural tube defects: second report of the Collaborative Acetylcholinesterase Study', *Prenat. Diagn.*, 9: 813–29.

Wald, N., Cuckle, H., Haddow, J. et al. (1991), 'Sensitivity of ultrasound in detecting spina bifida' (correspondence), *New Engl. J. Med.*, 324: 769–70.

Waller, L. (1989), 'UNESCO-WFMH Workshop on Fetal Tissue Transplantation', Mercy Maternity Hospital, Melbourne, Australia, 17 August. Unpublished discussion.

Walters, J. (1989), 'Anencephalic infants as sources for organs: gravity and the steepness and slipperiness of slopes' (letter to the editor), *JAMA*, 262: 2093.

Wanzer, S., Federman, D., Adelstein, S. et al. (1989), 'The physician's responsibility toward hopelessly ill patients', *New Engl. J. Med.*, 320: 844–9.

Warnock Report (1984), *Report of the Committee of Enquiry into Human Fertilization and Embryology*, UK Dept. of Health and Social Security, HMSO: London.

Watt, N., Anthony, J., Wynne, L. and Rolf, J. (1984), *Children at Risk for Schizophrenia: A Longitudinal Perspective*, Cambridge University Press: Cambridge.

Weir, R. and Gostin, L. (1990), 'Decisions to abate life-sustaining treatment for nonautonomous patients: ethical standards and legal liability for physicians after *Cruzan*', *JAMA*, 264: 1846–53.

Welch, C. (1989), 'Electroconvulsive therapy', in Section 17, 'Mood Disorders', in *Treatments of Psychiatric Disorders: A Task Force Report of the American Psychiatric Association*, Vol. 3, pp. 1803–13, American Psychiatric Association: Washington, DC.

Welkowitz, L., Papp, L., Coitre, M. et al. (1991), 'Cognitive-behavior therapy for panic disorder delivered by psychopharmacologically oriented clinicians', *J. Nerv. Ment. Dis.*, 179: 473–7.

Wennberg, J. (1990), 'Outcomes research, cost containment, and the future of health care rationing', *New Engl. J. Med.*, 323: 1202–4.

Wennberg, J., Freeman, J., Shelton, R. et al. (1989), 'Hospital use and mortality among Medicare beneficiaries in Boston and New Haven', *New Engl. J. Med*, 321: 1168–73.

Wertz, D., Rosenfield, J., Janes, S. and Erbe, R. (1991), 'Attitudes toward abortion among parents of children with cystic fibrosis', *Am. J. Public Health*, 81: 992–6.

Wexler, B. and Cicchetti, D. (1992), 'The outpatient treatment of depression: implications of outcome research for clinical practice', *J. Nerv. Ment. Dis.*, 180: 277–86.

White, L. (1938), 'Science is *Sciencing*', *Philosophy of Science*, 5: 369–89.

Wilfond, B. and Fost, N. (1990), 'The cystic fibrosis gene: medical and social implications for heterozygote detection', *JAMA*, 263: 2777–83.

Wilkerson, I. (1991a), 'Prosecutors seek to ban doctor's suicide device', *New York Times*, 5 January.

Wilkerson, I. (1991b), 'Talk of suicide and a search for death', *New York Times*, 9 January.

Wilkerson, I. (1991c), 'Blacks assail ethics in medical testing', *New York Times*, 3 June, p. A12.

Williams, B. (1971), 'The idea of equality', in Bedau, H. (ed.), *Justice and Equality*, Prentice Hall: New Jersey.

Williams, J., Sankay, H., Foster, P. et al. (1989), 'Splanchnic transplantation: an approach to the infant dependent on arenteral nutrition who develops irreversible liver disease', *JAMA*, 261: 1458–62.

Winslade, W., Liston, E., Ross, J. et al. (1984), 'Medical, judicial and statutory regulation of ECT in the United States', *Am. J. Psychiatry*, 141: 1349–55.

Winslow, R. (1989), 'Hospitals rise to transplant organs', *Wall Street Journal*, 29 August, p. 81.

World Federation for Mental Health (1948), *Mental Health and World Citizenship*, Report of Interprofessional Preparatory Commission for 3rd International Congress on Mental Health, WFMH: London.

World Federation for Mental Health (1989), *Declaration of Human Rights and Mental Health*, Office of the WFMH Secretary General: Baltimore.

World Health Organization, Annual Assembly (1987), Resolution 40.13, 'Development of Guiding Principles for Human Organ Transplants'.

World Health Organization, Division of Mental Health (1987), *Care for the Mentally Ill: Components of Mental Health Policies Governing the Provision of Psychiatric Services*, WHO: Geneva.

World Health Organization Regional Office for Europe (1989), *Draft European Declaration on the Rights of Patients*, WHO: Copenhagen.

World Health Organization Study Group Report (1973), *Health Education in Health Aspects of Family Planning*, World Health Organization Technical Report Series, No. 483, WHO: Geneva.

World Medical Association (1987), *The Declaration on Human Transplantation*, 39th Assembly, World Medical Association: Madrid.

Zeichner, C. (ed.) (1988), *Modern and Traditional Health Care in Developing Societies: Conflict and Cooperation*, University Press of America: Lanham, Md.

Index

301